Recent Advances in
SEXUALLY TRANSMITTED DISEASES

J. D. ORIEL MD
Senior Consultant Physician, Department of Genito-Urinary Medicine, University College Hospital, London, UK

J. R. W. HARRIS FRCP DTM & H
Senior Consultant Physician, Department of Genito-Urinary Medicine, St Marys Hospital, London, UK

Recent Advances in
SEXUALLY TRANSMITTED DISEASES

EDITED BY

J. D. ORIEL
J. R. W. HARRIS

NUMBER THREE

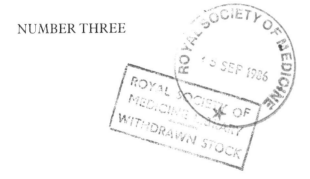

CHURCHILL LIVINGSTONE
EDINBURGH LONDON MELBOURNE AND NEW YORK 1986

CHURCHILL LIVINGSTONE
Medical Division of Longman Group Limited

Distributed in the United States of America by
Churchill Livingstone Inc., 1560 Broadway, New York,
N.Y. 10036, and by associated companies, branches and
representatives throughout the world.

First published 1986

ISBN 0 443 03325 0
ISSN 0143–6805

British Library Cataloguing in Publication Data
Recent advances in sexually transmitted diseases.
No. 3
　1. Venereal diseases
　I. Harris, J R W
　616.9'51　　　RC200　　　80–40969

Printed in Great Britain at The Bath Press, Avon

Preface

During the last five years the problems caused by sexually transmitted diseases have continued to increase. It is now increasingly realised that these conditions are not only a major cause of morbidity, but that they may cause serious illness or, sadly, death in young people. Previous complacent opinions that sexually transmitted diseases were of little importance, not meriting allocation of scarce research resources, did not long survive the advent of the acquired immune deficiency syndrome and discoveries about the relationships between transmissible viral infections and genital tract malignancy. The challenges and responsibilities of those working in this field are now formidable.

For this edition we have invited a completely new team of contributors, and we are very grateful to our colleagues from Europe, America and the UK for providing such interesting and authoritative reviews. We have not attempted to cover the whole of genito-urinary medicine; we hope to consider diseases which we have had to omit in this volume in future editions.

J. D. O.
J. R. W. H.

London, 1986

Contributors

M. W. ADLER MD FRCP FFCM
Professor of Genito-Urinary Medicine, Academic Department of Genito-Urinary
Medicine, The Middlesex Hospital Medical School, London, UK

L. COREY MD
Professor, Laboratory Medicine, Microbiology & Immunology, Head, Virology
Division, University of Washington, Seattle, Washington, USA

J. W. CURRAN MD MPH
Chief, AIDS Branch, Center for Infectious Diseases, Center for Disease Control,
Atlanta GA, USA

D. DANIELSSON MD PhD
Consultant, Department of Clinical Microbiology & Immunology, Orebro Medical
Center Hospital, Regionsjukhuset, Orebro, Sweden

D. P. DROTMAN MD MPH
Medical Epidemiologist, AIDS Branch, Center for Infectious Diseases, Center for
Disease Control, Atlanta GA, USA

C. S. F. EASMON PhD MD FRCPath
Professor of Medical Microbiology, St Marys Hospital Medical School, London,
UK

A. C. S. KEAT MD MRCP
Senior Lecturer in Rheumatology, Charing Cross & Westminster Medical Schools,
Westminster Hospital, London, UK

G. R. KINGHORN MB ChB MRCP
Consultant Physician in Genito-Urinary Medicine, Royal Hallamshire Hospital,
Sheffield, UK

D. J. McCANCE PhD
Senior Lecturer, Department of Microbiology, Guys Hospital Medical School,
London, UK

A. McMILLAN MD FRCP
Consultant Physician in Genito-Urinary Medicine, The Royal Infirmary, Edinburgh,
UK

A. MEHEUS MD
Associate Professor of Epidemiology & Social Medicine, University of Antwerp, Belgium

D. M. NOVICK MD
Associate Attending Physician, Department of Medicine & Division of Chemical Dependency, Beth Israel Medical Center; Assistant Professor of Medicine, Mount Sinai's School of Medicine of the City University of New York, USA

J. D. ORIEL MD
Senior Consultant Physician, Department of Genito-Urinary Medicine, University College Hospital, London, UK

A. J. PINCHING BM BCh MA D Phil. MRCP
Senior Lecturer & Honorary Consultant in Clinical Immunology, St Marys Hospital Medical School, London, UK

P. PIOT MD
Professor of Microbiology, Institute of Tropical Medicine, Antwerp, Belgium

A. R. RONALD MD FRCP(c) FACP
Professor & Head, Departments of Medical Microbiology & Clinical Microbiology, University of Manitoba, Winnipeg, Canada

J. SCHACHTER PhD
Professor of Epidemiology, Department of Laboratory Medicine, University of California, San Francisco, USA

H. C. THOMAS BSc PhD MRCPath FRCP (Lond) FRCP (Glas)
Professor of Medicine & Consultant Physician, Royal Free Hospital & School of Medicine, London, UK

J. W. WARD MD
EIS Officer, AIDS Branch, Center for Infectious Diseases, Centers for Disease Control, Atlanta GA, USA

Contents

1. Biology of *Neisseria gonorrhoeae*   *D. Danielsson*   1

2. Epidemiology and treatment of penicillinase-producing *Neisseria gonorrhoeae*   *M. W. Adler*   23

3. *Chlamydia trachomatis* infections: epidemiology and disease spectrum   *J. Schachter*   39

4. Laboratory diagnosis of *Haemophilus ducreyi* infections   *A. R. Ronald*   59

5. Genital herpes simplex virus infections: natural history and therapy   *L. Corey*   71

6. Genital papillomavirus infections: virology   *D. J. McCance*   109

7. Genital papillomavirus infections: clinical manifestations   *J. D. Oriel*   127

8. Genital papillomavirus infections: treatment   *G. R. Kinghorn*   147

9. Chronic hepatitis B virus infection: treatment and prevention   *H. C. Thomas,   D. M. Novick*   157

10. Genital ulceration in the tropics   *P. Piot,   A. Meheus*   175

11. Bacterial vaginosis   *C. S. F. Easmon*   185

12. Reactive arthritis and Reiter's syndrome   *A. C. S. Keat*   195

13. Epidemiology and prevention of the acquired immunodeficiency syndrome (*AIDS*)   *D. P. Drotman,   J. W. Ward,   J. W. Curran*   209

14. Clinical aspects of *AIDS* and other HTLV-III related conditions   *A. J. Pinching*   223

15. Proctocolitis in homosexual men   *A. McMillan*   243

16. Provision of services for sexually transmitted diseases in developing countries   *A. Meheus,   P. Piot*   261

Index   273

1. Biology of *Neisseria gonorrhoeae*

D. Danielsson

INTRODUCTION

Neisseria gonorrhoeae are Gram-negative diplococci of the genus *Neisseria* and the causative organisms of gonorrhoea. They generally infect the mucous membranes of the genital tract, whereas the closely related *N. meningitidis* and commensal *Neisseria* organisms infect or colonise those of the upper respiratory tract. However, pharyngeal gonorrhoea is also well recognised and occasional findings of meningococci or commensal *Neisseria* in specimens from the genitourinary tract have been documented. It must therefore be stressed that Gram-negative diplococci are always properly speciated, in genital as well as in extragenital gonorrhoea.

Some basic facts should first be considered. Gonorrhoea is a disease with a wide clinical spectrum; primarily it is a localised mucosal and submucosal infection which may be asymptomatic but which usually includes urethritis, cervicitis, proctitis and pharyngitis, and secondarily, it is a more invasive infection which causes acute salpingitis (AS) and disseminated gonococcal infection (DGI), sometimes inducing a hypersensitivity state with inflammation in synovial membranes and conjunctiva (Reiter's syndrome — see Chapter 12). The human being is the only host for the gonococcus, which has to meet nutritional requirements in competition with human defence mechanisms and immune system. The organism can only survive for a short period outside the human body, and there are also very effective antibiotics against it. However, the millions of new cases of gonorrhoea each year prove that the gonococcus can overcome and circumvent hostile environments. So far we have failed to control gonorrhoea by diagnostic, therapeutic or public health measures.

Two interesting questions present themselves: how is it possible for the gonococcus to cope with the host's defence mechanisms and immune system, and what are the exact mechanisms through which the gonococcus invades mucosal epithelial cells to penetrate to submucosal tissues, and sometimes to disseminate to distant tissues or organs?

The need for an answer to these and other questions have resulted in an impressive amount of high-quality basic research on the gonococcus over the past 10 years. Improved and sophisticated laboratory techniques have been applied to dissect gonococcal organisms with regard to the ultrastructure, antigenicity and immunogenicity of various outer membrane components, and to study interactions with eucaryotic cells, and the development of monoclonal antibodies. Interesting work has also been undertaken to elucidate the basis for conjugation, transformation and exchange of genetic information, and to make use of DNA technology for cloning of genes coding for gonococcal surface components etc. Considerable efforts are at present being made to develop a gonococcal vaccine, which is considered a realistic approach to comple-

1

ment other remedies to control gonorrhoea. This has, however, proved difficult since important cornerstones are still missing. There are, for example, no clear indications of the development of natural immunity after an infection, and it is therefore far from obvious which antigen(s) should be selected for a vaccine; the epidemiology and genetic stability of these antigens among strains occurring in various infected populations is also uncertain. Although we do not have complete answers to all these questions, we now have more insight into the functions, genetics and phase variations of the gonococcus which help to explain its ability to meet different situations.

The aim of this chapter is to present some of the information on the biology of the gonococcus which is currently available. To give a complete coverage of all the pertinent works dealing with this issue is an immense task, particularly in view of the rapid progress of research, and the reader who is interested in more detailed information is referred to further studies in the current literature. Besides a book on the gonococcus (Roberts, 1977), published proceedings from recent international conferences and workshops deal with particular aspects of the immunobiology and genetics of pathogenic *Neisseria* (Brooks et al, 1978; Danielsson & Normark, 1980; Schoolnik et al, 1985). There are also recent review articles that relate to special issues as physiology (Morse, 1979), biochemistry (Gotschlich, 1984) and genetics (Cannon & Sparling, 1984).

GONORRHOEA AND GONOCOCCAL INFECTION AT MUCOSAL AND CELLULAR LEVEL

A knowledge of the pathogenetic mechanisms of the gonococcus is a prerequisite for understanding the pathogenesis of gonorrhoea and for a realistic approach to the development of vaccine(s) and other ways of supplementing antibiotics and preventive measures for the control of this disease. The lack of an accepted experimental animal model has hampered such studies, and we must therefore rely on observations and studies of human tissue cells or organs. Harkness (1948) studied acute gonorrhoea by light microscopy of paraffin-embedded tissue sections and described the patchy destruction of epithelial cells with accumulation of gonocci and polymorphs in the submucosa. Since then we have learnt a great deal through electron microscopy studies (Ward & Watt, 1972; Novotny et al, 1975, 1977), and through experimental infection with the use of the human fallopian tube organ culture (Ward et al, 1974; Johnson et al, 1977; McGee et al, 1983). The following essential events, depicted in Figure 1.1, can be recognised.

The columnar epithelial cell is the preferential target for the gonococcus. Adherence to the cells is aided by pili on the gonococcus, the ligands of which cling to receptors of the cells. The structure and nature of these assumed receptors and ligands are unknown. Pili do not seem to be essential for the attachment, but piliated gonococci are about 5–10 times more efficient than non-piliated ones in attaching to epithelial cells. This means that other components of the outer membrane of the gonococcus contribute to the establishment of intimate contact. Microcolonies may form on the cell surface after adherence, but the phagocytosis (endocytosis) now beginning is more essential for the continuance of the infection. Microvilli protrude from the host cell surface and embrace the gonococcal cell (love at cellular level); this may continue until the gonococcal cell is phagocytosed and enclosed in a membrane bound vesicle

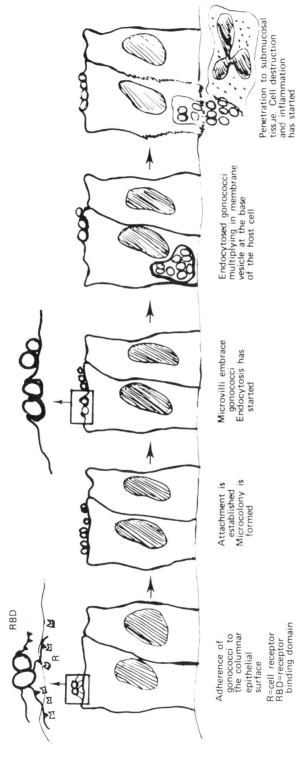

Fig. 1.1 Schematic drawing of the infection and invasion of columnar epithelial cells with gonococci.

RBD

R=cell receptor
RBD=receptor binding domain

Adherence of gonococci to the columnar epithelial surface

Attachment is established Microcolony is formed

Microvilli embrace gonococci Endocytosis has started

Endocytosed gonococci multiplying in membrane vesicle at the base of the host cell

Penetration to submucosal tissue. Cell destruction and inflammation has started in the epithelial cell. Gonococci then multiply within the phagocytic vesicle, which is transported to the basal surface of the cell. Lipopolysaccharides (LPS), enzymes and other components are liberated from gonococci and contribute to the destruction of cell boundaries and the killing of the host cell. Gonococci at the base of the cell penetrate submucosal tissue, the epithelial cell will be shed and some gonococci are expelled into the lumen of the mucosa ready to infect other epithelial cells. An inflammatory reaction with influx of polymorphonuclear leucocytes is evoked, and the symptoms of typical gonorrhoea then develop. These early events may be followed by an extension of the infection to accessory organs of the genitourinary tract (prostate, epididymis, endometrium of uterus, fallopian tube), and on some occasions an invasion of lymphatics and blood vessels for dissemination by the blood stream.

It is clear from these observations that surface components of the gonococcus must have particular characteristics to establish the intimate contact with human columnar epithelial cells and to transmit signals to the cell to start phagocytosis. A large number of research groups has made considerable efforts to clarify the biological properties of these organisms, and much knowledge has accumulated.

COLONY MORPHOLOGY AND CELLULAR FEATURES

Colony morphology in relation to virulence

Few bacteria grown in vitro have been subjected to such extensive studies of colonial morphology as *N. gonorrhoeae*. Differences were observed and described as early as 1904 by Lipschutz. This led to further observations by others (Hill, 1948). In 1963 Kellogg et al described the occurrence of four distinct colony morphology types (Fig. 1.2) which were designated T1, T2, T3 and T4. Gonococci from each of these colonial variants were inoculated into volunteers. Virulence was shown to be genetically linked

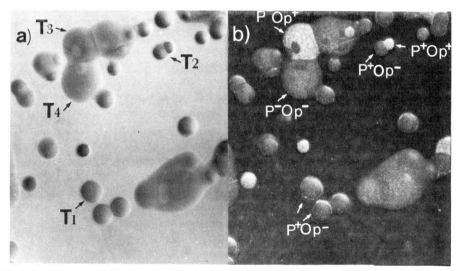

Fig. 1.2   Colony morphology variants of *Neisseria gonorrhoeae*. (a) Colony morphology types T1, T2, T3 and T3 as viewed in the stereomicroscope utilising transmitted light reflected from a diffusing substage mirror. (b) Piliated and non-piliated, opaque and transparent colonies as viewed utilising transmitted light reflected from a polished substage mirror. P + Op + = piliated opaque; P + Op − = pilated transparent; P − Op + = non-piliated opaque; P − Op − = non-piliated transparent.

to types T1 and T2, and pathogenicity was retained after passing them in vitro for 35 months (Kellogg et al, 1968). Sparling & Yobs (1967) found a predominance of T1 and T2 colonies in isolates from the urethra of males and endocervix of females with gonorrhoea, and this has been confirmed by several other workers.

Structure by electron microscopy

Following the definition of colony morphology and its relation to virulence (Kellogg et al, 1963, 1968) the structure of gonococci was extensively studied by electron microscopy (EM). Micrographs of thin sections of gonococci in gonorrhoeal pus (Novotny et al, 1975) and of cultured gonococci of various colony morphology types (Swanson et al, 1971) have revealed the corresponding basic structures, as in other Gram-negative bacteria; an undulating bilayered outer membrane (OM), an inner cytoplasmic membrane (CM) surrounding the bacterial cytoplasm, and between them a periplasmic space containing the peptidoglycan (PG) layer (Fig. 1.3). A fuzzy coat can also be seen, and a few research groups have claimed that this might be capsular material (Novotny et al, 1977; James & Swanson, 1977; Hendley et al, 1978) but this has never been defined with regard to its antigenic characteristics. The fuzzy coat is probably due to polyphosphate produced by the gonococcus which has no antigenic properties. The current consensus is that gonococci, as grown in the laboratory, are devoid of a capsule with antigenic properties. The most exciting findings of the EM studies were the demonstration of pili (fimbriae), i.e. hairlike structures on the external surface of the OM, which were present on cells from the virulent colony forms T1 and T2 but absent on those from the avirulent ones T3 and T4. These observations were made independently by Jephcott et al and Swanson et al in 1971. Pili were subsequently demonstrated on gonococcal cells in gonorrhoeal pus (Ward & Watt, 1972; Novotny et al, 1975).

Current nomenclature of piliated and non-piliated gonococcal cells

The definition of the four colonial variants was made possible by growing gonococci on a supplemented translucent agar medium which permitted examination of the colonies with a dissecting microscope, using transmitted light reflected from a diffusing substage surface. Size, colour and shape were the main characteristics of the typing scheme by Kellogg et al (1963); T1 and T2 colonies were small and dome shaped, T2 usually darker and with a much sharper rim than T1; T3 and T4 colonies were large and flatter, T3 dark and T4 light (Fig. 1.2). The typing scheme of Kellogg et al was modified after extensive studies by Swanson (1977, 1978, 1982) who related the differences to physical and chemical characteristics. The dark and light coloured variants of piliated and non-piliated colonies were characterised as opaque and transparent (Fig. 1.2), respectively, and differentiated by using light reflected from a polished substage mirror. Swanson showed that opacity was associated with the presence of particular proteins, so-called opacity proteins, which will be further discussed below. The observations by Swanson and his group have been confirmed by several other research groups, and the use of these markers has proved useful in everyday work with gonococci. Accordingly, piliation is indicated by Pil +, non-piliation by Pil −, and the presence or absence of opacity protein by Op+ and Op− respectively. Piliated opaque or transparent colonies are written as Pil + Op+ and Pil + Op− respectively, and non-piliated opaque or transparent colonies as Pil − Op+ and Pil − Op −.

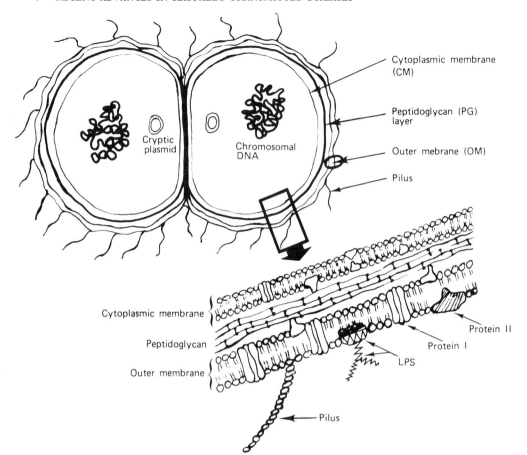

Cytoplasmic membrane (CM)

Peptidoglycan (PG) layer

Outer mebrane (OM)

Pilus

Cryptic plasmid

Chromosomal DNA

Cytoplasmic membrane

Peptidoglycan

Outer membrane

Protein II

Protein I

LPS

Pilus

Fig. 1.3 Ultrastructure of the gonococcal cell with particular regard to various surface components.

Sometimes only P or O are used, but these can cause confusion with other markers. It must also be stressed that absolutely homogeneous cultures of a particular phenotype, whether piliated/opaque, piliated/transparent, non-piliated/opaque or non-piliated/transparent, are impossible to obtain because of the phase variations to which both piliation and opacity are subject. This is not due to spontaneous mutations, but rather to genomic rearrangements of the structural genes coding for these proteins (Meyer et al, 1982, 1984).

The demonstration of colonial morphology and piliation related to virulence of the gonococcus has had a considerable influence on subsequent research efforts.

ULTRASTRUCTURE AND BIOLOGICAL SIGNIFICANCE OF THE CELL ENVELOPE

The ultrastructure of the gonococcal cell envelope (indicated by CM, PG and the OM components in the close up of Figure 1.3) conforms to that of other Gram-negative bacteria. The various structural components can be isolated by procedures applicable to other Gram-negative organisms (Johnston et al, 1976; Wolf-Watz et al, 1975).

Cytoplasmic membrane (CM)

This membrane delineates the cytoplasm of the gonococcal cell. From investigations by different research groups it is evident that this lipid bilayer contains the usual membrane enzymes, i.e. succinate, lactate, NADH dehydrogenases and ATPase (Morse et al, 1977; Morse, 1979).

Peptidoglycan (PG) layer

Chemical analyses have shown that the PG layer is composed of muramic acid, glutamic acid, alanine, diaminopimelic acid and glucosamine, which is a chemical composition found in most Gram-negative bacteria (Wolf-Watz et al, 1975). The PG layer is the target for penicillin, and several penicillin-binding components are present in the cell envelope. The most important among these is the D-alanine carboxy-peptidase, with characteristics of other DD-carboxy peptidases sensitive to beta-lactam antibiotics (Salton, 1977). Cross linking of the PG layer will not take place when these enzymes are inactivated, and the bacterial cell will lyse.

An interesting observation is the arthritopathic property in rats caused by hydrolase resistant O-acetylated PG from invasive gonococcal strain (Rosenthal & Fleming, 1984). PG might therefore play a role in the pathogenesis of gonococcal arthritis.

Outer membrane (OM)

It is obvious that the OM plays a major role in the establishment of intimate contact between gonococcal cells and the eucaryotic cells of the host, primarily the mucous membrane epithelial cells and leucocytes, and also for interaction with various humoral factors of the host's defence system. The three major components of the OM, i.e. the various membrane proteins, LPS and pili, have been and are still being subjected to intense research. The biological significance of the more important findings will be discussed below.

Lipopolysaccharides (LPS)

The endotoxic activity of gonococci as well as of other Gram-negative bacteria is confined to the lipid A moiety of the LPS molecule. This relatively complex molecule also contains the core oligosaccharide (composed of several monosaccharides and 3-deoxy-D-manno-octulosonic acid = KDO bound to lipid A) and the O-antigenic polysaccharide chain made up of oligosaccharide repeating units. Complete LPS, termed S type, is obtained from bacterial S (smooth) forms and has a high molecular weight O-chain (for example *Salmonellae*) whereas incomplete LPS, termed R type, has an incomplete O-antigenic polysaccharide chain. The general consensus is that gonococcal LPS of organisms cultured in vitro is of the R type, but whether or not S type LPS is produced in gonococcal infections is still unclear (Perry et al, 1977). It is located on the external surface of the OM (Fig. 1.3), as in other Gram-negative bacteria, and is often seen in EM photographs as membrane blebs external to the cells (Ward & Watt, 1975). LPS is easily extracted from the OM, but often difficult to obtain in pure form. This difficulty is connected with the fact that lipid A has hydrophobic character whereas the other parts of the LPS molecule, the core and the O-chain, are the hydrophilic polar region; because of this special precautions must be taken when LPS is being prepared in order to avoid formation of complexes.

Gonococcal LPS has been subjected to many studies because of its possible relationship to virulence, pathogenesis and immunity, and because of its potential use in serotyping and serodiagnosis. Previous work was reviewed by Perry et al (1977) and by Danielsson & Maeland (1978).

The endotoxic activity of gonococcal LPS can be demonstrated with the limulus lysate test, and with this shows activity which corresponds to those of meningococci and *E. coli* (Danielsson, Moi & Hagman unpublished observations). With the use of the human fallopian tube in vitro model McGee et al (1983) demonstrated that nonciliated epithelial cells were infected but not ciliated cells; the latter were sloughed off from the mucosa owing to the effect of LPS. With this model it would be of interest to study possible preventive effects of anti LPS antibodies against tissue destruction. However, studies by Maeland (1969, 1971) and by Apicella (1974) have demonstrated several antigenic specificities of the gonococcal LPS, varying among different strains, which might help to explain why possible anti LPS antibodies acquired in a previous gonococcal infection do not produce any significant protection against reinfection. This does not exclude protection against complications; Buchanan et al (1980) found that an episode of gonococcal salpingitis provided protection against recurrence with the same strain but not with a different one, but whether these patients had anti LPS antibodies was not investigated.

LPS was used by several workers to detect human antibodies in gonococcal infection with the aim of using such a test for serodiagnosis (Chacko & Nair, 1959; Maeland & Larsen, 1971; Watt et al, 1971; Ward & Glynn, 1972). The tests have varied considerably with regard to sensitivity, in one work varying from 27–84% according to the strain used for the preparation of LPS. The tests also showed low specificity, since cross reacting antibodies were present in many sera from uninfected controls.

Some of these findings may be explained by the fact that LPS of many gonococcal strains react with non-immune IgM of normal serum, complement is activated via the classical pathway, and gonococci are killed. Such strains are called serum sensitive (SerS) because they are sensitive to the bactericidal activity of normal serum (Schoolnik et al, 1979). Invasive strains, i.e. those associated with DGI, are serum resistant (SerR) (Schoolnik et al, 1976). OM antigens of these strains, probably OM proteins, react with non-immune IgG so that this complex exerts a blocking effect for IgM (Brooks et al, 1980; Rice et al, 1980). Further studies with monoclonal antibodies have shown that blocking non-bactericidal IgG also binds a C5b-9 complex but that this complex has a different configuration from the C5b-9 complex bound by bactericidal IgG and IgM (Joiner & Frank, 1984).

Gonococcal LPS seems to have receptors for pyocins, which are bacteriocins derived from *Pseudomonas aeruginosa* and which have an inhibitory effect on the growth of gonococci (Morse et al, 1976; Sadoff et al, 1978). Pyocin-resistant mutants can be derived, and it was shown that LPS of these mutants differed from the parent strain with regard to chemical characteristics and biological properties (Guymon et al, 1980). Pyocin typing was suggested by Sadoff et al (1978), and Blackwell et al (1983) showed that such typing could be used to differentiate SerS strains from SerR strains. Blackwell et al (1984) also showed that none of 34 sera from patients with gonorrhoea produced antibodies that were bactericidal for pyocin resistant strains.

The available data thus indicate that LPS can be of great importance in the pathogenesis of gonorrhoea, and also that expression and regulation of LPS itself and of

LPS antigens may vary from strain to strain and in different environments. Factors influencing these changes are at present being subjected to further investigation (Apicella et al, 1984).

Pili

The presence of pili (fimbriae) is clearly correlated to the ability of pathogenic bacteria to cause disease (Brinton, 1977; Brinton et al, 1978). Ever since 1971, when pili were first demonstrated on gonococci of the virulent T1 & T2 colonial morphology types but not on those of the avirulent T3 & T4 (Jephcott et al, 1971; Swanson et al, 1971), considerable attention has been paid to their role in the pathogenesis of gonorrhoea. It was soon reported that piliated gonococci attach more readily than non-piliated organisms to cervical and buccal epithelial cells (Mårdh & Weström, 1976; Tramont & Wilson, 1977), to the mucosal surface of human fallopian tube organ cultures (Ward et al, 1974), to human sperm (James-Holmquest et al, 1974) and to human red blood cells (Waitkins, 1974; Buchanan & Pearce, 1976). They were also shown to be more resistant to phagocytosis by human polymorphonuclear leucocytes (Thongthai & Sawyer, 1973). Genetic studies showed that transformation of gonococci by the transfer of DNA occurred at optimal rates only if the recipient was piliated (Sparling et al, 1977). Methods were described for the preparation of pili, and subsequent studies showed them to be immunogenic for rabbits and humans (Buchanan et al, 1973; Reimann & Lind, 1977).

Following these basic observations of gonococcal pili many studies have been made of their structures, physiochemical properties, antigenicity, immunogenicity and attachment to human cells, mostly because pili are potential candidates for a vaccine. Some of the more important results will be discussed below.

Physicocochemical studies indicate that each pilus is an assembly of up to 10 000 identical protein units, termed pilins, which aggregate to form filamentous structures approximately 6 nm in diameter and 1000 to 4000 nm in length. The subunit MWs of the purified pilus proteins from different strains vary between 17.5 and 21 kilodaltons (kd) as determined by sodium dodecyl sulphate polyacrylamide gel electrophoresis (SDS-PAGE) (Robertson et al, 1977; Hermodson et al, 1978; Brinton et al, 1978). Tryptic peptide maps of pili from various strains showed homology, but also differences related to the physicochemical diversity (Schoolnik et al, 1982). The antigenic heterogeneity of pili from various strains has been demonstrated by serologic studies with human and rabbit anti pilus antibodies (Buchanan, 1975; Novotny & Turner, 1975), Lind & Reimann, 1980) and extensive studies by Brinton et al (1982) showed that all the pili from more than 50 strains were of different serotypes. There were, however, obvious cross reactions which indicated common antigens. This cross reactivity between pairs of pilus types was arranged in a senior-junior order, where the senior was defined as the pilus type that induced the most cross reacting antibodies. Pilus variations were described by Lambden et al (1980, 1981) who identified in an isogenic strain four types of pili with different MWs, physiohemical characteristics and biological properties. Meyer et al (1982) cloned the gene encoding gonococcal pilus protein into *E. coli* and showed that pilus expression in *Neisseria gonorrhoeae* involves chromosomal rearrangement, which may explain the appearance of different pili in the same gonococcal strain. It seems likely that this might help the gonococcus to escape host defence mechanisms.

GONOCOCCAL PILUS VACCINE

It is assumed that each pilus unit possesses a receptor binding domain which, when expressed in an assembled state, results in a linear array of binding regions along the longitudinal axis of the intact pilus, promoting adherence to host cells. Blocking of this receptor binding domain with specific antibodies might therefore be protective, and consequently a pilus vaccine might be useful against gonorrhoea. Studies of the human immune response to gonococcal pili indicated antibody production against cross reactive antigens (Buchanan et al, 1973; Reimann & Lind, 1978), and adherence of gonococci to human cells, was inhibited by homologous and heterologous anti pilus antibodies (Tramont et al, 1979). Following these observations, which indicated that pilus antibodies might give protection, a pilus vaccine from a gonococcal strain, Pittsburgh 3-2, was developed and described by Brinton et al (1982). Human volunteers immunised with this vaccine were protected when challenged for experimental gonorrhoea. The protection was related to the injected vaccine dose, antibody levels to pili, and the challenge dose of gonococci of the same strain from which pilus vaccine had been produced. Challenges with heterologous gonococci were not tried. Based on the observations of protection in volunteers and the demonstrated safety of the vaccine a field trial was performed, but the results were disappointing as no protection could be demonstrated in vaccinated individuals compared with controls. (Report by Dr Tramont at the 4th International Conference on Pathogenic *Neisseria*, October 21–25, 1984, Asilomar, California, USA.)

Schoolnik et al (1982, 1983) have studied the antigenic properties of the domain of gonococcal pili responsible for the agglutination of human erythrocytes, with the aim of making a pilus vaccine. Pili preparations agglutinated red blood cells at concentrations of 0.2 to 82.5 mg/l pilus protein, with significant differences between strains and between various phenotypes of isogenic strains from which pili were prepared. This is in accord with the antigenic and biologic heterogeneity of gonococcal pili demonstrated by others. Chemical cleavage of the pilin with cyanogen bromide (CNBr) at the methionine residues resulted in two major fragments, CNBr-2 and CNBr-3. Schoolnik and his group showed that the CNBr-2 fragment inhibited the agglutination of erythrocytes by native pili from homologous and heterologous gonococcal strains. The CNBr-2 fragment of pili from different strains also showed considerable homology by peptide mapping and amino acid analysis, and marked serological cross reactivity, whereas the heterogeneity seemed to be preserved in the CNBr-3 fragment. It was therefore suggested that the CNBr-2 fragment might be superior to native pili as a vaccine for the immunoprophylaxis of gonorrhoea, because this domain seems to be highly conserved in Op+ and Op− clones of serologically unrelated gonococcal pili (Stephens et al 1984). Results of the protective activity of such a vaccine are, however, not yet available.

Outer membrane (OM) proteins

Proteins of the OM can be extracted from envelope preparations by different methods, for example by lithium acetate, ethanoldiamine or sarkosyl (Johnston et al, 1976; Buchanan et al, 1978). The most commonly used way to analyse these extracts is by SDS-PAGE after the method by Laemmli (1970), by which the molecular weight of the separated protein bands can be estimated (Fig. 1.4). (Treatment with SDS gives the proteins a globular structure with similar charge, and they will move according to size in PAGE.) The two best characterised OM proteins are protein I and protein II, abbreviated PI and PII respectively. These proteins were previously labelled with different names by various research groups. The present nomenclature was proposed and agreed at the EMBO Workshop on Genetics and Immunobiology of Pathogenic Neisseria in 1980 (Swanson & Heckels, 1980).

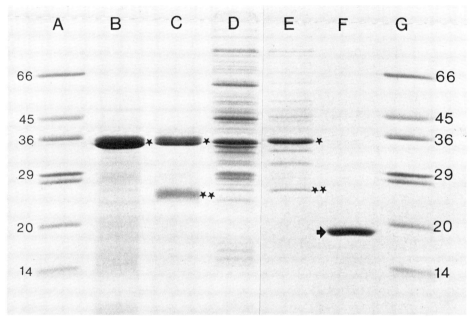

Fig. 1.4 Comparative SDS-PAGE banding patterns of some surface proteins of *Neisseria gonorrhoeae*. Lanes A and G: MW markers expressed in kd (kilodaltons). Lanes B, C, D and E with protein I = ★ (MW about 34 kd); Lanes C and E with protein II = ★★ (MW about 24 kd); Lane F with purified pilus protein (MW about 18 kd).

PROTEIN I

Represents about 30–40% of the OM proteins and was previously called the major or principal outer membrane protein (MOMP or POMP) (Johnston et al, 1976; Buchanan et al, 1978). It has a MW in the range of 32–40 kd and is present with the same MW on gonococcal cells regardless of colony morphology phenotype. It is heat resistant: its MW does not change with solubilisation in SDS by boiling versus 37–60°C. It is largely retained in sedimentable form after extraction of isolated OM with deoxycholate, and can be ^{125}I-labelled on intact gonococci by lactoperoxidase and H_2O_2, which proves that it is a surface protein (Swanson & Heckels, 1980). PI is located on both the inner and outer surface of the OM and thus has the structure of a transmembrane protein with porin function for transport of hydrophilic compounds over the OM barrier (Blake, 1983). It has great genetic and antigenic stability, and is present on both piliated and non-piliated cells whether they have opacity proteins or not.

By an Elisa inhibition test 9 serotypes of PI were defined with rabbit antibodies, and these were correlated with various gonococcal disease syndromes (Buchanan & Hildebrandt, 1981). The serological classification of gonococci by co-agglutination with polyclonal rabbit antibodies or mouse monoclonal antibodies into WI and WII/III serogroups is based on specific antigens of PI (Sandström & Danielsson, 1980; Tam et al, 1982). With the help of peptide mapping of PI two principal patterns, designated A and B respectively, were demonstrated (Sandström et al, 1982). Epitopes of PI/A corresponded to strains of serogroup WI and those of PI/B to strains of WII/III. The role of PI in the interaction of gonococci with eucaryotic cells is unclear, but infected patients produce antibodies against it (Lammel et al, 1984). Buchanan et al (1980) showed that an episode of gonococcal salpingitis provided protection against recurrence with the same but not against a different PI serotype, but whether this was due to antibodies to PI antigens or other OM components was not shown.

PROTEIN II

Protein II represents the opacity proteins which make the gonococcal colonies appear opaque in the stereomicroscope with a polished substage mirror, or dark or very dark with a diffusing substage mirror (Swanson 1977, 1978, 1982) (Fig. 1.2). PII has MWs in the range of 24–30 kd and differs from PI with regard to physicochemical characteristics (Swanson & Heckels, 1980; Heckels, 1981).

Opacity proteins were shown to be related to the leucocyte association (LA) factor (Swanson, 1977). They might also be important for the adherence of gonococci to host cells (Heckels, 1982), and in fact more organisms of Pil + Op + attached to vaginal epithelial cells and the mucosal cells of the fallopian tube than did organisms of Pil + Op − (Forslin & Danielsson, 1980; McGee et al, 1983). Draper et al (1984) also showed that purified opacity proteins had a high affinity to tissue culture cells.

Several subclasses of PII with different antigenic properties may be variably present on phenotypes of Pil+ or Pil− cells of an isogenic strain (Lambden et al, 1979; Heckels, 1981; Black et al, 1984). The opacity proteins are thus the components mainly responsible for the antigenic variations observed by many researchers in the past (Wilson, 1954; Danielsson & Sandström, 1980). The observation of a higher frequency of Pil + Op + gonococcal phenotypes in the urethra of men with gonorrhoea and in the cervix of women in the mid-term of the menstrual cycle is interesting. However, Pil + Op − phenotypes dominate around the time of menstruation and in isolates from the fallopian tubes in acute salpingitis. These variations can be demonstrated in one and the same patient (James et al, 1980). The PII changes occur in vitro in either direction, or to new Op variants at a random rate of approximately once in 1000 to 5000 cell divisions (Mayer, 1982) which is too high for a mutation. Recently Meyer et al (1984) showed that a single gonococcus may have several different Op genes and that the opacity phase variations are probably due to a genetic rearrangement of the structural genes coding for these proteins. Moroever, these genes map near the pilus expression locus, which may explain observed covariation. It seems very likely that the phase variations of the opacity proteins might serve the function of helping the gonococcus to escape from host defence mechanisms, since antibodies to some of the subclasses of PII have a bactericidal action whereas others do not have such an activity (Black et al, 1984). It is unclear what role these proteins might play in a vaccine.

OTHER OM PROTEINS

Several proteins other than PI & PII can be demonstrated by SDS-PAGE of OM extracts. One of these, with a MW of 30 kd, is designated PIII and is present on all gonococci and probably in other *Neisseria* as well (Swanson, 1982). Antigens on this protein might be of importance for the bactericidal action of anti gonococcal IgG (Rice et al, 1984).

A group of proteins is expressed under iron starvation in vitro (Norquist et al, 1976). These iron regulated proteins (FeRP) have apparent MWs in SDS-PAGE of about 100 kd, 70 kd and 37 kd (West & Sparling, 1985) and seem to be analogous to iron-repressible proteins in many other bacteria, some of which are known to be receptors involved in iron uptake. Various research groups are at present investigating the functions, regulations and antigenic properties of the FeRPs since they might be of importance in pathogenicity and virulence (Dyer et al, 1984; Morse et al, 1984). These proteins are therefore also of interest as vaccine candidates. Cannon et al (1984) have identified an additional protein antigen that is present on all gonococci and meningococci tested but not on commensal *Neisseria*. The function and role of this OM protein in pathogenic *Neisseria* is unclear. Bactericidal antibodies against it might be protective. The structural gene coding for this antigen has been cloned in *E. coli*.

IGA PROTEASE AND OTHER ENZYMES

Plaut et al (1975, 1977) and Mulks & Plaut (1978) demonstrated that both gonococci and meningococci elaborate a unique enzyme, IgA protease, which cleaves human serum and secretory IgA1 subclass into intact Fab2 and Fc2 fragments. Mulks et al (1980) also showed that secretory IgAl inhibited the adherence of genococci to human cells, but this inhibition was significantly reduced after cleavage with IgAl protease. These observations might have implications in vivo since IgA protease activity is found in vaginal secretions of woman with gonorrhoea (Blake et al, 1979). The enzyme has been purified and characterised and the structural gene coding for it in the gonococcus has been cloned in *E. coli*. Research studies are now under way to localise the active site of IgA protease and to determine whether specific antibodies can be produced against it which will inactivate it (Blake & Gotschlich, 1984).

Chen & Buchanan (1980) reported the identification of four different hydrolysases, one of which, an endopeptidase termed gonosin, was able to cleave succinylated elastin. The pathogenic potential of these enzymes was considered to play a role in the invasiveness of gonococci during ophthalmia neonatorum and contribute to the tenosynovitis of DGI.

PHENOTYPING OF GONOCOCCI — CLINICAL AND EPIDEMIOLOGICAL IMPLICATIONS

For a long time gonococcal epidemiology was hampered by the lack of reliable methods for such studies. During the last 10 years auxotyping and serological classification by co-agglutination have come into use for phenotyping of gonococcal isolates.

Auxotyping

Nutritional requirements of gonococci were extensively studied by Catlin (1973, 1977, 1978) who described a complete, chemically defined protein free medium, called

NEDA medium, which supports growth of most gonococci. By omitting the amino acids, vitamins or the bases (uracil and hypoxanthine) one at a time or in combination and examining the growth of gonococci it is possible to divide the isolates into distinct groups according to their nutritional requirements. In this way (Catlin, 1973; Carifo & Catlin, 1973) auxotype patterns are determined by the requirements, Pro- for proline, Arg- for arginine etc. Gonococci able to grow on all media of an auxotyping set are called prototrophic (Prot). Thus far 35 auxotypes have been identified by tests of clinical isolates (Catlin, 1978).

Table 1.1   Auxotyping of *Neisseria gonorrhoeae*. Comparison of frequencies of some of the auxotypes found by three different investigators

Auxotypes	Milwaukee[a] 251 isolates %	Stockholm[b] 166 isolates %	Swedish survey[c] 245 isolates %
Prototrophic	25.5	15.7	28.4
Pro$^-$	33.8	12.8	18.8
Arg$^-$	17.5	1.9	3.3
Arg$^-$Hyx$^-$Ura$^-$	9.6	40	19.2
Pro$^-$Arg$^-$Hyx$^-$Ura$^-$	2.0	6.0	16.7

(a) Carifo & Catlin, 1973
(b) Moberg, 1975
(c) Danielsson et al, 1983

Auxotyping has proved valuable in characterising strains in relations to clinical disease syndromes and antibiotic susceptibility, and in characterising PPNG strains. A high susceptibility to penicillin, ≤0.015 mg/l, was typical for AHU- and Pro- strains associated with DGI (Knapp & Holmes, 1975). Great geographical variations have been demonstrated, and also changes with time as illustrated by results from three different investigations in Table 1.1. Very little is known about the physiological and genetic differences that underlie the various nutritional requirements of gonococci, but they clearly reflect the development of very elaborate mechanisms to meet various nutritional situations.

Serological classification
In 1980 Sandström & Danielsson described the basis for serological classification of gonococci by co-agglutination. With the help of specific polyclonal rabbit anti gonococcal antibodies laboratory strains and clinical isolates were separated into three main serogroups designated WI, WII and WIII. Antigens of protein I were responsible, and by peptide mapping two principal PI molecules designated A and B were demonstrated (Sandström et al, 1982). WI strains possessed antigens of PI/A and WII/III strains antigen of PI/B. Monoclonal antibodies were developed against epitopes of PI/A and PI/B, respectively (Tam et al, 1982). Most strains of serogroup WI and WII/III reacted with more than one of the monoclonals against PI/A and PI/B, respectively. Two sets of monoclonals with six in each one were selected, and the reaction pattern observed with a particular strain was designated 'serovar' to denote a variety serologically defined by these monoclonal antibodies (Bygdeman et al, 1983; Knapp et al, 1984).

Many papers have been published in which serological classification has been used to characterise PPNG strains and various types of clinical isolates with regard to auxotype, antibiotic susceptibility, clinical disease syndromes and geographic distribution (for references see Bygdeman et al, 1983; Danielsson et al, 1983; Knapp et al, 1984), and also with regard to genomic fingerprinting (Falk et al, 1984; Falk et al, 1985). Geographical variations have been demonstrated, and nearly all the strains (96–98%) of auxotype AHU belong to serogroup WI whereas no particular serogroup or serovar specificity has been shown for other auxotypes. Invasive strains, i.e. those associated with DGI, have been shown to belong to particular serovars of serogroup WI whether they are of auxotype AHU- or Pro-. Of particular interest both from

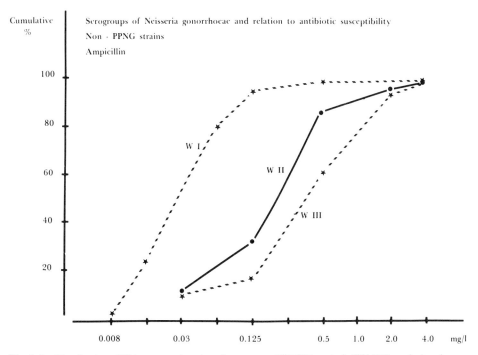

Fig. 1.5 Distribution of 726 gonococcal strains of serogroups WI (427 strains), WII (281 strains) and WIII (18 strains), respectively, with regard to susceptibility to ampicillin (data from Danielsson et al, 1983).

clinical and epidemiological points of view is the fact that practically all the strains of serogroup WI are sensitive to penicillin and tetracycline, whereas approximately 2/3 of those of serogroup WII and still more of those of WIII show decreased sensitivity (Fig. 1.5). A genetic linkage was in fact demonstrated between serogroup specificity and antibiotic susceptibility (Bygdeman et al, 1982).

Serological classification of gonococci with co-agglutination is feasible for monitoring clinical, epidemiological and laboratory studies. The tests are easy to perform and show good reproducibility between various laboratories, which indicates stability of the epitopes of protein I. However, with the use of a set of 12 monoclonal antibodies, six against PI/A and six against PI/B, a considerable number of serovars were shown to occur in a study of strains from Scandinavia (Bygdeman et al, 1983). In a world wide survey of strains 18 serovars of serogroup WI and 28 of serogroup WII/III were identified (Knapp et al, 1984). The reason for this great diversity of serovars is not yet known, but it might be due to genetic variation. In a recent study of in vitro transformation of chromosomal DNA with mutations to increased resistance to penicillin cotransformation of serogroup and serovar specificity was obtained, on some occasions with new serovar specificities indicating chromosomal recombinations under some conditions, for example, mutations to increased resistance to penicillin (Danielsson, Faruki & Sparling: to be published).

CONCLUDING REMARKS

Most of the basic research so far carried out on the gonococcus has been restricted to a few single strains. However, even the organisms of a single, apparently uniform strain have been shown to possess great diversity, seemingly influenced by various host and environmental factors. The ability of an isogenic strain to express opacity protein phase changes and different pili types is an excellent example of this. Though not quite essential for adherence to host cells the presence of pili potentiates this process by a factor of 5 to 10, and something similar is probably true for the opacity proteins. There is much evidence that the immune and non-specific defence mechanisms of the human host are activated and react against them, but the phase changes of various surface components clearly demonstrate that the gonococcus has developed delicate mechanisms to circumvent hostile environments. One may well be pessimistic about these phenomena, and also about the diversity of auxotypes and serovars. However, molecular biology and genetic research now being performed at several laboratories will certainly give us more detailed insight into the elaborate mechanisms of the gonococcus, and hopefully this knowledge will result in our finding the Achilles' heel of this organism. Until then, however, we have to continue to combat gonorrhoea with conventional methods, and there is every reason that these should be refined as well.

REFERENCES

Apicella M A 1976 Serogrouping of *Neisseria gonorrhoeae*: identification of four immunologically distinct acidic polysaccharides. Journal of Infectious Diseases 134: 377–383

Apicella M A, Morse S A, Mandrell R E, Griffis J M 1984 Factors influencing the antigenic structure of the lipooligosaccharides of *Neisseria gonorrhoeae*. Presented at the 4th International Conference on Pathogenic Neisseria, Asilomar (Stanford University Medical Center) Abstract 82

Black W J, Schwalbe R S, Nachamkin I, Cannon J G 1984 Characterization of *Neisseria gonorrhoeae* protein II phase variation by use of monoclonal antibodies. Infection and Immunity 45: 453–457

Blake M, Holmes K K, Swanson J 1979 Studies on gonococcus infection. XVII. IgA1 cleaving protease in vaginal washings from women with gonorrhoea. Journal of Infectious Diseases 139: 89–92

Blake M, Gotschlich E C 1983 Gonococcal membrane proteins — speculations on their role in pathogenesis. Progress in Allergy 33: 298–313

Blake M S, Gotschlich E C 1984 Studies on the IgA1 protease: improved methods of enzyme purification and detection, production of polyclonal and monoclonal antibodies, and localization of active site of the enzyme molecule. Poster presented at the 4th International Conference on Pathogenic Neisseria, Asilomar, Stanford University Medical School, Abstract 34

Blackwell C C, Kowolik M, Winstanley F P, Kinane D F, Weir D M, Law J A, HowangChork Y L 1983 ABO blood group and suceptibility to gonococcal infection. I. Factors affecting phagocytosis of Neisseria gonorrhoeae. Journal of Clinical and Laboratory Immunology 4: 173–178

Blackwell C C, Winstanley F P, Weir D M, Kinane 1984 Absence of bactericidal antibodies against group-I lipopolysaccharide determinants of Neisseria gonorrhoeae during human infection. Journal of Medical Microbiology 17: 353–356

Brinton C C 1977 The piliation phase syndrome and uses of purified pili in disease control. In: Miller C E (ed) XIIIth US Japan Conference of Health, Bethesda, Md, p 34–60

Brinton C C, Bryan J, Dillon J, Guerina N, Jacobsen L J, Labik A, Lee S, Levine A, Lim S, McMichael J, Polen S, Rogers K, To A, To S 1978 Uses of pili in gonorrhoea control: role of bacterial pili in disease, purification and properties of gonococcal pili, and progress in the development of a gonococcal pilus vaccine for gonorrhoeae. In: Brooks G F, Gotschlich E C, Holmes K K, Sawer W D, Young F E (eds) Immunobiology of Neisseria gonorrhoeae, American Society for Microbiology, Washington, DC p 155–178

Brinton C C, Word S W, Brown A, Labik A, Bryan J R, Lee S W et al 1982 The development of a Neisserial pilus vaccine for gonorrhoea and meningococcal meningitis. In: Robbins J B, Hill J C, Sadoff J C (eds) Seminars in infectious disease, volume IV: bacterial vaccines, Thieme, New York, p 140–159

Brooks G F, Lammel C J, Burns E Z, James J F 1980 Confounding factors affecting normal serum killing of *Neisseria gonorrhoeae* colony phenotype variants. In: Danielsson D, Normark S (eds) Genetics and Immunobiology of Pathogenic Neisseria, EMBO Workshop, Hemavan, University of Umeå, Sweden, p 251–254

Buchanan T M, Swanson J, Holmes K K, Kraus S J, Gotschlich E C 1973 Quantitative determination of antibody to gonococcal pili. Changes in antibody levels with gonococcal infection. Journal of Laboratory and Clinical Investigations 52: 2896–2909

Buchanan T M 1975 Antigenic heterogeneity of gonococcal pili. Journal of Experimental Medicine 141: 1470–1475

Buchanan T M, Pearce W A 1976 Pili as mediator of the attachment of gonococci to human erythrocytes. Infection and Immunity 13: 1483–1489

Buchanan T M, Chen K C S, Jones R B, Hildebrandt J F, Pearce W A, Hermodsen M A, Newlan J C, Luchtel D L 1978 Pili and principal outer membrane protein of *Neisseria gonorrhoeae*: immunochemical, structural and pathogenetic aspects. In: Brooks G F, Gotschlich E C, Holmes K K, Sawyer W D, Young F E (eds) Immunobiology of *Neisseria gonorrhoeae*. American Society for Microbiology, Washington, DC p 145–154

Buchanan T M, Eschenbach D A, Knapp J S, Holmes K K 1980 Gonococcal salpingitis is less likely to recur with *Neisseria gonorrhoeae* of the same principal outer membrane antigenic type. American Journal of Obstetrics and Gynecology 138: 978–980

Buchanan T M, Hilderbrandt J F 1981 Antigenspecific serotyping of Neisseria gonorrhoeae. Characterization based upon principal outer membrane protein. Infection and Immunity 32: 985–994

Bygdeman S, Bäckman M, Danielsson D, Norgren M 1982 Genetic linkage between serogroup specificity and antibiotic resistance in Neisseria gonorrhoeae. Acta pathologica et microbiologica scandinavica, Section B 90: 243–250

Bygdeman S, Danielsson D, Sandström E 1983 Gonococcal W serogroups in Scandinavia. A study with polyclonal and monoclonal antibodies. Acta pathologica et microbiologica scandinavica, Section B 91: 293–305

Cannon J G, Sparling P F 1984 The genetics of the gonococcus. Annual review of microbiology 38: 111–133

Cannon J G, W J, Nachamkin I, Stewart P W 1984 Monoclonal antibody that recognizes an outer membrane antigen common to the pathogenic Neisseria species but not to most nonpathogenic Neisseria species. Infection and Immunity 43: 994–999

Carifo K, Catlin B W 1973 *Neisseria gonorrhoeae* auxotyping: differentiation of clinical isolates based on growth responses on chemically defined media. Applied Microbiology 26: 223–230

Catlin B W 1973 Nutritional profiles of *Neisseria gonorrhoeae*, *Neisseria meningitidis*, and *Neisseria lactamica* in chemically defined media and the use of growth requirements for gonococcal typing. Journal of Infectious Diseases 128: 178–194

Catlin B W 1977 Nutritional requirements and auxotyping. In: Roberts R B (ed) The Gonococcus, New York, Wiley, p 92–109

Catlin B W 1978 Characteristics and auxotyping of *Neisseria gonorrhoeae*. In: Bergan T, Norris J R (eds) Methods in Microbiology, Academic Press, London, New York, San Francisco, p 345–380

Chacko C W, Nair G M 1959 Sero-diagnosis of gonorrhoea with a microprecipitin using a lipopolysaccharide antigen from *Neisseria gonorrhoeae*. British Journal of Venereal Diseases 45: 33–38

Chen K C S, Buchanan Tm 1980 Hydrolases from Neisseria: Pathogenesis and diagnostic implications. In: Danielsson D, Normark S (eds) Genetics and immunobiology of pathogenic Neisseria. EMBO workshop, Hemavan, University of Umeå, Sweden, p. 229

Danielsson D, Maeland J A 1978 Serotyping and antigenic studies of *Neisseria gonorrhoeae*. In: Bergan T, Norris J R (eds) Methods in Microbiology, volume 10, Ch. XII, Academic Press, London, New York, San Francisco, p 315–344

Danielsson D, Sandström E 1980 Serology of *Neisseria gonorrhoeae*. Demonstration by co-agglutination and immunoelectrophoresis of antigenic differences associated with colour/opacity colonial variants. Acta pathologica et microbiologica scandinavica, Section B 88: 39–46

Danielsson D, Bygdeman S, Kallings I 1983 Epidemiology of gonorrhoea: serogroup, antibiotic susceptibility and auxotype patterns of consecutive gonococcal isolates from ten different areas of Sweden. Scandinavian Journal of Infectious Diseases 15: 33–42

Draper D L, Lammel C J, Sweet R L, Brooks G F 1984 Attachment of gonococcal outer membranes containing protein II variants to HELA 229 cells. Presented at the 4th International Conference on Pathogenic Neisseria, Asilomar (Stanford University Medical Center), Abstract 92

Dyer D W, Blackman E, West S, Sparling P F 1984 Genetic approaches to understanding the mechanisms of iron utilization by the pathogenic Neisseria. Presented at the 4th International Conference on Pathogenic Neisseria, Asilomar (Stanford University Medical Center), Abstract 66

Falk E S, Bjorvaln B, Danielsson D, Kristiansen B E, Melby K, Sorensen B 1984 Restriction endonuclease fingerprinting of chromosomal DNA of *Neisseria gonorrhoeae*. Acta pathologica et microbiologica scandinavica, Section B 92: 271–278

Falk E S, Danielsson D, Bjorvaln B, Melby K, Sorensen B, Kristiansen B E, Lund S, Sandström E 1985 Phenotypic and genotypic characterization of penicillinase producing strains of *Neisseria gonorrhoeae*. Acta Pathologica et Microbiologica Scandinavica, Section B93: 91–97

Forslin L, Danielsson D 1980 In vitro studies of the adherence of *Neisseria gonorrhoeae* and other urogenital cells, with special regard to the menstrual cycle. Gynecologic and Obstetric Investigation 11: 327–340

Guymon L F, Esser M, Daly J, Sparling P F, Shafter W 1980 Characterisation of lipopolysaccharide mutants of *Neisseria gonorrhoeae*. In: Danielsson D, Normark S (eds) Genetics and immunobiology of pathogenic Neisseria, EMBO Workshop, Hemavan, University of Umeå, Sweden, p 33–36

Gotschlich E C 1984 Gonorrhoea. In: Germanier R (ed) Bacterial vaccines, Academic Press, New York, p 351–373

Harkness A H 1948 The pathology of gonorrhoea. British Journal of Veneral Diseases 24: 137–147

Heckels J E 1981 Structural comparison of *Neisseria gonorrhoeae* outer membrane proteins. Journal of Bacteriology 145: 736–742

Heckels J E 1982 Role of surface proteins in the adhesion of *Neisseria gonorrhoeae*. In: Schlessinger D (ed) Microbiology 1982, American Society for Microbiology, Washington, DC p 301–304

Hendley J O, Powell K R, Jordan J R, Rodewald R D, Volk W A 1978 Capsules of Neisseria gonorrhoeae. In: Brooks G F, Gotschlich E C, Holmes K K, Sawyer W D, Young F E (eds) Immunobiology of *Neisseria gonorrhoeae*. American Society for Microbiology, Washington, DC p 116–120

Hermodsen M A, Chen K C S, Buchanan T M 1978 Neisseria pili proteins: amino terminal amino acid sequence and identification of an unusual amino acid. Biochemistry 17: 442–445

Hill J H 1948 Fundamental problems for laboratory research on *Neisseria gonorrhoeae* and gonococcal infection. American Journal of Syphilis, Gonorrhoea and Venereal Diseases 32: 165–176

James J F, Swanson J 1977 The capsule of the gonococcus. Journal of Experimental Medicine 145: 1082–1086

James J F, Lammel C J, Draper D L, Brooks G F 1980 Attachment of N. *gonorrhoeae* colony phenotype variants to eucaryotic cells and tissues. In: Danielsson D, Normark S (eds) Genetics and immunobiology of pathogenic Neisseria, EMBO Workshop, Hemavan, University of Umeå, Sweden p 213–216

James-Holmquest A N, Swanson J, Buchanan T M, Wende R D, Williams R P 1974 Differential attachment of piliated and nonpiliated Neisseria gonorrhoeae to human sperm. Infection and Immunity 9: 897–899

Johnson A P, Taylor-Robinson D, McGee Z A, Melly M A, Camey F E 1977 Preliminary studies on the mechanism by which *Neisseria gonorrhoeae* damages host tissue. FEMS Microbiology Letters 1: 247–249

Johnston K H, Holmes K K, Gotschlich E C 1976 The serological classification of *Neisseria gonorrhoeae*. I. Isolation of the outer membrane complex responsible for serotypic specificity. Journal of Experimental Medicine 143: 741–758

Joiner K A, Frank M M 1984 Mechanisms of serum resistance in Neisseria gonorrhoeae. Presented at the 4th international conference on pathogenic *Neisseria*. Asilomar (Stanford University Medical Center) Abstract 84

Jephcott A E, Reyn A, Birch-Andersen A 1971 *Neisseria gonorrhoeae*. III. Demonstration of presumed appendages to cells from different colony types. Acta pathologica et microbiologica scandinavica, Section B 79: 437–439

Kellogg D S, Peacock W L, Deacon W E, Brown L, Pirkle C I 1963 *Neisseria gonorrhoeae*. I. Virulence genetically linked to clonal variation. Journal of Bacteriology 85: 1274–1279

Kellogg D S, Cohen I R, Norins L C, Schroeter A L, Reising G 1968 *Neisseria gonorrhoeae*. II. Colonial variation and pathogenicity during 35 months in vitro. Journal of Bacteriology 96: 596–605

Knapp J S, Holmes K K 1975 Disseminated gonococcal infection caused by *Neisseria gonorrhoeae* with unique nutritional requirements. Journal of Infectious Diseases 132: 204–206

Knapp J S, Tam M R, Nowinski R C, Holmes K K, Sandström E G 1984 Serological classification of *Neisseria gonorrhoeae* with use of monoclonal antibodies to gonococcal outer membrane protein I. Journal of Infectious Diseases 150: 44–48

Lambden P R, Heckels J E, James L T, Watt P J 1979 Variations in surface protein composition associated with virulence properties in opacity types of *Neisseria gonorrhoeae*. Journal of General Microbiology 114: 305–312

Lambden P R, Heckels J E, McBride H, Watt P J 1981 The identification and isolation of novel pilus types produced by variants of *N. gonorrhoeae* P9 following selection in vivo. FEMS Microbiology Letters 10: 339–341

Laemmli U K 1970 Cleavage of structural proteins during the assembly of the head of bacteriophage T4. Nature (London) 227: 680–685

Lammel C J, De Kay V J, Knapp J S, Sweet R L, Brooks G F 1984 Men and women infected with the same strain of *Neisseria gonorrhoeae* often have antibody responses to different gonococcal antigens. Presented at the 4th International Conference on Pathogenic Neisseria, Asilomar (Stanford University Medical Center) Abstract 101

Lind I, Reimann K 1980 Studies on the antigenic heterogeneity of Neisseria gonorrhoeae pilus antigens. In: Danielsson D, Normark S (eds) Genetics and immunobiology of pathogenic Neisseria, EMBO Workshop, University of Umeå, Sweden, p 95–97

Lipschutz B 1904 Über einen einfachen Gonokokkennahrboden, Zentralblatt für die Bakteriologie 36: 743–749

Maeland J A 1969 Antigenic determinants of aqueous ether extracted endotoxin from *Neisseria gonorrhoeae* Acta pathologica et microbiologica scandinavica 76: 475–483

Maeland J A, Kristoffersen T, Hofstad T 1971 Immunochemical investigations on *Neisseria gonorrhoeae* endotoxin. Acta pathologica et microbiologica scandinavica Section B 79: 233–238

Maeland J A, Larsen B 1971 Human serum antibodies reacting with endotoxin from *Neisseria gonorrhoeae*. British Journal of Venereal Diseases 47: 269–272

Mayer L W 1982 Rates of in vitro changes in gonococcal opacity phenotypes. Infection and Immunity 37: 481–485

McGee Z A, Stephens D S, Hoffman L H, Schlech W F, Horn R G 1983 Mechanisms of musocal invasion by pathogenic Neisseria. Review of Infecious Diseases Vol 5, Supplement 4, The University of Chicago, p S708–S714

Meyer T F, Mlaver N, So M 1982 Pilus expression in Neisseria gonorrhoeae involves chromosomal rearrangement. Cell 30: 45–52

Meyer T F, Stern A, Nickel P, So M 1984 Molecular genetics of the gonococcal opacity protein. Presented at the 4th International Conference of Pathogenic Neisseria, Asilomar (Stanford University Medical Center), Abstract 61

Morse S A, Vaughan P, Johnson D, Iglewski B H 1976 Inhibition of *Neisseria gonorrhoeae* by a bacteriocin from *Pseudomonas aeruginosa*. Antimicrobial Agents and Chemotherapy 10: 354–362

Morse S A, Miller R D, Hebeler B H 1977 Physiology and metabolism of *Neisseria gonorrhoeae*. In: Roberts R B (ed) The Gonococcus, New York, Wiley, p 213–253

Morse S A, Cacciapuoti A F, Lysko P G 1979 Physiology of *Neisseria gonorrhoeae*. Advances in Microbiology and Physiology, 20: 251–320

Morse S A, Mietzner T A 1984 Iron-regulated membrane proteins of *Neisseria gonorrhoeae*: Isolation and characterization of a major 37 000 dalton iron-regulated protein. Presented at the 4th International Conference on Pathogenic Neisseria, Asilomar (Stanford University Medical Center) Abstract 85

Moberg I 1975 Auxotyping of gonococcal isolates. In: Danielsson D, Juhlin L, Mårdh P A (eds) Genital infections and their complications, Almqvist & Wiksell International, Stockholm, p 271–273

Mulks M H, Plaut A G 1978 IgA protease production as a characteristic distinguishing pathogenic from harmless Neisseriae. New England Journal of Medicine 299: 973–976

Mulks M H, Plaut A G, Lamm M 1980 Gonococcal IgA protease reduces inhibition of bacterial adherence by human secretory IgA. In: Danielsson D, Normark S (eds) Genetics and immunobiology of pathogenic Neisseria. EMBO Workshop, Hemavan, University of Umeå, Sweden, p 217–220

Mårdh P A, Weström L 1976 Adherence of bacteria to vaginal epithelial cells. Infection and Immunity 13: 661–666

Norquist A, Davies J, Norlander L, Normark S 1978 The effect of iron starvation on the outer membrane protein composition of Neisseria gonorrhoeae. FEMS Microbiology Letters 4: 71–75

Novotny P, Short J A, Walker P D 1975 An electron-microscope study of naturally occurring and cultured cells of *Neisseria gonorrhoeae*. Journal of Medical Microbiology 8: 413–427

Novotny P, Turner W H 1975 Immunological heterogeneity of pili of *Neisseria gonorrhoeae*. Journal of General Microbiology 89: 87–92

Novotny P, Short J A, Hughes M, Miller J J, Syratt C, Turner W H, Harris J R W, McLennan I

P B 1977 Studies on the mechanism of pathogeneicity of *Neisseria gonorrhoeae*. Journal of Medical Microbiology 10: 347–365

Perry M B, Diena B B, Ashton F E 1977 Lipopolysaccharides of *Neisseria gonorrhoeae*. In: Roberts R B (ed) The Gonococcus, Wiley, New York, p 285–301

Plaut A G, Gilbert J V, Artenstin M S, Capra J D 1975 *Neisseria gonorheae* and *Neisseria meningitidis*: Extracellular enzymes cleaves human immunoglobulin A. Science 190: 1103–1105

Plaut A G, Gilbert J V, Wistar R 1977 Loss of antibody activity in human immunoglobulin A exposed to extracellular immunoglobulin A protease of *Neisseria gonorrhoeae* and *Streptococcus sanguis*. Infection and Immunity 17: 130–135

Reimann K, Lind I 1977 An indirect haemagglutination test for demonstration for gonococcal antibodies using gonococcal pili as antigen. I. Methodoogy and preliminary results. Acta pathologica et microbiologica scandinavica, Section C 85: 115–122

Rice P A, Huff P M, Lamb K J, O'Brien J P 1980 *Neisseria gonorrhoeae* surface antigens: their interaction with human sera. In: Danielsson D, Normark S (eds) Genetics and immunobiology of pathogenic *Neisseria*. EMBO Workshop, Hemavan, University of Umeå, Sweden, p 255–259

Rice P A, Tam M R, Blake M S 1984 IgG antibodies in normal human serum directed against PIII block killing of serum resistant *N. gonorrhoeae* by immune serum. Presented at the 4th International Conference on Pathogenic Neisseria, Asilomar (Stanford University Medical Center), Abstract 108

Rosenthal R S, Fleming T J 1984 Arthropathic properties of gonococcal peptidoglycan. Presented at the 4th International Conference on Pathogenic Neisseria, Asilomar (Stanford University Medical Center), Abstract 86

Robertson J N, Vincent P, Ward M E 1977 The preparation and properties of gonococcal pili. Journal of General Microbiology 102: 169–177

Sadoff J C, Zollinger W D, Sidbersky H 1978 Cell surface structures of *Neisseria gonorrhoeae*. In: Brooks G F, Gotschlich E C, Holmes K K, Sawyer W D, Young F E (eds) Immunobiology of Neisseria gonorrhoeae. American Society for Microbiology, Washington, DC p 93–100

Salton M R J 1977 Enzymatic basis for β-lactam antibiotic activity. In: Roberts R B (ed) The Gonococcus, Wiley, New York, p 177–196

Sandström E, Danielsson D 1980 Serology of *Neisseria gonorrhoeae*. Classification with co-agglutination. Acta pathologica et microbiologica scandinavica, Section B 88: 27–38

Sandström E G, Chen K C S, Buchanan T M 1982 Serology of *Neisseria gonorrhoeao*: Co-agglutination serogroups WI and WII/III correspond to different outer membrane portein I molecules. Infection and Immunity 38: 462–470

Schoolnik G K, Buchanan T M, Holmes K K 1976 Gonococci causing disseminated gonococcal infection are resistant to the bactericidal action of normal human sera. Journal of Laboratory and Clinical Investigations 58: 1163–1173

Schoolnik G K, Ochs H D, Buchanan T M 1979 Immunoglobulin class responsible for gonococcal bactericidal activity in normal human sera. Journal of Immunology 122: 1771–1779

Schoolnik G K, Tai J Y, Gotschlich E C 1982 The human erythrocyte binding domain of gonococcal pili. In: Robbins J B, Hill J C, Sadoff J C (eds) Seminars in infectious disease, volume IV: bacterial vaccines, Thieme, New York, p 172–180

Schoolnik G K, Tai J Y, Gotschlich E C 1983 A pilus peptide vaccine for prevention of gonorrhoea. Progress in Allergy 33: 314–331

Sparling P F, Yobs A R 1967 Colonial variation of *Neisseria gonorrhoeae* isolated from males and females. Journal of Bacteriology 93: 513–515

Sparling P F, Biswas G D, Sox T E 1977 Transformation of the Gonococcus. In: Roberts R B (ed) The Gonococcus, Wiley, New York p 155–176

Stephens D S, Whitney A M, Schoolnik G K 1984 Pilin subunits of *Neisseria meningitidis* contain an epitope in common with the receptor-binding domain of gonococcal pili. Presented at the 4th International Conference on Pathogenic Neisseria, Asilomar (Stanford University Medical Center), Abstract 51

Swanson J, Kraus S J, Gotschlich E C 1971 Studies on gonococcus infection. I. Pili and zones of adhesion: their role to gonococcal growth patterns. Journal of Experimental Medicine 134: 886–906

Swanson J 1977 Surface components associated with gonococcal cell interactions. In: Roberts R B (ed) The Gonococcus, Wiley, New York, p 369–401

Swanson J 1978 Cell wall outer membrane variants of *Neisseria gonorrhoeae*. In: Brooks G F, Gotschlich E C, Holmes K K, Sawyer W D, Young F E (eds) Immunobiology of Neisseria gonorrhoeae, American Society for Microbiology, Washington DC p 130–137

Swanson J, Heckels J 1980 Proposal: Nomenclature of gonococcal outer membrane proteins. In: Danielsson D, Normark S (eds) Genetics and immunobiology of pathogenic *Neisseria*, EMBO Workshop, Hemavan, University of Umeå, Sweden, p xxi–xxiii

Swanson J 1982 Colony opacity and protein II compositions of gonococci. Infection and Immunity 37: 359–368

Tam M R, Buchanan T M, Sandström E, Holmes K K, Knapp J S, Siadak A W, Nowinski R C 1982 Serological classification of Neisseria gonorrhoeae with monoclonal antibodies. Infection and Immunity 36: 1042–1053

Thongtai C, Sawyer W D 1973 Studies on virulence of *Neisseria gonorrhoeae*: I. Relation of colonial morphology and resistance to phagocytosis by polymorphonuclear leuococytes. Infection and Immunity 7: 373–379

Tramont E C, Wilson C 1977 Variations in buccal cell adhesion of *Neisseria gonorrhoeae*. Infection and Immunity 16: 709–711

Tramont E C, Ciak J, McChesney D, Boslego J, Brinton C C 1979 Cross-reactivity of epithelial cell attachment. In: Proceedings of the 11th International Conference on Antimicrobial Agents and Chemotherapy, Boston, p 1239–1240

Waitkins S 1974 Fimbrial hemagglutination by *Neisseria gonorrhoeae*. Journal of Clinical Pathology 25: 56–59

Ward M E , Glynn A A 1972 Human antibody response to lipopolysaccharides from *Neisseria gonorrhoeae*. British Journal of Veneral Diseases 50: 272–276

Ward M E, Watt P J 1972 Adherence of *Neisseria gonorrhoeae* to urethral mucosal: an electron microscopic study of human gonorrhoea. Journal of Infectious Diseases 126: 601–605

Ward M E, Watt P J, Robertson J N 1974 The human fallopian tube: a laboratory model for gonococal infection. Journal of Infectious Diseases 129: 650–659

Ward M E, Watt P J 1975 Studies on the cell biology of gonorrhoea. In: Danielsson D, Juhlin L, Mårdh P A (eds) Genital infections and their complications, Almqvist & Wiksell International, Stockholm, p 229–242

Watt P J, Ward M E, Glynn A A 1971 A comparison of serological tests for the diagnosis of gonorrhoea. British Journal of Venereal Diseases 47: 448–451

West S E H, Sparling P F 1985 Response of *Neisseria gonorrhoeae* to iron limitation: alterations in expression of membrane proteins without apparent siderophore production. Infection and Immunity 47: 388–394

Wilson J F 1954 A serological study of *Neisseria gonorrhoeae*. Journal of Pathology and Bacteriology 68: 495–514

Wolf-Watz H, Elmros T, Normark S, Blom G D 1975 Cell envelope of *Neisseria gonorrhoeae*: outer membrane and peptidoglycan composition of penicillin sensitive and resistant strains. Infection and Immunity 11: 1332–1341

2. Epidemiology and treatment of penicillinase-producing *neisseria gonorrhoeae*

M. W. Adler

EPIDEMIOLOGY

Historical background to PPNG development

Gonoccal strains, partially resistant to penicillin and other antibiotics, have long been recognised and infections caused by them have been treated with dose increases or with alternative antibiotics. The advent and decline in effectiveness of the sulphonamides for the treatment of gonorrhoea in the 1930s and 1940s illustrates this phenomenon. It is known, historically, that chromosomal antimicrobial resistance in *Neisseria gonorrhoeae* was present in the 1930s from the use of sulphonamides. An examination of gonococcal strains collected in Denmark before 1937 indicated that 8% were resistant at that time to 50 μg/ml of sulphapyridine (Reyn, 1961). This gonococcal resistance continued throughout the 1940s with a resulting decline in the usefulness of sulphonamides in the treatment of gonorrhoea. Thus, by the end of the 1940s, about 90% of gonococcal isolates showed increased resistance to sulphonamides and approximately the same proportion of patients with gonorrhoea failed to be cured with these types of drugs (Dunlop, 1949).

In the face of this increased resistance, penicillin started to be widely used for patients with gonorrhoea. Before this extensive use of penicillin for gonorrhoea, virtually all gonococci were susceptible to less than 0.03 units/ml of penicillin (Cohn & Seijo, 1944; Romansky, 1946). However, with the widespread availability and use of penicillin chromosomal mutations occurred with resulting increases in resistance to penicillins. One of the factors that played a part in the spread of resistance was the use of slow release penicillins such as PAM (procaine penicillin in oil with aluminium monostearate) given as a single dose. Such types of preparations did not provide high blood levels and gave a long sub-therapeutic 'tail' which could convert patients with gonorrhoea 'into living test tubes for producing resistant strains of gonococci . . .' (Curtis & Wilkinson, 1958). The increased resistance has resulted in the necessity to use larger curative doses of penicillin for gonorrhoea. It has been demonstrated in the United States that in 1955 only 0.6% of gonococcal isolates required more than 0.05 units/ml of penicillin to inhibit the growth of the organism and that this proportion had increased to 42% by 1965 (Martin & Price, 1970). In the Far East and Vietnam the proportion of strains requiring 1 unit/ml of penicillin in the early 1970s was 15% and 61% respectively (Watko & Brownlow, 1975; Hart, 1973).

Initial reports of PPNG

Despite this forty years of increasing resistance to penicillin in certain parts of the world, few people anticipated total resistance. However, Falkow's prediction in early 1975 of the possible emergence of a gonococcus that would eventually acquire total resistance to penicillin was all too quickly fulfilled (Falkow et al, 1976). Strains of PPNG first emerged in the Far East and West Africa. By late 1975 to early 1976 the first reports of this occurrence had also emerged from North America and the United Kingdom.

In the United States the first two cases were identified in March and April 1976 in two men who had had sexual contacts in East Asia before returning by plane to the USA. Both were picked up as a result of treatment failure with penicillin and eventually responded to spectinomycin (Ashford et al, 1976; Mareck, 1976).

The first British case was described by Phillips in the *Lancet* in September 1976 and was a report of a B-lactamase producing gonococcus isolated from a woman with pelvic inflammatory disease (Phillips, 1976). This case was followed two months later by a description of an outbreak in Liverpool (Percival et al, 1976). This was a well defined epidemic of 80 cases, infected males were usually under 30 and black, whereas the females were white and slightly younger. The type of plasmid identified and the fact that isolates were of the same auxotype pointed to a single, but unidentified source, probably from West Africa.

Plasmid types
The Far Eastern isolates were originally found to contain both a 4.4 and 24.5 mega dalton plasmid. Originally the African strains of PPNG contained a smaller sized plasmid of 3.2 mega daltons. More recently, cases in Africa (Ghana & Kenya) have been described with isolates containing the 4.4 mega dalton (Asian) plasmid. The 3.2 and 4.4 mega dalton plasmids are resistance (R) factors which code for beta-lactamase production. The larger (24.5 mega dalton) plasmid is a conjugative or transfer factor which enables resistance to be transferred to other gonococci and other organisms. The R plasmids are readily lost on subculture in vitro unless this is carried out in the presence of penicillin or ampicillin. The picture became further complicated with the report from Van Embden and his colleagues in Holland that they were isolating African strains which, in addition to the conventional 3.2 mega dalton plasmid, also carried one that was 24 mega dalton in size (Van Embden et al, 1981). Finally, an analysis of plasmid types of PPNG isolates in Liverpool showed that even though all the cases in 1976 and 1977 only contained the 3.2 M.D. plasmid this had changed by 1982. In that year 54 cases were found with the following plasmids — 4.4 alone (31 cases), 3.2 alone (15), 3.2 + 24.5 (5) and 4.4 + 24.5 (3) — (Arya et al, 1984). The features of different plasmid types are described in more detail by Danielson in the first half of this section (Biology of *N. gonorrhoeae*).

Originally all cases of PPNG were responsive to treatment with spectinomycin, but recently cases of PPNG that are resistant to this drug have appeared (see treatment). As indicated above PPNG strains develop their resistance through plasmids. Recently, however, beta-lactamase negative strains have been described which developed chromosomally mediated resistance. The first of such cases were recognised in the United States in 1983 in North Carolina (Centers for Disease Control, 1983a). This was an outbreak of 200 cases and, since that time, a further 16 states within America have reported this same phenomenon (Centers for Disease Control, 1983b). Cases are reported in both heterosexuals and homosexuals. The strains are sensitive to spectinomycin and the cephalosporins. Most of the cases reported so far were picked up after treatment with routine penicillin or tetracycline had failed. Most of these cases have been endemic, in contrast to PPNG where foreign importation is responsible for the majority of cases.

Prevalence of PPNG

Following the reports from America and the United Kingdom, it appeared that no country wished to be without the status symbol of its own PPNG isolates. These strains have now been identified in 56 countries and epidemiological evidence suggests their presence in at least another 40 countries (Table 2.1). It is probably true to

Table 2.1   Countries with identified strains of Beta-lactamase producing *Neisseria gonorrhoeae*

Africa	Africa	Americas	East Asia	Europe	South East Asia
Morocco	Mauritus	Canada	Philippines	France	Indonesia
Ghana	Sudan	United States	Hong Kong	Belgium	Singapore
Mali	Malawi	Mexico	Taiwan	Netherlands	Malaysia
Nigeria	Uganda	Panama	Guam	United Kingdom	Thailand
Central African		Argentina	Japan	West Germany	India
Republic					
Gabon	Togo	Colombia	Republic of Korea	Denmark	Sri Lanka
Zaire	Benin		New Zealand	Switzerland	
Madagascar	Algeria		New Hebrides	Sweden	
Zambia	Sierra Leone		Australia	Norway	
Senegal	Gambia			Finland	
				Poland	
Ivory Coast	Kenya			Spain	
Chad	Niger				
Egypt	Cameroon				
	S. Africa				

say that 'the number of countries where PPNG has been identified appears to be limited only by the capacity of local laboratory services to isolate and test for these strains' (Centers for Disease Control, 1982a).

(i) Far East and Africa

The prevalence of PPNG is highest in South East Asia and Africa. This prevalence has been changing in an alarming fashion in these two endemic areas (Table 2.2).

Table 2.2   % PPNG strains — prevalence in endemic areas

	1977	1978	1980	1981	1982
	%	%	%	%	%
Asia					
Philippines	30		30		
Singapore	0.3		19.2	30	
Thailand		8.6	28.8	42	
Africa					
Nigeria	3		20		
Ghana					32
Kenya			0		20

In Singapore most PPNG are isolated from prostitutes, with their predominantly foreign clientele distributing PPNG throughout the world. The same picture is to be found in Bangkok (Thailand) and the Philippines. Surveys in the latter have reported that 30–40% of isolates were PPNG, largely among bar girls or prostitutes.

Recent data from the Philippines are not available, but in Singapore and Thailand the increases have been very marked. In the former, an increase from 0.3% of isolates to 30% in just 4 years and, in the latter, from 8.6 to 42% in only 3 years (Rajan et al, 1981; Brown et al, 1982) have been reported. The African data are more sparse but support the general trend of an increasing prevalence of PPNG (Osoba, 1981). Ratnam and colleagues, reporting a low prevalence of PPNG (3.2%) in Lusaka, Zambia, make the point that this figure, and others in different African countries, are probably higher than realised. Special facilities for the diagnosis and treatment of

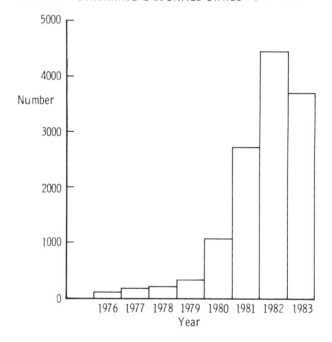

Fig. 2.1

sexually transmitted diseases (STDs) are only found in a few teaching centres; 'in general, diagnosis remains largely presumptive on clinical presentation alone and treatment practices are suboptimal. Furthermore, follow up is poor and neither treatment failures nor sexual contacts are identified' (Ratnam et al, 1982).

(ii) The United States
Since the original case reports in the United States in 1976 the number of cases has increased (Fig. 2.1). From 1976 to 1979 the number of cases rose slowly, most occurring in people or their sexual partners who had travelled to the Far East. After 1979 the number of cases started to rise rapidly; thus in that year there were only 328 reported cases but this has risen to 4457 by 1982 with a slight decline to 3720 for 1983. (Table 2.3) Despite this alarming increase the proportion of PPNG isolates to non-PPNG was less than 0.5%.

Naturally this low overall prevalence hides the fact that rates vary throughout the United States and that short lived local, usually urban, outbreaks do occur (Jaffe et al, 1981, Centers for Disease Control 1980). One such outbreak occurred during 1980 and 1981 in Los Angeles, during which an average of 50 cases per month were being notified (Centers for Disease Control 1983c). In some areas of America, endemic transmission is mainly responsible for the continued prevalence of PPNG (e.g. New York City, California and Florida) These three centtres alone account for nearly 60% of all PPNG in the States. In contrast to endemic transmission leading to a sustained high prevalence, outbreaks may be due to importation of strains as occurred in Washington and Shreveport (Handsfield et al, 1982).

Table 2.3   Proportion of PPNG isolates in relation to all cases of gonorrhoea in the United States 1976–1983

Year	Gonorrhoea	PPNG	
		N	% of all G.
1976	1,001,994	98	0.09
1977	1,002,219	185	0.01
1978	1,013,436	202	0.01
1979	1,004,058	328	0.03
1980	1,004,029	1099	0.10
1981	990,864	2734	0.27
1982	960,633	4457	0.46
1983	900,435	3720	0.41

(iii) The United Kingdom

Since the first case reports in the United Kingdom (UK) in 1976 the number of cases and prevalence rate have increased (Public Health Laboratory Service Communicable Disease Centre, 1982; Jephcott et al, 1981; Johnston & Kolator, 1981). Figure 2.2 illustrates the annual doubling and exponential growth in the number of cases from 1977 to 1982. The 1983 figures (latest available numbers) show that this doubling has now ceased. (Public Health Laboratory Service Communicable Disease Centre, 1983). The proportion of PPNG isolates in relation to all isolates of *N. gonorrhoeae* in the UK is currently below 2% (Table 2.4). These national data, however, hide regional differences. The mean rate for the three years 1979–1981 inclusive was highest in ports and tourist areas (Adler & McCutchan, 1984). Even regional differences hide the very dramatic fluctuations that can occur from month to month in large clinics. McManus et al (1982) reported monthly rates ranging from 0.95 to 10.2 over a seven month period in a central London clinic.

A national surveillance system for PPNG exists in the UK which allows for an examination of the geographical source of infections. Table 2.5 shows the percentage of cases acquired abroad and imported into the UK as well as indigenous cases where the consort was infected within the UK and, lastly, indirect importation. Until 1980 the rise in PPNG had resulted largely from directly imported cases and the ratio of these to indigenous cases was constantly running at about 2:1. This suggests that increasing importation, not sustained transmission within the country was the reason for the substantial increase in incidence. In 1980 a shift from imported to indigenous or endemic transmission started to appear and a cross over between the two types actually took place in the second half of the year and has been maintained ever since (Fig. 2.3). Between 1980 and 1981 indigenous cases increased by 230% while imported cases increased by only 53% (McCutchan et al, 1982).

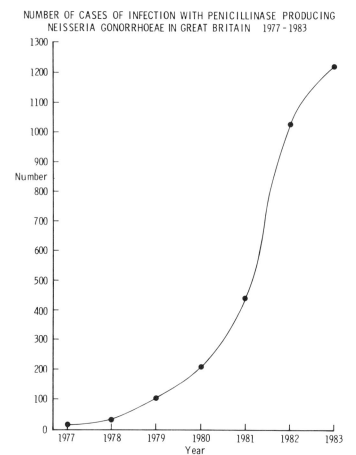

NUMBER OF CASES OF INFECTION WITH PENICILLINASE PRODUCING
NEISSERIA GONORRHOEAE IN GREAT BRITAIN   1977 - 1983

Fig. 2.2

Table 2.4 Proportion of PPNG isolates in relation to all cases of
gonorrhoea in the United Kingdom

Year	1977–1983 All cases of gonorrhoea	PPNG	Isolates
		N	% of all G.
1977	65,963	15	0.02
1978	63,569	31	0.05
1979	61,616	104	0.17
1980	60,850	211	0.3
1981	58,301	443	0.8
1982	58,782	1033	1.7
1983	N.A.	1223	

An examination of the characteristics of the people who were infected with PPNG
shows that these strains are mainly imported by male airline passengers who had
recently been infected in endemic areas. It was found that directly imported strains
had occurred predominantly in men at a ratio of 9:1 but indigenous strains, like
other strains of gonorrhoea in Great Britain were divided nearly equally between

Table 2.5   PPNG — presumed place of infection — United Kingdom 1977–1983

Place of Infection	1977		1978		1979		1980		1981		1982		1983	
	n	%	n	%	n	%	n	%	n	%	n	%	n	%
Abroad	7	(47)	18	(58)	55	(53)	110	(52)	168	(38)	236	(23)	252	(21)
Consort infected abroad	1	(7)	3	(10)	13	(13)	21	(10)	46	(10)	65	(6)	88	(7)
Consort infected in UK	5	(33)	8	(26)	21	(20	50	(24)	165	(37)	517	(50)	610	(50)
Not known	2		2		15		30		64		215		273	
TOTAL	15		31		104		211		443		1033		1223	

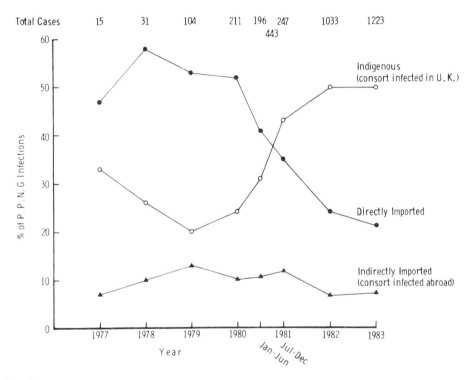

SOURCE OF PPNG IN GREAT BRITAIN

Fig. 2.3

the sexes at a ratio of 1.7:1. The short incubation period of gonorrhoea and the slow and infrequent rail or sea connections to the endemic areas made air travel the only plausible mode of transmission. It was also found that men and women who import PPNG are typically older than those infected with indigenous PPNG and older than patients with gonorrhoea in the UK.

The predominance of PPNG found amongst men, and the age distribution of those importing such strains, may be partly explained by more frequent travel to endemic areas by men (2:1) and by older people. Since older men travel more often to endemic regions than other groups in the population they are more likely to be exposed to PPNG than younger men and women. Most PPNG reaches the UK from two primary endemic regions (Table 2.6). Over the last seven years 42% of the cases were derived from the Far East, 35% from Africa and the remaining 22% from Europe and other sources.

Table 2.6 Geographical origins of 851 cases of PPNG imported into Great Britain (1977–1983)

Region	Annual number of imported cases							Total imported cases	
	1977	1978	1979	1980	1981	1982	1983	n	%
Far East	2	7	31	49	79	102	90	360	42.3
Africa	5	9	17	37	54	71	109	302	35.5
Europe	0	0	4	15	20	30	35	104	12.2
Others	0	2	3	9	15	34	22	85	10.0
All regions	7	18	55	110	168	237	256	851	100.0

The increased importation of PPNG seen originally in the UK could have resulted from an increase in (a) importation of gonorrhoea (b) travel to endemic areas or finally (c) prevalence in endemic areas. Cases of gonorrhoea (not PPNG) imported into the UK have increased from 3.25 to 4.03% of all cases, an increase of 24%. During this same period PPNG has increased from 0.33 to 4.50, a 13 fold or 1300% increase. Airline travel between Great Britain and West Africa has increased by 60% from 1979 to 1981. South East Asian arrivals and departures increased by only 5% and travel to and from Thailand, from which 56% of all Asian cases arose, decreased by 5% during the same period. Thus, neither importation of gonorrhoea nor travel to endemic areas have increased sufficiently to account for more than a small amount of the large increase in PPNG in the UK. The most likely explanation is that there has been an expansion of PPNG strains within endemic areas of Africa and Asia and that this is the major reason that the disease doubled annually in Great Britain from 1977–1982.

The UK picture of a predominence of endemic to imported cases of PPNG since 1980 is not always reflected at the same point in time in special local situations. Thin et al (1983) noted that, in their population in South London, this switch from imported to indigenous did not occur until 1982.

(iv) Europe

Holland is the only European country, apart from the United Kingdom, that has reported a substantial number of cases, in particular in The Hague and Amsterdam. Other countries in Europe have few cases with a low prevalence. In Zurch, Switzerland, for example, the prevalence of PPNG in 1980 was 1.7% and in 1982 stood at 2.9% (Eichman & Piffaretti, 1984). All the Swiss strains (30 in all) were imported.

In Holland the first cases of PPNG were reported in 1977 (Stolz, 1977). The prevalence has been found to vary throughout the country. The highest rates in 1982 were found in The Hague (23%) and Amsterdam (11%) (Ansink-Schipper et al, 1984). Four plasmid patterns were described. The isolation rate from homosexuals was low, 2.6% of all the strains occurring in this group of patients.

In Scandinavian countries the prevalence is on the low side. Denmark reported its first cases in 1977 (3 cases), rising to 129 by 1983. This represents 1.2% of all gonorrhoea notified during that year. Sixty-eight per cent of cases occurred in males.

Apart from 12 cases (9%) of pharyngeal gonorrhoea, all were cases of genital gonorrhoea. Twenty-two per cent of the infections had been acquired in the Far East, but the majority were acquired within Denmark (Lind et al, 1984). Other Scandinavian countries show similar low prevalence rates for PPNG (Table 2.7).

Table 2.7   Prevalence of PPNG strains in the nordic countries

Country	Population (millions)	Number of strains							
		1976	1977	1978	1979	1980	1981	1982	1983
Denmark	5.1	0	3	14	37	59	104	100	129
Finland	4.7	0	10	35	9	22	54	21	28
Iceland	0.2	0	0	0	0	0	2	16	5
Norway	4.0	2	10	14	37	68	77	99	130
Sweden	8.2	0	12	29	79	199	156	121	?

Factors encouraging the development of PPNG

The development of B lactamase producing strains and the subsequent development of spectinomycin resistance is in large part due to the use of sub optimal doses of antibiotics. The indiscriminate use of antibiotics tends to occur in countries with poor medical services lacking an infra-structure of a comprehensive STD service run by specialists in that field. In the United Kingdom, for example, 90% of STD care is provided by specialists, in the United States 20%, and in developing countries about 1% of cases. 'In many areas, drugs important in the treatment of STD are available over the counter. Such practices should be terminated. Use of regimens achieving less than 95% cure rates have been historically associated with rapid increases in the prevalence of resistant organisms. Practitioners are therefore cautioned not to use less than recommended dosages' (World Health Organisation, 1983).

In the same way that freely available antibiotics, bought on the open market without any attempt at examination and diagnosis, is ill advised so is the practice of chemoprophylaxis. This approach is often used by prostitutes. Goh (1984) and his colleagues studied 777 prostitutes in Singapore and found that in 99 (12.7%) penicillin could be detected in the urine and that the rate of gonococcal infections in these women was half (5.1%) that of those not using prophylactic penicillin (11.2%). Of particular significance was the fact that those taking penicillin and developing gonorrhoea were more likely to be infected with PPNG strains than those women not using chemprophylaxis and developing gonorrhoea (40% compared with 26.5%) (Table 2.8). The sources for purchase of penicillin and other antibiotics were private doctors (23%), unlicensed medicinal shops (22%), drug peddlers within brothels (9%) and the remainder from friends and colleagues.

Table 2.8   Urinary antibiotics in prostitutes and effect on PPNG infection

Urinary antibiotics	Number	%	N. gonorrhoeae isolated	PPNG isolated	% PPNG
Not detected	611	78.6	68	18	26.5
Penicillin detected	99	12.7	5	2	40.0
Non-penicillin detected	67	8.6	4	1	25.0
Total	777	100.0	77	21	

[Source — Goh et al, 1984]

Other reasons are postulated for the emergence of PPNG, such as the use of selective media containing vancomycin in the laboratory diagnosis of gonorrhoea and environmental factors. One of the environmental factors postulated is that the gonococcus in the male rectum is exposed to bile salts and fatty acids and that resistance to these is genetically linked to resistance to penicillin as well as other antimicrobial agents (World Health Organisation, 1983).

Clinical manifestations of infections with PPNG
The same sites (urethra, rectum, cervix and pharynx) are infected as with ordinary *N. gonorrhoeae* infections, and the clinical manifestations are similar. It is of interest, however, that the prevalence of PPNG infections is low in homosexuals and that some reports indicate that pelvic inflammatory disease occurs relatively more frequently with this type of infection. The low rate of PPNG in homosexuals is not fully understood. Two explanations are postulated. Firstly, that the infection started and has remained, heterosexual in nature and has not spread outside this group because of lack of sexual contact to any large extent between heterosexual and homosexual populations. The second possibility is that PPNG are less able to infect rectal mucosa (McCormack, 1982). This lower rate of PPNG has also been documented in two series in the United Kingdom (McManus et al, 1982; Thin et al, 1983).

The higher rate of PID in some series is difficult to interpret, especially since other workers have shown that this complication is no higher than in those women suffering from straightforward gonococcal infections (Arya et al, 1978). In an outbreak of PPNG in Los Angeles in 1980, 21.2% of women infected had PID. This is higher than the expected rate of between 10 to 18% normally seen with ordinary *N. gonorrhoeae* infections. (Eschenbach & Holmes, 1975; Westrom, 1980). Finally, cases of ophthalmia neonatorum caused by PPNG have been reported in the Far East and United Kingdom. (Pang et al, 1979; Dunlop et al, 1980; Thirumoorthy et al, 1982) These were case reports, and it is not possible to say whether this complication is greater than one would expect with non-beta-lactamase producing strains.

TREATMENT AND CONTROL

The treatment and control of isolated cases or outbreaks of PPNG infections will vary in different parts of the world, depending upon the availability of antibiotics and medical care services.

Antibiotics
Spectinomycin was the original drug used in the treatment of patients with PPNG infections and is still the mainstay of treatment in such instances. Most of the original cases and outbreaks were contained with spectinomycin. The dosage used and failure rate varied. The lowest dose (1 gram) intramuscularly was used by Beddard & Harrison (1978) in 189 female patients with a failure rate of 4.8%. Arya and his colleagues (1978) reported a similar failure rate (4.3%) using 2 grams in 23 patients (18 men, 5 women). Also, in 1978, Siegel et al, studying 134 patients of both sexes reported a failure rate of 3.7% using 2 grams and no failures in 17 patients when 4 grams were used. Further studies since then have shown failure rates of zero using 2 grams when used in the Far East and the Philippines (Wighall et al, 1981; Tupasi et al,

1980). With such good cure rates there is no indication for using either 3.2 grams (Nayyar et al, 1980) or 4 grams (Siegel et al, 1978). Spectinomycin is an excellent drug. One big advantage is that it is hardly used except for treating gonorrhoea and in vitro the mutation rate of gonococci to resistance to it is very low. If its use could be restricted to treating proven or epidemiologically probable infections with PPNG it would retain its effectiveness longer than if it were used generally as a first line treatment for gonorrhoea (Wilkinson 1984, personal communication).

The cephalosporins (particularly cefoxitin, cefuroxime and cefotaxime) have also been used especially once it was realised that some strains were developing a resistance to spectinomycin. Even though the cephalosporins are useful they should not be used widely. The failure rates using various new cephalosporins at various doses are extremely low, ranging from 0–1.8%. Cefoxitin can be administered in a dose of 1–2 grams in combination with 1 gram of probenecid. A small series (12 patients) in which the lower dose was used in the Far East (Sanchez et al, 1981) showed no failures. Other studies with the use of 2 grams also show no failures (Berg et al, 1979; Hamson & Berg personal communication, 1980). Currently 2 grams is considered the most appropriate dose of Cefoxitin for the treatment of uncomplicated infections with PPNG.

Similarly good cure rates have been achieved using a dose of 1.5 grams of Cefuroxime (Nayyar et al, 1980; Tupasi et al, 1980). Finally, Cefotaxime has been used effectively in PPNG infections at doses ranging from 0.5–1.0 grams intramuscularly. In England no failures were recorded using 0.5 grams (Boakes et al, 1981). In Singapore (Rajan et al, 1980) a dose of 1 gram resulted in a failure rate of 1.8%, and with the same dose no failures were found in 31 patients in the Western Pacific. (Lancaster et al, 1981). The lower dose of 0.5 grams is suitable in most instances, Other newer cephalosporins are being developed and show equally good efficacy to the three mentioned above in the treatment of PPNG infections.

In summary, there is little to choose on clinical grounds between Spectinomycin and the various new cephalosporins when deciding upon treatment. In vitro studies indicate minor differences between the efficacy of the drugs, but not enough to alter the choice between spectinomycin and cefotaxime to which isolates were most susceptible (Piot et al, 1980). The cost difference again is marginal between most of the cephalosporins and spectinomycin for comparable courses (Table 2.9). In view of equal clinical efficacy and marginal cost differences, spectinomycin is still the drug of choice in PPNG infections.

In certain instances or special circumstances first line therapy with spectinomycin may not be so effective. In pelvic inflammatory disease spectinomycin can be used

Table 2.9   Costs of different drugs for the treatment of infections due to PPNG

Drug		Cost	
		Pounds*	Dollars†
Spectinomycin	(2 grams)	4.49	9.20
Cefoxitin	(2 grams)	9.83	14.30
Cefuroxime	(1.5 grams)	5.88	
Cefotaxime	(1 gram)	4.95	11.45

*Monthly Index of Medical Specialities (MIMS) November 1984
†Washington 1982— from Drug Topics Red Book 1982

(2 grams intramuscularly twice a day) but many authorities favour the cephalosporins, an example of a suitable regime being cefuroxime 1.5 g with 1 gram probenecid followed by 0.75 grams 8 hourly. A disseminated gonoccocal infection due to PPNG could also be treated with this regime, or with 0.5 grams cefotaxime four times a day intramuscularly for five days (Lancet, 1982), or finally as recommended by Centers for Disease Control (1982), with cefoxitin 1 gram or cefotaxime 500 mgs four times a day intravenously for at least seven days.

Pharyngeal infections are often hard to eradicate, whether the organism is B lactamase producing or not. In PPNG infections spectinomycin is not as effective as the cephalosporins and its use can give failure rates as high as 80%. In view of this either trimethoprim-sulfamethoxazole, 9 tablets as a single dose daily for 5 days (Jaffe 1981), or a long course of a cephalosporin, for example cefuroxime 0.75 g daily for 3 days (Lindberg et al, 1982) have been recommended.

Other regimes have been or are being evaluated in the treatment of PPNG infections, for example gentamicin, kanamycin and a combination of clavulanic acid and amoxycillin, moxalactam, thiamphenicol and rosaramicin. (Rajan et al, 1979; Tan et al, 1980; De Koning et al, 1981; Lao et al, 1981; Tight et al, 1981; Alexander, 1981).

Spectinomycin resistant PPNG are now recognised (Ashford et al, 1981; Easmon et al, 1982, Centers for Disease Control, 1982c and 1983d; Ison et al, 1983) but are not usually prevalent enough to suggest a switch away from this first line drug. It illustrates the importance of continued microbiological surveillance of all cases of gonorrhoea, PPNG producing or not, and the use of adequate doses of the chosen antibiotic preferably given under supervised conditions.

Medical care services

Antibiotic therapy for the sexually transmitted diseases (STDs) should not be divorced, in ideal circumstances, from a comprehensive service which in addition to correct diagnosis and treatment provides follow up and tracing of sexual contacts.

The treatment of an infection caused by PPNG requires far more than the provision of a diagnosis and treatment of one individual. Adequate control must incorporate a number of features, including contact tracing. In ideal circumstances the following methods for the control of PPNG need to be considered.

(1) Microscopy and culture of all cases of urethral, vaginal and rectal discharge or exposed sites in a symptomatic and asymptomatic 'at risk' patient.

(2) Sensitivity testing of all isolates and routine testing of all gonococcal isolates for B-lactamase production.

(3) Insistence on follow up. It must be explained to patients with a presumptive diagnosis of straightforward gonorrhoea treated on microscopic grounds that treatment must be monitored since it is not always successful. Tests of cure should be performed at follow up.

(4) Contact tracing must be carried out; failure to do such is failure of control. Such contacts should be treated initially with spectinomycin or a B-lactamase-resistant antibiotic.

(5) Pragmatism and not elitism in treatment. In countries with a low prevalence of PPNG, penicillin is the first line of treatment for gonorrhoea. It is often suggested that the first line therapy should be switched to spectinomycin once the prevalence level of PPNG reaches 5% or more of all gonococcal isolates.

There does not appear to be any scientific basis for this recommendation, and to some extent the level chosen should depend upon the medical care system available for the diagnosis, treatment and follow up of STDs. If this is good and patients attend for follow up the 5% level might be increased. In contrast, in countries with poor facilities and with little hope of performing follow up, this level might be a suitable cut off point. Clearly in many countries the prevalence levels of PPNG are so high (Far East) that spectinomycin is used for all cases of gonorrhoea. Likewise patients returning from endemic areas who develop gonorrhoea should be treated with spectinomycin in preference to penicillin at the initial consultation, as should their contacts.

Slightly different approaches can be used in well defined outbreaks of PPNG. In the United States such outbreaks have been well contained by the setting up of special task forces. This involves active aggressive contact tracing. In an outbreak in Norfolk, Virginia, 74 contacts of eight index cases were named, and fell within the jurisdiction of the local health department (Pariser, 1983). Of these, 69 were traced and treated if this had not previously occurred. This involved tracing five generations of contacts. Another similar outbreak occurred in Los Angeles between August 1980 and March 1981 (Centers for Disease Control, 1983c). This large outbreak reached 50 cases per month and was eventually contained and controlled by an extensive campaign which included the use of spectinomycin for all patients with gonorrhoea living in high prevalence districts, screening high risk groups, aggressive contact tracing and involvement of the media.

Conclusions
The development of PPNG should act as a lesson for the future management of the STDs. It is entirely possible that similar drug resistant organisms could develop with the indiscriminant use of antibiotics and antivirals. For example, the recent discovery of Acyclovir for the treatment of herpes simplex virus infections could be entirely put at risk by its widespread use and the development of resistant strains of the virus.

PPNG has been reasonably well controlled in developed countries through surveillance, accurate diagnosis and selection of an appropriate antibiotic. It is saluatory that the indiscriminate use of a cheap antibiotic, such as penicillin, has meant that the first line of therapy for gonorrhoea in many countries is now an expensive drug such as spectinomycin or one of the cephalosporins.

I am grateful to Professor Ian Phillips and Dr A. E. Wilkinson for their advice in the preparation of this chapter.

REFERENCES

Adler M W, McCutchan J A 1985 Survey of cases of penicillinase producing Neisseria gonorrhoeae in the United Kingdom. Genitourinary Medicine 61: 36–38

Alexander W J, DeShazo W F, Cassell G H 1981 Treatment of urethritis with rosarmicin and tetracycline (abstract no. 617). In program and abstracts of the 21st Interscience Conference on Antimicrobial Agents and Chemotherapy. American Society for Microbiology, Washington DC

Ansink-Schipper M C, Van Klingeren B, Huikeshoven M H, Woudstra R K, Dessens-Kroon M, Van Wijngaarden L J 1984 Epidemiology of PPNG infections in the Netherlands: analysis by auxanographic typing and plasmid identification. British Journal of Venereal Diseases 60: 141–146

Arya O P, Rees E, Percival A, Alergant C D, Annels E H, Turner G C 1978 Epidemiological treatment of gonorrhoea caused by penicillinase producing strains in Liverpool. British Journal of Venereal Diseases 54: 28–35

Arya O P, Rees E, Turner G C, Percival A, Bartzokas C A, Annels E H, Carey P B, Ghosh A K, Jephcott A E, Johnston N A 1984 Epidemiology of penicillinase producing Neisseria gonorrhoeae in Liverpool from 1977 to 1982. Journal of Infection 8: 70–83

Ashford W A, Golash R G, Hemming V G 1976 Penicillinase producing Neisseria gonorrhoeae. Lancet ii: 657–658

Ashford W A, Potts D W, Adams H J U et al 1981 Spectinomycin resistant penicillinase producing Neisseria gonorrhoeae. Lancet ii: 1035–1037

Beddard J R, Harrison W O 1978 One gram spectinomycin therapy of penicillinase producing Neisseria gonorrhoeae. Abstract 18th Interscience Conference on Antimicrobial Agents and Chemotherapy, Atlanta October 1–4 1978. American Society for Microbiology

Berg J W, Kilpatrick M E, Harrison W O, McCutchan J A 1979 Cefoxitin as a single dose treatment for urethritis caused by penicillinase producing Neisseria gonorrhoeae. New England Joural of Medicine 301: 509–11

Boakes A J, Barrow J, Eykyn S J, Phillips I 1981 Cefotaxime for spectinomycin resistant Neisseria gonorrhoeae. Lancet ii: 96

Brown S, Warnuisson T, Biddle J, Panikabutra K, Traisupa A 1982 Antimicrobial resistance of Neisseria gonorrhoea in Bangkok: Is single drug treatment phasse. Lancet ii: 1366–1368

Centers for Disease Control 1980 An outbreak of penicillinase producing Neisseria gonorrhoeae — Shreveport, Louisianna Morbidity and Mortality Weekly Report 29: 241–243

Centers for Disease Control 1982a Global distribution of penicillinase producing Neisseria gonorrhoeae (PPNG). Morbidity and Mortality Weekly Report 32: 1–3

Centers for Disease Control 1982b Sexually Transmitted Diseases: treatment guidelines. Morbidity and Mortality Weekly Report 31: 405

Centers for Disease Control 1982c Spectinomycin resistant Neisseria gonorrhoeae — World wide. Morbidity and Mortality Weekly Report 31: 632–682

Centers for Disease Control 1983a Penicillin resistant gonorrhoea North Carolina. Morbidity and Mortality Weekly Report 32: 273–275

Centers for Disease Control 1983b Chromosomally mediated resistant Neisseria gonorrhoea United States. Morbidity and Mortality Weekly Report 33: 408–410

Centers for Disease Control 1983c Penicillinase producing Neisseria gonorrhoeae — Los Angeles. Morbidity and Mortality Weekly Report 32: 181–182

Centers for Disease Control 1983d Spectinomycin resistant penicillinase producing Neisseria gonorrhoeae. Morbidity and Mortality Weekly Report 32: 51–52

Cohn A, Seijo I H 1944 The in vitro effect of penicillin. Journal of American Medical Association 124: 1125–1126

Curtis F R, Wilkinson A E 1958 A comparison of the in vitro sensitivity of gonoccoci to penicillin with the results of treatment. British Journal of Venereal Diseases 34: 70–79

DeKoning G A J, Tio D, Coster J F, Coutinho R A, Ansink-Schipper M C 1981 The combination of clavulanic acid and amoxycillin (Augmentin) in the treatment of patients infected with penicillinase producing gonococci. Journal of Antimicrobial Chemotherapy 8: 81–82

Dunlop E M C 1949 Gonorrhoea and the sulphonamides. British Journal of Venereal Diseases 25: 81–83

Dunlop E M, Rodin P, Seth A D, Kolator B 1980 Opthalmia neonatorum due to Beta-lactamase producing gonococci. British Medical Journal 279: 483

Easmon C S F, Ison C A, Bellinger C M et al 1982 Emergence of resistance after spectinomycin treatment for gonorrhoea due to beta-lactamase producing strains of Neisseria gonorrhoeae. British Medical Journal 284: 1064–1065

Eichmann A R, Piffaretti J C 1984 Penicillinase producing Neisseria gonorrhoeae in Zurich, Switzerland. British Journal of Venereal Diseases 60: 147–150

Eschenbach D A, Holmes K K 1975 Acute pelvic inflammatory disease; current concepts of pathogenesis, aetiology and management. Clinical Obstetrics and Gynaecology 18: 35–36

Falkow S, Elwell L P, De Graaff J 1976 A possible model for the development of plasmid mediated penicillin resistance in the gonococcus. In Sexually Transmitted Diseases. Ed. Catterall R D, Nicol C S. Academic Press, London 1976

Goh C L, Meija P, Sng E H, Bajan V S, Thirumoorthy T 1984 Chemoprophylaxis and gonococcal infection in prostitutes. International Journal of Epidemiology 13: 344–446.

Handsfield H H, Sandstrom E G, Knapp J S, Perine P L, Whittington W L, Sayers D E, Holmes K K 1982 Epidemiology of penicillinase producing Neisseria gonorrhoeae infections: analysis by auxotyping and serogrouping. New England Journal of Medicine 306: 950–954

Hart G 1973 Penicillin resistance of the gonococcus in South Vietnam. Medical Journal of Australia 2: 638

Ison C A, Littleton K, Shannon K P, Easmon C S F, Phillips I 1983 Spectinomycin resistant gonococci. British Medical Journal 287: 1827–1829

Jaffe H W, Biddle J W, Johnson J R, Wiesner P J 1981 Infections due to penicillinase producing Neisseria gonorrhoeae in the United States 1976–1980. Journal of Infectious Diseases 144: 191–197

Jephcott A E, Dickgiesser N, McClean A N 1981 Penicillinase producing gonococci in Britain. Lancet ii: 247–248

Johnston N A, Kolator B 1981 Emergence in Britain of beta-lactamase producing gonococci with new plasmid combination. Lancet i: 445

Lancaster D J, Berg S W, Harrison W O, Ockrermann K O 1981 Treatment of penicillin resistant gonorrhoea with Cefotaxime. In Cefotaxime sodium, a new cephalosporin. Current Research Bio Medical Information Corporation, New York 8/–90

Lancet Leader 1982 Penicillinase producing gonococci further complications ii: 912–913

Lao L M, Lao M L M 1981 Amoxycillin 3 g + clauvulanic acid 0.25 mg in the treatment of acute male penicillin resistant gonorrhoea in the Philippines. Proceedings of International Congress of Chemotherapy, Florence, Italy, July 19–24

Lind I, Bollerup A C, Gadeberg O V, Reimann K, Bentzon M W 1984 Activities of the WHO collaborating Centre for reference and research in gonococci, Copenhagen, for the year 1983. WHO/VDT/Res/Gon 84: 144

Lindberg M, Ringertz O, Sandstrom E 1982 Treatment of pharyngeal gonorrhoea due to beta-lactamase producing gonococci. British Journal of Venereal Diseases 58: 101–104

McCormack W M 1982 Penicillinase producing Neisseria gonorrhoeae — a retrospective. New England Journal of Medicine 307: 438–439

McCutchan J A, Adler M W, Berrie J R H 1982 Penicillinase producing Neisseria gonorrhoeae in Great Britain, 1977–1981 alarming increase in incidence and recent development of endemic transmission. British Medical Journal 285: 337–340

McManus T J, Harris J R W, Ison C A, Easmon C S F 1982 Penicillinase producing Neisseria gonorrhoeae. Letter New England Journal of Medicine 307: 1706

Martin J E, Lester A, Price E V 1970 Comparative study of gonococcal susceptibility to penicillin in the United States 1955–1969. Journal of Infectious Diseases 122: 459–463

Nayyar K C, Michel M F, Stolz E 1980 Antibiotic sensitivities of gonococci isolated in Rotterdam and results of treatment with Cefuroxime. British Journal of Venereal Diseases 56: 249–251

Nayyar K C, Noble R C, Michel M F, Stolz E 1980 Gonorrhoea in Rotterdam caused by penicillinase producing gonococci. British Journal of Venereal Diseases 56: 244–248

Osoba A O 1981 Sexually transmitted diseases in tropical Africa: a review of the present situation. British Journal of Venereal Diseases 57: 89–94

Pang R, Teh L B, Rajan V S, Sng E H 1979 Gonococcal ophthalmia neonatorum caused by beta-lactamase producing Neisseria gonorrhoeae. British Medical Journal 1: 380

Pariser H, Marino A F, Hana C 1982 Analysis of a recent epidemic due to penicillinase producing Neisseria gonorrhoeae: epidemiologic and medical considerations. Sexually Transmitted Diseases 9: 132–134

Percival A, Corkhill J E, Arya O P et al 1976 Penicillinase producing gonococci in Liverpool. Lancet ii: 1379–1382

Phillips I 1976 Beta-lactamase producing, penicillin resistant gonococcus. Lancet ii: 656–657

Piot P, Van Dyck E, Colaert J, Ursi J 1980. In vitro activity of cefotaxime and other cephalosporins against Neisseria gonorrhoeae. Journal of Antimicrobial Chemotherapy 6 (Suppl A): 47–50

Public Health Laboratory Service Communicable Disease Centre and the Communicable Diseases (Scotland Unit) 1983 Penicillinase producing Neisseria gonorrhoeae in Britain 1982. British Medical Journal 286: 1628–1629

Public Health Laboratory Service Communicable Disease Centre and the Communicable Diseases (Scotland Unit) 1984 Penicillinase producing Neisseria gonorrhoeae in Britain 1983. British Medical Journal 288: 1746–1745

Rajan V S, Pang R, Tan N J, Sng E H 1979 Kanamycin in the treatment of penicillinase producing gonococcal infections. Asian Journal of Infectious Diseases 3: 37–39

Rajan V S, Sng E H, Pang R, Tan N J, Thirumoorthy T, Yeo K L 1980 HR 756-new cephalosporin in the treatment of gonorrhoea caused by ordinary and penicillinase producing strains of Neisseria gonorrhoeae. British Journal of Venereal Diseases 56: 255–258

Rajan V S, Thirumoorthy T, Tan N J 1981 Epidemiology of penicillinase producing Neisseria gonorrhoeae in Singapore. British Journal of Venereal Diseases 57: 158–161

Ratnam A V, Patel M I, Mubenga R C, Hira S K 1982 Penicillinase producing gonococcal strains in Zambia. British Journal of Venereal Diseases 58: 29–31

Reyn A 1961 Sensitivity of N. gonorrhoeae to antibiotics. British Journal of Venereal Diseases 37: 145–157

Romansky M J 1946 The current status of calcium penicillin in Beeswax and peanut oil. American Journal of Medicine 1: 395–411

Sandez P L, Wignall F S, Harrison W O, Berg J W 1981 One gram Cefoxitin cures uncomplicated gonococcal urethritis caused by penicillinase producing Neisseria gonorrhoeae (PPNG) Abstract 21st Interscience Conference on Antimicrobial agents and Chemotherapy. American Society for Microbiology Washington DC

Siegel M S, Thornsberry C, Biddle J W et al 1978 Penicillinase producing Neisseria gonorrhoeae: Results of surveillance in the United States. Journal of Infectious Diseases 137: 170–175

Stolz E 1977 Mede nammeus de Werkgroep voor gonorrebestrijding. Ned Tijdshr Greneeskd 121: 620

Tan N J, Rajan V S, Pang R, Sng E H 1980 Gentamicin in the treatment of infections due to penicillinase-producing gonococci. British Journal of Venereal Diseases 56: 394–396

Thin R N, Barlow D, Eykyn S, Phillips I 1983 Imported penicillinase producing Neisseria gonorrhoeae becomes endemic in London. British Journal of Venereal Diseases 59: 364–368

Thirumoorthy T, Rajan V S, Goh C L 1982 Penicillinase producing Neisseria gonorrhoeae opthalmia neonatorum in Singapore. British Journal of Venereal Diseases 58: 308–310

Tight R, Jones R 1981 Moxalactam for the treatment of gonococcal urethritis (abstract no. 323). In Program and abstracts of the 21st Interscience Conference on Antimicrobial Agents and Chemotheray. American Society of Microbiology, Washington DC

Tupasi T E, Cusologi L B, Torres C A, Calubiran O V, de Jesus I 1980 Single dose alternative therapy for uncomplicated gonorrhoea in women with special reference to beta-lactamase producing strains. WHO Report No. VDT/80/1424 WHO, Geneva

Van Embden J D A, Van Klingeren B, Dessens-Kroon M, Van Wijngaarden L J 1981 Emergence in the Netherlands of penicillinase producing gonococci carrying 'Africa' plasmid in combination with transfer factor. Lancet i: 938

Washington E A 1982 Update on treatment recommendations for gonococcal infections. Review of Infectious Diseases 4: suppl, Nov–Dec, S: 758–771

Watko L P, Brownlow W J 1975 Antibiotic sensitivity related to Neisseria gonorrhoeae isolated in the Western Pacific in 1971. British Journal of Venereal Diseases 51: 34–37

Westrom L 1980 Incidence, prevalence and trends of acute pelvic inflammatory disease and its consequences in industrial countries. American Journal of Obstetrics and Gynaecology 138: 880–892

Wignall F J, Lancaster D J, Harrison W O, Kerbs S B J, Berg S W 1981 Oral rosoxacin versus parenteral spectinomycin in treatment of gonococcal urethritis caused by penicillin resistant and sensitive strains. Abstract 21st Interscience Conference on Antimicrobial agents and Chemotherapy American Society for Microbiology. Washington DC

World Health Organisation 1983 Current treatments in the control of sexually transmitted diseases WHO/VDT/83. 433

3. *Chlamydia trachomatis* infections: epidemiology and disease spectrum

Julius Schachter

THE ORGANISM

Chlamydia trachomatis is a gram-negative, obligate, intracellular bacterium (Moulder, 1984). The chlamydiae are differentiated from all other microorganisms by a unique life cycle. It involves infection of susceptible cells by induced phagocytosis. The organism, in a phagosome, undergoes a morphological change from the infectious elementary body (EB, approximately 350 nm in diameter) to the initial body or reticulate body (RB) form (approximately 1μ in diameter) which represents the replicative and metabolically active form of the organism. The RB is not infectious. It divides by binary fission. Towards the end of the growth cycle (approximately 48 hours) the RB condenses to the EB form which is then released from the host cell.

There are only two species within the genus *Chlamydia*. *Chlamydia psittaci* is a natural parasite of birds and lower mammals and causes the human disease psittacosis (Schachter & Dawson, 1978). It is not a natural human parasite as it appears to infect humans only as a result of exposure to infected avian or other mammalian species. *Chlamydia trachomatis*, on the other hand, is almost exclusively a human pathogen. Those strains that are known to infect humans have no known animal reservoir. By the use of serologic procedures 15 serovars of *Chlamydia trachomatis* have been identified (Grayston & Wang, 1975). The A through C serovars are commonly associated with endemic blinding trachoma. The D through K serovars are associated with oculogenital infections, while the L serovars represent the lymphogranuloma venereum (LGV) strains. These latter organisms are biologically more invasive and can be differentiated in vitro rather readily from the other *C. trachomatis* biovars which have a more restricted host range and are less capable of serial growth in cell culture systems. Although LGV is a sexually transmitted disease, it will not be discussed in this chapter, nor will ocular trachoma, which is not currently recognised to have any relationship to sexual transmission.

The D and E serovars are generally recognised to be the most common of the sexually transmitted *C. trachomatis* strains (Kuo et al, 1983). It is likely that research using new methodology such as monoclonal antibody probes will identify more serovars.

INFECTION OF THE MALE GENITAL TRACT

Urethral infection

The most common manifestation of sexually transmitted *Chlamydia trachomatis* infections is non-gonococcal urethritis (NGU) in men (Schachter, 1978; Oriel & Ridgway, 1982a). This syndrome is defined by exclusion, i.e. the failure to find *Neisseria gonor-*

rhoeae in urethral specimens from a man with urethritis. NGU is more common than gonococcal urethritis (GU). The age distribution is quite similar for NGU and GU with most cases being found in the 15–25 year age group, although NGU is more common than GU in men of higher socioeconomic class and in heterosexual males.

The disease is characterised by pyuria and there is usually a mucoid to mucopurulent discharge which is less purulent than the typical discharge in GU. The incubation period of NGU is in the 1–3 week range. Onset often follows a change in sex partners. The clinical findings in NGU have sufficient overlap with those of GU as to render diagnosis purely on clinical grounds inaccurate. Men without overt discharge can have NGU and a common method of diagnosing the condition is to demonstrate a 'significant' number of polymorphonuclear leukocytes (PMN) in either first-catch urine (FCU) or a smear prepared from a urethral swab. If a Gram stain of discharge shows many PMN but no intracellular diplococci, a presumptive diagnosis of NGU is made. There is no unanimity as to what is a 'significant' number of PMN. For resuspension of the centrifuged sediment of a 10–15 ml sample of FCU the usual criterion is $\geqslant 15$ PMNs per $400 \times$ high power field and for a smear obtained by urethral swabbing the cut off is $\geqslant 5$ PMNs seen on oil immersion field at $1000 \times$ (Swartz & Kraus, 1979; Bowie, 1978; Holmes et al, 1975).

Transmission

The transmissibility of chlamydial infections is not known. Crude estimates have been made on the basis of infection rates in partners of incident cases, but these studies are difficult to interpret. In one study it was found that 28% of male partners of women with chlamydial cervicitis were infected, in contrast with an 81% recovery rate for gonococci, when that was the infecting organism in the female cervix (Lycke et al, 1980). Similar results were obtained for the partners of those women who had dual infections. The obvious conclusion derived from these data would be that *Neisseria gonorrhoeae* is more infectious than *Chlamydia trachomatis* but unfortunately, this conclusion would not be valid because of the differences in the natural history of the disease (for example, longer incubation period for chlamydial infection), lower sensitivity of chlamydial isolation and the potential impact of the immune status on the host (Schachter et al, 1983).

It is impossible with certainty to document the time trends for chlamydial infections in men or women since these infections are rarely accurately diagnosed. If, however, one looks at the incidence of non-gonococcal urethritis in England or in selected clinics in the United States it is clear that NGU has been rising markedly over the past decade as compared to gonococcal infections (Oriel & Ridgway, 1982a). If one assumes that 40–50% of NGU is caused by *Chlamydia trachomatis* and 60–70% of female partners of men with chlamydial infection acquire the infection, one must conclude that it is likely that chlamydial infections have also been rising in a dramatic fashion. The most reasonable explanation for this increase is that there are no clearcut chlamydial control programmes in effect. Most STD control has been aimed at syphilis and gonorrhoea and the drugs of choice have, for most of the recent past, been penicillins or other beta-lactams. These drugs are ineffective in treating chlamydial infections; there would be a selection in the population for penicillin-resistant organisms. The coincident infection rate for *C. trachomatis* (20% for men, 40% for women) in gonorrhoea is one measure of the potential reservoir for accumulation. Since the signs and symptoms of chlamydial infection are relatively non-specific, clinical grounds would not provide adequate criteria for presumptive treatment of *Chlamydia* (this is now, of course, the standard for managing NGU in males; recently it has been suggested that this might be a prudent approach in selected female populations). Thus, it is clear that chlamydial infections had to accumulate within the population. It is also obvious that as time goes by we will recognise more of the late consequences of these infections that have become epidemic within the past two decades.

Treatment of NGU

Although a purist would like to see a specific aetiologic diagnosis established, it is clear that the diagnosis of chlamydial infection will not determine the first line management of NGU. NGU can and should be treated before a specific aetiologic diagnosis can be established. It is clear that somewhere between 35–50% of NGU is caused by *Chlamydia trachomatis* (Oriel & Ridgway, 1982a; Taylor-Robinson & Thomas, 1980). It is as yet uncertain as to what the other causes of NGU are, although *Ureaplasma urealyticum* is a leading candidate for causation in perhaps 25% of cases.

In the past NGU was considered a trivial condition. It was often not treated on the assumption that it would resolve spontaneously. In addition, some physicians tended not to treat NGU because treatment often failed and the patient was then faced with a series of courses of therapy, none of which were curative. Those views reflected the uncertainty inherent in the term, 'non-specific urethritis'. Now that management of NGU has been put on a rational basis, it is clear that the earlier outlook was misguided. Although NGU is clearly the most trivial of the chlamydial genital tract infections, it is not a trivial condition. It is important to the male because of the potentially serious complication of epididymitis (Berger et al, 1978). More important is the risk that the male transmits chlamydiae to the female contact who is at risk for the most serious complications of chlamydial infection. Therefore, not only is a man with NGU a candidate for immediate therapy with tetracycline, but the sex partners are as well. More than one-third of female partners of men with NGU have a chlamydial infection (Oriel & Ridgway, 1982b). If the male has a chlamydial urethritis the infection rate in the consort is >65%.

Thus once a presumptive diagnosis of NGU is made on the basis of a Gram stained smear, immediate therapy with tetracyclines is called for (CDC, 1982). The generally accepted treatment regimens are 1 g of tetracycline per day (250 mg 4 times daily) to be given for 2 weeks, or 2 g/day (500 mg 4 times daily) to be given for 1 week. Shorter courses of therapy have not been shown to be effective and longer courses are not needed. If a patient is unable to tolerate tetracycline, erythromycin (stearate, ethylsuccinate or base) should be substituted at the equivalent dosage and duration.

These treatment regimens will provide cure rates for chlamydial infections well in excess of 90% and will result in cure of NGU in appproximately 85% of cases. There is both symptomatic relief and objective response (loss of PMNs in the urethra) which can be monitored. Some treated men develop an asymptomatic pyuria, in the absence of chlamydial infection, as they are followed for longer periods of time. The meaning of this observation is not clear. It is also clear that some men with NGU do not respond to these treatment regimens and the aetiology of their disease remains obscure. There are anecdotal reports of tetracycline-resistant chlamydiae causing NGU. To the author's knowledge, no tetracycline-resistant *Chlamydia trachomatis* have ever been recovered. There is a small (2–5%) tetracycline treatment failure rate for chlamydial urethritis as there is for virtually any well accepted treatment modality for most infectious diseases. Some of the reasons for treatment failures include (a) taking tetracyclines when milk products or other food products are being eaten, (b) a failure to treat sex partners resulting in reinfection, or (c) poor compliance. The problem of chelation of tetracycline by calcium in milk products can be overcome by the use of the longer acting tetracyclines. Thus, doxycycline or minocycline at 100 mg twice daily for 7–14 days is considered as effective as the other regimens.

One reason for immediate treatment of NGU with tetracycline rather than awaiting a microbiology report is that ureaplasmas and other potential pathogens for most NGU are also tetracycline and/or erythromycin sensitive. Thus, the microbiologic diagnosis will not provide therapeutic guidance.

Diagnosis
For a specific diagnosis of chlamydial urethritis the only recommended methods are isolation of the organism, or perhaps the use of the newly described antigen detection methods (Schachter, 1980; Tam et al, 1984). Serology does not play a role in diagnosis as there are high background prevalence rates of antichlamydial antibody in sexually active young men. Seroconversion is rarely demonstrated except for that small subset of cases that are having their first chlamydial infection (Bowie et al, 1977). Giemsa stain of urethral smear is not a sensitive procedure for diagnosing chlamydial infection.

Postgonococcal urethritis
Postgonococcal urethritis (PGU) is a specific subset of NGU which appears shortly after a male has been successfully treated for gonorrhoea. Most cases of PGU are caused by *C. trachomatis* (Richmond et al, 1972; Oriel et al, 1975). Many men have a concomitant chlamydial infection at the time they are diagnosed as having a gonococcal infection. If gonorrhoea is treated with penicillin or other beta-lactam drugs that are not effective against *C. trachomatis*, the chlamydial infection persists. Many of these men have a brief period of symptomatic relief followed by an exacerbation of their symptoms. The likeliest explanation of this sequence is that both infections are acquired at the same time and that while the gonococcal infection has a typical incubation period of 2–5 days, the chlamydial infection more typically has an incubation period of 1–3 weeks. Thus, the gonococcal infection has resolved in the face of therapy during the incubation period of the chlamydial infection, which then becomes clinically manifest. In the United States approximately 20% of men with gonorrhoea have concomitant chlamydial infection, while in Europe rates twice that are common (Oriel & Ridgway, 1982a).

In recognition of the importance of this double infection a common treatment now used for gonorrhoea involves the immediate administration of an effective beta-lactam, such as 3 g of amoxycillin or 3.5 g of ampicillin, taken orally with 1 g probenecid (benamid) while the patient is being seen. This is then followed with a week of tetracycline, as is used for treating NGU (CDC, 1982). This treatment has been shown to reduce the incidence of PGU. Because the reported attack rates for PGU have ranged from 60–100% of men with double infection and are probably 85–90%, such a presumptive therapy for chlamydial infection in men with gonorrhoea is warranted.

Epididymitis

Epididymitis is the most important complication of NGU in males. *C. trachomatis* is recognised as the leading cause of epididymitis in young (<35 years of age) sexually active men, causing approximately 60% of epididymitis in this age group (Berger et al, 1978). Most of these men have urethral signs or symptoms and *Chlamydia* can be recovered from urethral specimens as well as epididymal aspirates. Those men usually have very high levels of antichlamydial antibody. *Neisseria gonorrhoeae* is the other most common cause of epididymitis in men of this age.

Urethral stricture and prostatitis

Urethral stricture and prostatitis are other complications of NGU but the role of *C. trachomatis* in these conditions is not clear. Since the advent of effective chemotherapy for NGU there are few documented cases of new urethral stricture developing after NGU. Because invasive diagnostic procedures to look for strictures are not commonly used, one would not be detecting small strictures. The assumption that *Chlamydia trachomatis* can cause strictures is based on cystoscopic examinations performed in studies in the early 1960s and because *Chlamydia trachomatis* is commonly associated with scarring in conjunctival infection (Schachter & Dawson, 1978). While strictures may have been an important manifestation in the past they are not seen often enough to allow a meaningful statement concerning their development.

While there is a growing literature suggesting that *C. trachomatis* is an important cause of prostatitis, this author is not aware of any study which is free from serious objections that render any such conclusions as unproven. The most common problem with studies associating *Chlamydia* with prostatitis is a failure to exclude chlamydial infection of the urethra as the source of the agent that is presumably being isolated from the prostatic expressates. Some studies have serious technical flaws. For example, inoculation of cell cultures with undiluted prostatic fluid results in sufficient damage to the cell sheets to render them incapable of growing chlamydiae. Thus some reports have obviously been based on identification of artifacts in the cultures as *Chlamydia*. Since *Chlamydia trachomatis* infects columnar epithelial cells and the organism can reach the epididymis, it is obviously an attractive hypothesis to consider that this organism is also involved in acute prostatitis. At this point, however, that conclusion must remain as a speculation, as no acceptable evidence has yet been brought forth.

Proctitis

It is clear that proctitis is a polymicrobial disease with potential for multiple aetiologies. In some clinic settings chlamydiae have been recovered from rectal swabs from men, but no related clinical findings could be usefully associated (Munday & Taylor-Robinson, 1983). In one study at a Seattle STD clinic *C. trachomatis* was recovered from the rectums of 12% of homosexual men with proctitis (Quinn et al, 1981). Asymptomatic homosexual men had a 6% rectal recovery rate for *Chlamydia*. It is likely that here too both clinically apparent and inapparent infections can occur.

It should be noted that a more severe form of proctitis is associated with the lymphogranuloma venereum (LGV) biovars of *C. trachomatis*. LGV will not be discussed in this review but it is a disease of varying endemicity and has long been recognised as a cause of severe proctocolitis with a pathologic response in the colon which may be similar to that seen in Crohn's disease. Chlamydiae are not the cause of Crohn's disease but pathologists should be alert to the possibility that homosexual male being evaluated for Crohn's disease or ulcerative colitis may actually have a treatable LGV infection. In studies performed in San Francisco on men being seen for severe proctitis (where common causes such as gonorrhoea, herpes and syphilis had already been excluded), we recovered *C. trachomatis* from biopsies in approximately 25% of the homosexual men studied. Approximately 70% of the isolates in these men, who were seen in the gastrointestinal disease clinic, were LGV strains.

Inapparent infection

It is obvious that asymptomatic chlamydial infections will only be diagnosed by micro-biologic procedures. Just as we now recognise that case finding from symptomatic individuals will reveal asymptomatic gonococcal infections in either men or women, it is predictable that the same will often be found for *C. trachomatis*. Asymptomatic infections are a hallmark of chlamydial infections in general. There are few studies relevant to this subject but two that have focused on this point frequently found asymptomatic chlamydial infections in sexually active military men or in men being examined at a VD clinic (Podgore et al, 1982; Stamm et al, 1984).

This is particularly important in any effort to deal with the public health impact of chlamydiae. Current control methods for STD are often based on contact tracing after the diagnosis of cases identified by screening tests or by diagnosis of symptomatic individuals. Much of the emphasis is placed on routine screening of sexually active young women because they are readily accessible through birth control clinics and other settings where pelvic examinations are routine. It is clear that these types of screening studies which often find high prevalence rates of chlamydial infection in asymptomatic females, are not going to be truly successful in controlling STD because the asymptomatic male reservoir is largely ignored. The reason for this is most likely because there is no readily applicable non-invasive screening test for STD in men. My colleagues and I have been investigating this problem in adolescent males. We became concerned with studies that indicate that 14–18% of sexually active female teenagers seen in our clinics had chlamydial infection but the only males being treated were those who were named contacts or symptomatic males seeking treatment (Shafer et al, 1984). A study performed on sexually active adolescent males demonstrated that approximately 20% of them in the same clinic setting had asymptomatic pyuria and in this pilot project, of the 23 men with pyuria, 21 (91%) yielded either chlamydiae or gonococci (Adger et al, 1985). Thus, it is possible in selected settings that screening for pyuria may be a useful procedure for STD control if predictive values for gonococcal or chlamydial infection are anywhere near as high as observed in the preliminary study.

GENITAL TRACT INFECTIONS IN WOMEN

Cervical infection

The cervix is the most commonly infected site in the female genital tract. A number of studies have suggested that there are typical signs and symptoms for chlamydial infection of the cervix. This includes the finding of a mucopurulent endocervicitis (Rees, 1980; Brunham et al, 1984). It should be noted that most of these studies have been performed in clinics for symptomatic women and in STD clinics. Screening studies on women who are appearing for birth control advice or routine Papanicolaou smears have provided a somewhat different picture, suggesting more than half of the infections in those settings are clinically inapparent (Schachter et al, 1983).

There are some common features that can be associated with chlamydial infection among symptomatic women. *C. trachomatis* is a parasite of columnar epithelium; as yet it has not been found to be capable of growth in squamous cells. Thus the organism does not cause vaginitis. The major sites within the lower genital tract that would be susceptible would be in the endocervical os within the squamocolumnar junction and in the urethra. Careful study of signs and colposcopic examination of the cervix have shown that chlamydial infection of the cervix in asymptomatic women is regularly associated with inflammatory changes (Hare & Thin, 1983). The signs that have been statistically associated with the infection are leukorrhoea, mucopurulent discharge within the endocervical canal which could be detected by a 'swab test' (insertion of a white swab within the endocervical canal which appears yellow on visual examination after removal from the cervix) (Brunham et al, 1984). There is also hyperaemia and oedema of the ectopy which is commonly found in association with chlamydial infection. The friability associated with the infection can also be demonstrated by the use of a swab. Rotation of a swab firmly within the squamo-columnar junction will result in bleeding. This presumably results from hyperaemia and is also a common finding in chlamydial infections of the conjunctiva. This syndrome which is termed 'mucopurulent endocervicitis' is a suggested basis for presumptive therapy for chlamydial infection in the absence of chlamydial cultures.

The accuracy of the diagnosis of mucopurulent endocervicitis in predicting chlamydial infection appears to vary with the population being studied. Most women with this finding in an STD clinic had culture proven chlamydial infection. In another study only 35% of women who were diagnosed as having endocervicitis (although without the swab tests referred to above) yielded chlamydiae from the cervix (Schachter et al, 1983). Thus it appears likely that a presumptive diagnosis can be made in some populations with the application of highly selective diagnostic criteria. The predictive value of this diagnosis for chlamydial infection is at best 50–60%. In the absence of culture this may be a useful guide to therapy.

Histologically the cervical infections are often characterised by non-specific inflammatory reactions but in some studies specific lymphoid follicles have been seen in association with chlamydial infection (Hare & Thin, 1983). It is likely that this is a specific response to antigenic stimulus resulting from chlamydial infection. Chlamydial infection in the eye causes a follicular conjunctivitis.

There are other analogies between urethral infection in the male and cervical infection in the female. Rees has shown the regular presence of 'mucopus' within the endocervix of Chlamydia infected women (Rees et al, 1982). She has also shown that this finding, which often accompanies gonococcal infection, will persist after treatment with beta-lactam drugs which eradicate the gonoccoccal infection in women who have chlamydial infection coincident with GC. Thus this may be a postgonococcal cervicitis quite analogous to the PGU seen in males. It is clear that if gonococcal infections are treated simply with penicillin, that a higher rate of salpingitis will be seen in the treated women than will develop if these women had received tetracycline originally (Rees, 1980). The likelihood is that the penicillin does not affect the chlamydial infection and thus these women are left with chlamydial infection of the cervix which may ascend, producing salpingitis. Because tetracycline is not effective enough in treating gonococcal infection, current recommendation calls for use of a beta-lactam drug immediately (ampicillin or amoxycillin given with probenacid) followed by a week of tetracycline. This should provide adequate therapy for both the gonococcal infection identified and the initial reason for therapy, as well as for the concomitant chlamydial infection that is found in approximately 40% of these women.

The many similarities between cervical infection in the female and urethral infection in the male are sufficient to tempt one to consider the cervix to be the analogue of the urethra in the male and cervicitis to be analogous to urethritis in the male. While this may well be true in some selected populations, this is a dangerous extrapolation to make as a general conclusion. It is clear that there are many more common potential pathogens within the cervical environment and more complicated tissue responses than one can readily diagnose for the male urethra. Thus the analogy may be appropriate in some settings but is probably too simplistic for universal application.

The prevalence of chlamydial cervical infection appears to be quite high and in STD clinics is often equivalent to or exceeded only by the prevalence of gonococcal infection. Approximately 40% of women with gonorrhoea have concomitant chlamydial infection (Oriel & Ridgway, 1982a). However, as soon as one begins screening of symptomatic individuals in other settings, the chlamydial infection rate usually far exceeds the gonococcal infection rate. The general determinants or demographic characteristics of the high risk populations are quite similar. Thus high rates of chlamydial infection are found in young unmarried sexually active women living under poor socioeconomic conditions. Age is clearly the highest risk factor for chlamydial infection and the highest rates are found in sexually active teenagers. It is relatively common to find such infection rates for teenagers in urban areas ranging from 15–20%; these are usually 4–5 times higher than the recovery rates observed for gonococci in the same populations. In higher socioeconomic classes and in older women, chlamydial infection rates tend to be much lower and recovery rates of 2–5% are usually found in such settings.

There have also been a number of studies in pregnant women indicating a wide range of chlamydial prevalence. Some studies found no *Chlamydia* at all, others had a range from 2% to more than 30%. The prevalence followed the socioeconomic conditions described above, with the low rate occuring in older and usually middle income populations while the highest rate was observed in teenage pregnant women seen in a ghetto population.

Other lower genital tract infections

Although *Chlamydia* have been recovered from the ducts of Bartholin glands, most of the cases reported also had gonococcal infections (Davies et al, 1978) and thus it is not clear whether *Chlamydia* alone causes Bartholinitis, although this seems to be a reasonable supposition.

Chlamydial infections appear to occur in the female urethra at a relatively high but as yet ill-defined rate (Paavonen, 1979). The great majority of women who yield the organism from the urethra have concomitant cervical infection and it is difficult to identify any population that has infection only in the urethra. Some studies identified a subset of women (perhaps 10–20%) among those found to have chlamydial infection that had agent recovery only from the urethra and not from the cervix. However some of this finding could simply reflect the enhanced sensitivity of testing multiple specimens with cervical contamination of the genital tract environment. There is one convincing study associating chlamydial infection with the urethral syndrome (Stamm et al, 1980). Many studies have found that *Chlamydia* were commonly found in women who presented with cervical discharge, dysuria and urinary frequency. However, these are common findings in STD clinics and many of these women also have multiple pathogens, so it is somewhat difficult to attribute these conditions to the chlamydial infection. Stamm and colleagues, however, studied women with the acute urethral syndrome and found that chlamydial infection from the cervix was specifically associated with a group of women who had sterile pyuria. This rigorous study was performed with the use of suprapubic aspiration to determine the presence of bacteria in the urine. It is the most convincing demonstration that *Chlamydia trachomatis* can be associated with the urethral syndrome in women. However, it would be unwise to assume that the results of this study which was performed on young college women can be extrapolated to the urethral syndrome in other populations. It is entirely possible that older women with more exposure to *Chlamydia* may be responding differently. The *Chlamydia* recovered were obtained by cervical and not urethral culture. It is uncertain that one can make a universal statement that *Chlamydia* are major causes of the urethral syndrome in all demographic settings.

Dysplasia

Like other sexually transmitted infections, *Chlamydia trachomatis* has been suggested as a potential cause of cervical dysplasia (Hare & Thin, 1983; Schachter et al, 1982b; Paavonen & Purola, 1980). It is clear that the most common response to chlamydial infection in the cervix is that of acute inflammatory changes, repair and metaplasia. A suggestion has been made that metaplastic atypia may also result. An association has also been found between follicular cervicitis demonstrated by biopsy and dysplasia and it is assumed that follicular cervicitis is an indicator of chlamydial infection. A number of case control studies and retrospective serologic studies have also shown high rates of previous exposure to *C. trachomatis* in women with dysplasia as compared to controls. None of the data available prove a causative role. Prospective studies have not been reported nor have appropriately designed treatment trials which would show that early cytologic changes could be reversed by effective antichlamydial therapy.

Upper genital tract infection

Acute salpingitis (AS) is clearly the most important complication of chlamydial genital tract infection (Westrom & Mardh, 1982). Some workers have suggested that one of the few reasons for doing chlamydial cultures in men with NGU is to determine the prevalence of chlamydial infection in the population as an indirect indicator of risks presented to women who may develop AS. Eilard was the first to point out that *Chlamydia* could be recovered from the fallopian tubes of women with AS (Eilard et al, 1976). The leading students of this condition have been Westrom and his colleagues at Lund, Sweden who have been studying the role of *Chlamydia* in AS for at least a decade. Their report in 1977 that 30% of women with AS yielded *C. trachomatis* from needle aspirates of fallopian tubes focused attention on chlamydiae as potentially important pathogens in AS (Mardh et al, 1977). *C. trachomatis* has also been regularly recovered from the cervix and endometrium of women with acute salpingitis (Mardh et al, 1981).

It is clear that AS is a polymicrobial disease and a number of pathogens make important contributions to the condition (Eschenbach et al, 1975). In many settings the gonococcus is the leading cause of AS and *Mycoplasma hominis* has also been implicated in some cases. Anaerobes are also recognised as important causes of AS, as are facultative aerobes. The contributions of these different pathogens appear to vary in different geographic locations. There also are some demographic differences. For example, the sexually transmitted infections such as *Chlamydia* and gonococci are more commonly found in young sexually active women, while anaerobes are more often found in older women.

For a number of years it was somewhat disconcerting to note that chlamydiae were often recovered from cervical cultures done in the United States but evidence that the organism contributed to salpingitis was scant. In contrast, in Scandinavia many studies implicated chlamydiae in AS. A number of possible explanations for the differing results were made. These included different patient populations and selection by use of different clinical criteria, and perhaps even simply geographic differences in the distribution of pathogens. Specimen collection was one obvious problem since many of the studies performed in Scandinavia were based on biopsy specimens collected by laparoscopy, while this procedure was not a common one in the United States. It was also somewhat disconcerting for investigations in the United States regularly to show high seroconversion rates or high levels of IgM antibody (studies using these criteria indicated infection rates of 20–25%) with relatively low cervical infection rates or cervical infection rates that did not differ between cases and controls (Eschenbach et al, 1975; Sweet et al, 1980).

Recently, however, when more invasive procedures were used to collect specimens from the upper genital tract, rather than simply from the cervix, it has been shown that chlamydial infection rates do actually parallel the serologic rates found earlier. Thus, in one earlier study in San Francisco, only 5% of women with AS yielded chlamydiae from the cervix, but 24% of patients seroconverted (Sweet et al, 1980). When endometrial cultures were introduced the recovery rate rose, with 24% of endometrial cultures yielding chlamydiae, compared to 14% from the cervix (Sweet et al, 1983).

The Swedish group has defined the clinical spectrum of AS on the basis of the pathogens recovered and has shown that women with chlamydial salpingitis tended not to be severely ill (Svensson et al, 1981). The clinical findings were relatively mild compared to those seen in gonococcal and anaerobic AS. The women with chlamydial AS usually have a chronic course and were seen after having symptoms of lower abdominal pain for more than a week. They were usually afebrile. Paradoxically, women with chlamydial AS appeared to have higher sedimentation rate, which could indicate a greater degree of tissue involvement. In fact, it is quite likely that the relatively mild disease seen in 'pure' chlamydial salpingitis has a deleterious effect on outcome because the women may have a longer period of fallopian tube inflammation which leads to a poor prognosis for their fertility. It is clear that women with AS are at relatively high risk of involuntary infertility and the infertility rates following gonococcal and chlamydial salpingitis appear to be quite similar.

In studies in San Francisco it has been found that multiple infections in women with AS are quite common. Indeed in a recently published report, there were no women who had single infections (Sweet et al, 1983). Of particular interest in that study was the finding that women who were treated with newer cephalosporins as single drug therapy for AS virtually always had a good clinical response. However those who had *Chlamydia* recovered from the endometrium maintained persistent infection in the absence of any symptoms. It is feared by the investigators that such women would be at risk for sterilizing complications, such as tubal occlusion. It should be noted that the findings relative to the presence of multiple pathogens are in conflict with results reported from Sweden. It is uncertain as to whether this is a reflection of different populations being studied or more rigorous efforts made to identify the anaerobes that were commonly recovered in the San Francisco study.

It is clear that the finding of the failure of beta-lactam drugs to eradicate *Chlamydia* despite good clinical response means that clinical response cannot be used to assess the microbiological response to therapy. The finding also validates the treatment recommendations made by the Centers for Disease Control in the United States that multiple drug therapy is required and that every patient with AS should be treated with a regimen that would be effective against gonococci, aerobes, anaerobes and chlamydiae (CDC, 1982). It is clear that there is no single drug that would be active against this multiplicity of pathogens and suggested treatment regimens for inpatient therapy included combinations such as cefoxitin and a tetracycline or clindamycin and tobramycin. Each of these regimens has shortcomings in terms of efficacy against the different pathogens and it is clear that controlled treatment trials are necessary to determine which, if any, of these combinations will be superior. Since maintenance of fertility is the obvious goal of any treatment modality for AS (over and above obtaining initial responses), it is clear that it will be years before a clearcut mandate for an optimal regimen will be delivered.

Endometritis has also been associated with chlamydial infection (Mardh et al, 1981; Paavonen et al, 1982). There are few studies relevant to this point, and the diagnosis of endometritis is a difficult one to establish. However, the likelihood that the organism causes endometritis is probably great. *C. trachomatis* is an important cause of acute salpingitis and the spread appears to be canalicular. It is quite reasonable to consider that this may be an ascending infection which involves the endometrium.

Perihepatitis or the Fitz-Hugh-Curtis syndrome, once thought to be exclusively due to gonococcal infection is now recognised to be usually of chlamydial aetiology (Muller-Schoop et al, 1978). The earlier assumption that it was due to gonorrhoea was actually based on the fact that gonococci were recovered from cervices of some women with this condition. We now recognise that cervical cultures need not reflect tubal pathogens and serologic and other studies have suggested that chlamydiae are a common cause.

Infertility

Involuntary infertility is the most important consequence of AS and a number of studies being performed on women being evaluated for infertility have shown a great excess of antibody to *C. trachomatis* in those who have tubal-factor infertility. While it is easy to criticise these studies, particularly on the basis of selection of controls, the general consistency of the results obtained in studies from several countries is quite compelling (Cates, 1984). On balance one must accept the conclusion that *C. trachomatis* is an important cause of tubal occlusion. Of considerable interest is that many of the women with tubal occlusion do not have a previous history of AS. This is consistent with the findings that chlamydial salpingitis can be relatively benign and the clinical findings and symptoms may be rather non-specific. This suggests that many cases of chlamydial salpingitis will not be diagnosed unless there is a greater index of suspicion on the part of gynaecologists, but even in that case it is likely that many cases will go undiagnosed and untreated. Thus, it is imperative that greater efforts be made to reduce the reservoir for *Chlamydia* in an effort to reduce the complications seen in women.

Complications of pregnancy

Because *C. trachomatis* is commonly found in the cervix of pregnant women, it has also been reasonable to consider that this organism may also be associated with complications of pregnancy. Although one study associated chlamydial infection with foetal wastage (Martin et al, 1982), this has not been confirmed in other studies performed in different populations (Thompson et al, 1982; Harrison et al, 1982). The balance of the evidence would suggest that no complications of pregnancy outcome can be attributed to uncomplicated chlamydial infections. Neither stillbirths nor low birth weight can be attributed to *Chlamydia*. Postpartum endometritis does occur and this is not an unexpected complication of chlamydial infection (Wager et al, 1980). More studies are needed to estimate the importance, or frequency, of this complication.

Risk factors for chlamydial infection

As mentioned above, it is clear that the most important risk factor for chlamydial infection is age, with higher infection rates being found in younger women. Race may be a factor as a number of studies have found higher infection rates in black women. This may reflect socioeconomic status. Multiple partners are also associated with chlamydial infection as is the use of oral contraceptives (OC) (Oriel & Ridgway, 1982a). The rationale for this latter finding is not clear. Many women who use OC are found to have ectopy and this finding is also significantly associated with chlamydial infection. It is uncertain whether *Chlamydia* induce ectopy (unlikely) or whether *Chlamydia* are more often recovered from women with ectopy because specimen collection is more efficient, or whether women with ectopy are more susceptible to chlamydial infection since the cells that the organism parasitises are more exposed. On a pragmatic basis, young sexually active women using OC are at high risk for *C. trachomatis* infection.

A number of studies have suggested that OC are protective for acute salpingitis. This may be too broad a statement since the available data suggests only that OC protect against gonococcal salpingitis. If the attack rates for chlamydial salpingitis are the same for OC users or non-users, the higher prevalence rate of chlamydial infection in OC users would produce a higher prevalence of chlamydial salpingitis in the population due to the oral contraceptive use (Washington et al, 1984).

Treatment

Uncomplicated chlamydial infection in the female genital tract will respond to the same treatment regimens mentioned above for treating males. In pregnant women, erythromycin would be the drug of choice and success rates approximating to 90% have been obtained using erythromycin ethylsuccinate at 1.6 g/day for 7 days or using the stearate at 1 g/day for 14 days (Schachter, 1984; Podgore et al, 1980).

CHLAMYDIAL INFECTION IN INFANTS

Conjunctivitis

A newborn infant exposed to an infected birth canal can acquire a chlamydial infection (Schachter & Dawson, 1978; Schachter & Grossman, 1981). The most common clinical manifestation is inclusion conjunctivitis of the newborn (ICN). This disease has an incubation period of approximately 6–19 days and approximately one-third of exposed infants will develop ICN. The clinical spectrum of the condition ranges from a mild conjunctivitis with oedema and hyperaemia to a mucopurulent conjunctivitis, then to a severe purulent conjunctivitis which is clinically indistinguishable from severe gonococcal ophthalmia neonatorum. In prospective studies where ocular samples have been collected regularly, inapparent infections have not been seen. Thus it appears that the newborn always reacts with some signs of conjunctivitis when the eye is infected. If pseudomembranes form, sheet scarring of the conjunctivae may develop. Persistent infection and blinding sequelae such as is seen in trachoma, although reported are rare. If untreated, most of these infants will resolve spontaneously with no signs of infection after a few months. If the disease lasts long enough a follicular conjunctivitis such as is seen in adults who have developed an immune response will be observed. Micropannus and keratitis occur if treatment is not initiated early.

In the past ICN was treated topically with tetracycline or erythromycin ointments or sulfonamide drops. These were accompanied by failure rates that were reported to be as high as 50% (Rowe et al, 1979). It is now clear that a perinatally exposed infant has extraocular infections and virtually all infants with conjunctivitis have naso-pharyngeal infection and are at risk for serious complications. Failure of topical therapy, previously attributed to compliance problems, is probably often due to reinfection from exogenously infected sites. Therefore, systemic treatment is recommended and erythromycin ethylsuccinate at 40 mg/kg in divided doses given 4 times daily for 2 weeks has been successful.

Chlamydial conjunctivitis can often be diagnosed on cytologic grounds. In severe cases the Giemsa stained conjunctival scrapings usually (>90%) show characteristic chlamydial inclusions. The organism can be readily isolated in tissue culture. Serology is not useful for this diagnosis. The predominant antibodies being measured at the age when the infants are usually seen (1 to 2 weeks) are maternally transmitted IgG antibody. Attempts to demonstrate chlamydial antigen in clinical specimens by use of fluorescein-conjugated monoclonal antibody or by enzyme immunoassay have not been well studied for ICN, but will probably be positive, since large amounts of agent are found in infants with active conjunctivitis.

Pneumonia

In recent years a characteristic pneumonia syndrome caused by *Chlamydia trachomatis* has been recognised to be a major problem in the United States (Beem & Saxon, 1977). The disease has not been as frequently seen in Europe. This is likely to be an artefact of the health care delivery systems in respective countries. The condition has been observed in Canada, England, Sweden, France and Israel and prospective studies have suggested that approximately one in six perinatally exposed infants develops pneumonia. The disease typically occurs when the infants are between 2 and 12 weeks of age. In studies in the United States, approximately 30–40% of the infants who are hospitalised with pneumonia in the first 6 months of life have chlamydial infection (Harrison et al, 1978). Many of these infants have concomitant viral infections but comparative studies, based on clinical findings, and the response to erythromycin, have suggested that the clinical findings in most of these infants can be attributed to the chlamydial infection (Tipple et al, 1979). The importance of the other infections suggests that here, as in many other chlamydial infections (trachoma, acute salpingitis, urethral and cervical infections) that the *Chlamydia* are accompanied by other potential pathogens and that there may be modifying effects on the immune response which allow one or the other agents to become clinically important.

Chlamydial pneumonia of the newborn is virtually always an afebrile disease which is characterised by a hacking cough reminiscent of pertussis but lacking the inspiratory whoop. The infants have radiologic findings of hyperinflation and often have a relative eosinophilia. Hypergammaglobulinaemia of the IgG class is regularly found and IgM levels are almost always elevated. While the disease is usually diagnosed by isolation of the organism from effected infants, recent studies have suggested that the most efficient method of diagnosing pneumonia may be determination of high ($\geqslant$1:32) levels of specific antichlamydial IgM antibody in the microimmunofluorescence test (Schachter et al, 1982a).

LABORATORY DIAGNOSIS OF CHLAMYDIAL INFECTIONS

Methods for diagnosing chlamydial infections are basically the same as those used for other bacteria (Schachter, 1980). These include direct isolation of the organism, cytology or demonstration of the presence of the organism in stained preparations collected from patient's tissue, or serologic means. Currently it would appear that the most sensitive method for detecting chlamydial infection is isolation. The sensitivity of the procedure is not known but it is likely to be of the order of 80–90% for symptomatic or clinically apparent infections of the lower genital tracts of men or women (urethra or cervix). The generally accepted system to isolate *C. trachomatis* uses cycloheximide-treated McCoy cells (Ripa & Mardh, 1977).

Isolation
Chlamydial infection usually occurs at superficial mucous membrane layers. It is imperative that an appropriate specimen is collected. Sampling of urine or discharges is inadequate. Swabs must be collected from the involved site by vigorous rubbing against the tissue surface to collect an adequate cell specimen. In sites such as the cervix, where discharge is commonly found, the discharge should be cleaned away before the specimen is collected. All of these sites are contaminated with unwanted bacteria. Antibiotics that are inactive against *Chlamydia* are included in collection media to remove these unwanted bacteria. Streptomycin, gentamycin, vancomycin and antifungals such as amphotericin-B or nystatin are commonly used. Special transport media have been devised and the 2SP formulation is probably the most popular one. It may have some advantages, but tissue culture medium containing fetal calf

serum and antibiotics is also often used. The specimens should be kept refrigerated after they are collected and should be processed within 72 hours of collection. If they must be kept longer they should be frozen soon after collection. Swabs used for collection should be proven non-toxic to the McCoy cells and chlamydiae.

The clinical specimens are centrifuged on to McCoy cells (3000 g for 1 hour) which are then incubated in a cycloheximide containing medium (the cycloheximide stops the metabolism of the mammalian cell while having no effect upon the *Chlamydia*). After 48–72 hours incubation the cells are stained for the presence of typical chlamydial inclusions. The use of immunofluorescent procedures to demonstrate inclusions is clearly the most sensitive technique (Thomas et al, 1977; Stamm et al, 1983). These are also relatively expensive, and require special microscopes. The iodine stain is the simplest procedure, but it is less sensitive than other techniques. Giemsa stain is used by some, but it is more difficult for the microscopist. Negative specimens in the initial isolation attempt are often subjected to a blind passage. This will result in increased chlamydial recovery rate but the cost benefit ratio will be a function of the population being tested. For symptomatic patients in an STD clinic blind passage does not appear to add a large increment of positives (only 10%). In screening asymptomatic individuals the amplifying effect of the passage is more important, as 25% of isolates may be missed in first passage.

For most procedures the isolation attempts are performed in flat bottom vials which contain coverslips. Ninety-six well tissue culture plates are more efficient and less expensive but are less sensitive for recovery of the organism (Yoder et al, 1981). For testing patients from STD clinics, where relatively high amounts of agent are present, the flat bottom plates may well be preferred since they allow processing large numbers of specimens. In screening asymptomatic individuals, who have lower quantities of agent present, the 96-well plates are markedly less sensitive and should not be used.

Cytology

The direct examination of smears collected from the affected sites was the original means of demonstrating chlamydial infection before these organisms had been cultured. The Giemsa stain was the classic procedure but it is a time consuming and insensitive one. Immunofluorescent (IF) procedures using polyclonal antibodies were also used to demonstrate the typical chlamydial inclusions. Although IF is a more sensitive procedure than Giemsa it is less sensitive than cell culture and because the polyclonal antibodies suffer from problems of non-specific staining the procedure has largely been abandoned. More recently, fluorescein-conjugated, species-specific monoclonal antibodies have been made commercially available (Tam et al, 1984). These are far cleaner reagents and do not give the background of non-specific staining that is often seen with the polyclonal IF reagents. The procedure is approximately 90% as sensitive as culture and may well represent a reasonable alternative to culture in settings where isolation is not routinely performed. Specificity of the test appears to be quite good (>98%), in the hands of experienced microscopists. It is a procedure which does require training, and one cannot simply purchase the reagent and start to use it. It is imperative that microscopists standardise their slide reading by examining known positive and negative slides. This reagent, which is specific for antigenic determinants on the major outer membrane protein of *C. trachomatis* (Stevens et al, 1982), stains elementary bodies in the clinical specimens quite well but inclusions are not often seen. Thus a positive specimen is identified on detection of the elementary bodies. More confirmatory studies on the performance of this test are needed before recommendations on its use can be made.

It should be noted that some workers have claimed that chlamydial infections can be diagnosed by use of the Papanicolaou stain. On the basis of most studies the only conclusion that can be reached is that this is simply not true. The specific analysis of cytologic findings with Papanicolaou staining may allow identification of a subset of patients who have a higher recovery rate for *Chlamydia* (Dorman et al, 1983). Thus the technique may be used for screening populations but it should not be used for diagnosis. Chlamydial inclusions stain poorly by this method.

Other non-culture methods of chlamydial detection

Recently, enzyme immunossay has been used for detection of chlamydial antigen in clinical specimens (Herrman et al, 1983). Although such products have been licensed, they are not yet commercially available and only company supported studies are available. The test appears to be as sensitive as culture using first passage results, but as is true for any non-culture method, will have a certain number of false-positive results which become more important as the prevalence of infection in the population under study decreases.

Methods for detecting chlamydial DNA in clinical specimens are also being investigated (Palva et al, 1984). Probes have been developed for both plasmid and chromosomal DNA (Lovett et al, 1979). Preliminary results have been promising. As expected, the specificity has been high (chlamydial DNA does not show high levels of homology with other organisms) and the sensitivity seems to be similar to culture. Non-radioactive labels (such as biotin-avidin-peroxidase systems) will have to be developed before DNA probes can be evaluated as a routine diagnostic test.

Serology

The complement fixation test is used to diagnose systemic infection with *Chlamydia* and measures antibody response to a genus-specific determinant. It is not useful in the diagnosis of common genital tract infections. The microimmunofluorescence (Micro-IF) procedure developed by Wang and Grayston has been extensively used to study genital tract infections (Wang & Grayston, 1970). The Micro-IF test used is an indirect immunofluorescent test using chlamydial elementary bodies as antigens. Reticulate body antigens have also been used but do not appear to offer significant advantages over the EBs (Wang & Grayston, 1982).

Micro-IF has ben a most useful epidemiologic tool and has helped to provide clues to clinical conditions deserving of further investigation, but it is not a regularly useful diagnostic procedure. This is not due to any problems of the test but simply reflects the high prevalence of antibodies to *C. trachomatis* among the populations being studied for active infection. Thus the sensitivity of the test is quite high but the specificity is poor. Virtually all (>99%) women and most (>90%) men with proven chlamydial infections have IgG antibodies to *C. trachomatis* by the Micro-IF test. In the relatively uncommon instance of early study of patients having first chlamydial infections one can demonstrate seroconversion, but this is not particularly useful for patient management because of the time necessary to collect paired serum specimens. Single point determinations of IgM antibody levels are also not useful in diagnosing the infection. Here too, this is because of the relatively high prevalence found in populations at risk for STDs, and the fact that the IgM response is relatively short-lived in patients with current infection and thus will not be found in many patients with proven chlamydial infection.

Complications of chlamydial genital tract infections may be more readily diagnosed by serologic means. Very high titres are seen in women with acute salpingitis or the Fitz-Hugh-Curtis syndrome, or in men with epididymitis. Here too, serodiagnosis leaves something to be desired but it can be more useful because of the elevated levels.

While enzyme immunoassays have been described for measuring chlamydial antibody, there has not been a wide experience with this technology. It seems at least as sensitive as the Micro-IF but is not particularly useful in diagnosing current infection for the same reasons that the Micro-IF fails. There is, however, one instance where serology can be used routinely: diagnosis of chlamydial pneumonia in infants. In this condition there is a defined exposure and the detection of high levels ($>1:32$) of IgM antibody will support a diagnosis of *Chlamydia* pneumonia (Schachter et al, 1982a). It may even be preferred to isolation of the organism from the nasopharynx, because inapparent nasopharyngeal infection is relatively common in perinatally exposed infants who may develop pneumonia due to other organisms. IgG antibodies, which are often of maternal origin, are not as useful although they can provide some support for consideration of Chlamydia pneumonia; the incubation period of the pneumonia is often 2 months, which will allow for diminution of maternally transmitted IgG levels. Infants with pneumonia usually have IgG antibody levels $>1:256$.

REFERENCES

Adger H, Shafer M-A, Sweet R L, Schachter J 1985 Screening for Chlamydia trachomatis and Neisseria gonorrhoeae in adolescent males: value of first catch urine. Lancet 2(8409): 944–945

Beem M O, Saxon E M 1977 Respiratory tract colonization and a distinctive pneumonia syndrome in infants infected with Chlamydia trachomatis. New England Journal of Medicine 293: 306–310

Berger R E, Alexander E R, Monda G E, Ansell J, McCormick G, Holmes K K 1978 Chlamydia trachomatis as a cause of acute 'idiopathic' epididymitis. New England Journal of Medicine 298(6): 301

Bowie W R 1978 Comparison of gram stain and first-voided urine sediment in the diagnosis of urethritis. Sexually Transmitted Diseases 5(2): 39–42

Bowie W R, Wang S-P, Alexander E R, Floyd J, Forsyth P, Pollock H, Tin J-S, Buchanan T, Holmes K K 1977 Etiology of non-gonococcal urethritis: evidence for Chlamydia trachomatis and Ureaplasma urealyticum. Journal of Clinical Investigations 59: 735–742

Brunham R C, Paavonen J, Stevens C E, Kiviat N, Kuo C-C, Holmes K K 1984 Mucopurulent cervicitis— the ignored counterpart in women of urethritis in men. New England Journal of Medicine 311(1): 1–6

Cates W, Jr 1984 Sexually transmitted organisms and infertility: the proof of the pudding. Sexually Transmitted Diseases 11(2): 113–116

Centers for Disease Control 1982 Sexually transmitted diseases: treatment quidelines 1982. Reviews of Infectious Diseases 4 (supplement): S729–S746

Davies J A, Rees E, Hobson D, Karayiannis P 1978 Isolation of Chlamydia trachomatis from Bartholin's ducts. British Journal of Venereal Disease 54(6): 409

Dorman S A, Danos L M, Wilson D J, Noller K L, Malkasian G D, Goellner J R, Smith T F 1983 Detection of chlamydial cervicitis by Papanicolaou stained smears and culture. American Journal of Clinical Pathology 79(4): 421–425

Eilard T, Brorson J E, Hamark B, Forssman L 1976 Isolation of Chlamydia trachomatis in acute salpingitis. Scandanavian Journal of Infectious Diseases suppl: 82

Eschenbach D A, Buchanan T M, Pollock H M, Forsyth P S, Alexander E R, Lin J S, Wang S-P,

Wentworth B B, McCormack W M, Holmes K K 1975 Polymicrobial etiology of acute pelvic inflammatory disease. New England Journal of Medicine 293: 166

Grayston, T, Wang S-P 1975 New knowledge of chlamydiae and the diseases they cause. Journal of Infectious Diseases 132: 87–105

Hammerschlag M R, Anderka M, Semine D Z, McComb D, McCormack W M 1979 Prospective study of maternal and infantile infection with Chlamydia trachomatis. Pediatrics 64(2): 142

Hardy P H, Hardy J B, Nell E E, Graham D A, Spence M A, Rosenbaum R C 1984 Prevalence of six sexually transmitted disease agents among pregnant inner-city adolescents and pregnancy outcome. Lancet 2(8398): 333

Hare J M, Thin R N 1983 Chlamydial infection of the lower genital tract of women. British Medical Bulletin 39(2): 138

Harrison H R, Alexander E R, Weinstein L, Lewis M, Sim D A 1982 Epidemiologic correlations of genital infections and outcomes of pregnancy. In: Mardh P-A, Holmes K K, Oriel J D, Piot P Schachter J (eds) Chlamydial infections, Elsevier Biomedical, Amsterdam p 159–162

Harrison H R, English M G, Lee C K, Alexander E R 1978 Chlamydia trachomatis infant pneumonitis. comparison with matched controls and other infant pneumonitis: New England Journal of Medicine 298: 702–708

Herrman J E, Howard L V, Armstrong A S, Craine M C 1983 Immunoassays for detection of Neisseria gonorrhoeae and Chlamydia trachomatis in samples from a single specimen. In: Program and abstracts of the International Society for STD Research 5th International Meeting August 1–3 (abstract 44) p 76

Holmes K K, Handsfield H H, Wang S-P, Wentworth B B, Turck M, Anderson J B, Alexander E R 1975 Etiology of non-gonococcal urethritis. New England Journal of Medicine 292(23): 1199–1205

Kuo C-C, Wang S-P, Holmes K K, Grayston J T 1983 Immunotypes of Chlamydia trachomatis isolates in Seattle, Washington. Infection and Immunity 41(2): 865–868

Lovett M A, Kuo C-C, Holmes K K, Falkow S 1979 Plasmids of the genus Chlamydia. In: Program and abstracts of the 11th international congress of chemotherapy and 19th interscience conference on antimicrobial agents and chemotherapy. American Society for Microbiology, Washington DC (abstract 6)

Lycke E, Lowhagen G-B, Hallhagen G, Johannisson G, Ramstedt K 1980 The risk of transmission of genital Chlamydia trachomatis infection is less than that of genital Neisseria gonorrhoeae infection. Sexually Transmitted Diseases 7(1): 6–10

Mardh P-A, Moller B R, Ingerselv H J, Nussler E, Westrom L, Wolnerhanssen P 1981 Endometritis caused by Chlamydia trachomatis. British Journal of Venereal Diseases 57(3): 191

Mardh P-A, Ripa T, Svensson L, Westrom L 1977 Chlamydia trachomatis infection in patients with acute salpingitis. New England Journal of Medicine 296: 1377–1379

Martin D H, Koutsky L, Eschenbach D A, Daling J R, Alexander E R, Benedetti J K, Holmes K K 1982 Prematurity and perinatal mortality in pregnancies complicated by maternal Chlamydia trachomatis infections. Journal of the American Medical Association 247: 1585–1588

Moulder J W, Hatch T P, Kuo C-C, Schachter J, Storz J 1984 Chlamydiales Storz and Page 1971, 334. In: Krieg N R, Holt J G (eds) Bergey's manual of systematic bacteriology, Vol 1 Williams and Wilkins, Baltimore p 729

Muller-Schoop J W, Wang S-P, Munzinger J, Schlapfer H U, Knoblauch M, Ammann R W 1978 Chlamydia trachomatis as possible cause of peritonitis and perihepatis in young women. British Medical Journal 1(6119): 1022–1023

Munday P E, Taylor-Robinson D 1983 Chlamydial infection in proctitis and Crohn's disease. British Medical Bulletin 39(2): 155–158

Oriel J D, Reeve P, Thomas B J, Nicol C S 1975 Infection with Chlamydia group A in men with urethritis due to Neisseria gonorrhoeae. Journal of Infectious Diseases 131: 376–382

Oriel J D, Ridgway G L 1982a Genital infection by Chlamydia trachomatis. Arnold, London

Oriel J D, Ridgway G L 1982b Studies of the epidemiology of chlamydial infection of the human genital tract. In: Mardh P-A, Holmes K K, Oriel J D, Piot P, Schachter J (eds) Chlamydial infections, Elsevier Biomedical, Amsterdam p 425–428

Paavonen J 1979 Chlamydia trachomatis-induced urethritis in female partners of men with non-gonococcal urethritis. Sexually Transmitted Diseases 6: 69

Paavonen J, Brunham R C, Kiviat N, Stevens C, Kuo C-C, Stamm W Holmes K K, Eschenbach D A 1982 Clinical and histologic evidence of endometritis among women with cervicitis. In: Mardh P-A, Holmes K K, Oriel J D, Piot P, Schachter J (eds) Chlamydial infections, Elsevier Biomedical, Amsterdam p 163–165

Paavonen J, Purola E 1980 Cytologic findings in cervical chlamydial infection. Medical Biology 58(3): 174

Palva A, Jousimies-Somer H, Saikku P, Vaananen P, Soderlund H, Ranki M 1984 Detection of Chlamydia trachomatis by nucleic acid sandwich hybridization. FEMS Microbiology Letters 23: 83–89

Podgore J K, Belts R, Alden E, Alexander E R 1980 Effectiveness of maternal third trimester erythromycin in prevention of infant Chlamydia trachomatis infection. In: Program and abstracts of the 20th Interscience Conference on Antimicrobial Agents and Chemotherapy, American Society for Microbiology Washington DC (abstract 524)

Podgore J K, Holmes K K, Alexander E R 1982 Asymptomatic urethral infections due to Chlamydia trachomatis in male US military personnel. Journal of Infectious Diseases 146(6): 828

Quinn T C, Goodell S E, Mkrtichian E, Schuffler M D, Wang S-P, Stamm W E, Holmes K K 1981 Chlamydia trachomatis proctitis. New England Journal of Medicine 305(4): 195–200

Rees E 1980 The treatment of pelvic inflammatory disease. American Journal of Obstetrics and Gynecology 138(7): 1042–1047

Rees E, Davies J A, Bradley M G, Hobson D, Byng R E, Karayiannis P 1982 Chlamydia trachomatis in relation to post-gonococcal cervicitis. In: Mardh P-A, Holmes K K, Oriel J D, Piot P, Schachter J (eds) Chlamydial infections, Elsevier Biomedical Amsterdam p 147–150

Richmond S J, Hilton A L, Clarke S K R 1972 Chlamydial infection: Role of Chlamydia subgroup A in non-gonococcal and post-gonococcal urethritis. British Journal of Venereal Disease 48: 437–444

Ripa K T, Mardh P-A 1977 Cultivation of Chlamydia trachomatis in cycloheximide-treated McCoy cells. Journal of Clinical Microbiology 6(4): 328–331

Rowe S, Aicardi E, Dawson C, Schachter J 1979 Purulent ocular discharge in neonates: significance of Chlamydia trachomatis. Pediatrics 63: 628–632

Schachter J 1978 Chlamydial infections. New England Journal of Medicine 298: 428–435 & 490–495 & 540–549

Schachter J 1980 Chlamydiae (psittacosis-lymphogranuloma venereum-trachoma group). In: Lennette E H (ed) Manual of clinical microbiology, 3rd edn. American Society for Microbiology, Washington DC p 357–364

Schachter J 1984 Erythromycin treatment of chlamydial infection in pregnancy. Presented at the 57th Annual Meeting of the American Epidemiological Society, March 22–23, 1984 (abstract)

Schachter J, Cles L D, Ray R M, Hesse F E 1983 Is there immunity to chlamydial infection of the human genital tract? Sexually Transmitted Diseases 10(3): 123–125

Schachter J, Dawson C R 1978 Chlamydial infections, Publishing Sciences Group, Littleton

Schachter J, Grossman M 1981 Chlamydial infections. Annual Review of Medicine 32: 45–61

Schachter J, Grossman M, Azimi P H 1982a Serology of Chlamydia trachomatis in infants. Journal of Infectious Diseases 146(6): 530–535

Schachter J, Hill E C, King E B, Heilbron D C, Ray R M, Margolis A J, Greenwood S A 1982b Chlamydia trachomatis and cervical neoplasia. Journal of the American Medical Association 248(17): 2134–2138

Schachter J, Stoner E, Moncada J 1983 Screening for chlamydial infections in women attending family planning clinics: evaluations of presumptive indicators for therapy. Western Journal of Medicine 138(3): 375–379

Shafer M-A, Blain B, Beck A, Dole P, Irwin C E, Sweet R, Schachter J 1984 Chlamydia trachomatis: important relationships to race, contraception, lower genital tract infection, and Papanicolaou smears. Journal of Pediatrics 104(1): 141–146

Stamm W E, Wagner K F, Ansell R, Alexander E R, Turck M, Counts G, Holmes K K 1980 Causes of the acute urethral syndrome in women. New England Journal of Medicine 303(8): 409–415

Stamm W E, Koutsky L A, Benedetti J K, Jourden J L, Brunham R C, Holmes K K 1984 Chlamydia trachomatis: urethral infection in men. Annals of Internal Medicine 100(1): 47

Stamm W E, Tam M, Koester M, Cles L 1983 Detection of Chlamydia trachomatis inclusions in McCoy cell cultures with fluorescein-conjugated monoclonal antibodies. Journal of Clinical Microbiology 17(4): 666–668

Stevens R S, Tam M R, Kuo C-C, Nowinski R C 1982 Monoclonal antibodies to Chlamydia trachomatis: antibody specificities and antigen characterization. Journal of Immunology 128: 1083–1089

Svensson L, Westrom L, Mardh P-A 1981 Acute salpingitis with Chlamydia trachomatis isolated from the fallopian tubes: clinical, cultural and serologic findings. Sexually Transmitted Diseases 8(2): 51

Swartz S L, Kraus S J 1979 Persistent urethral leukocytosis and asymptomatic chlamydial urethritis. Journal of Infectious Diseases 140(4): 614–617

Sweet R L, Draper D L, Schachter J, James J, Hadley W K, Brooks G F 1980 Microbiology and pathogenesis of acute salpingitis as determined by laparoscopy: what is the appropriate site to sample? American Journal of Obstetrics and Gynecology 138(7): 985–989

Sweet R L, Schachter J, Robbie M 1983 Failure of beta lactam antibiotics to eradicate Chlamydia trachomatis in the endometrium despite apparent clinical cure of acute salpingitis. Journal of the American Medical Association 250(19): 2641–2645

Tam M R, Stamm W E, Handsfield H H, Stephens R, Kuo C-C, Holmes K K, Ditzenberger K, Crieger M, Nowinski R C 1984 Culture-independent diagnosis of Chlamydia trachomatis using monoclonal antibodies. New England Journal of Medicine 310(18): 1146–1150

Taylor-Robinson D, Thomas B J 1980 The role of C. trachomatis in genital tract and associated diseases. Journal of Clinical Pathology 33: 205–233

Thomas B J, Evans R T, Hutchinson G R, Taylor-Robinson D 1977 Early detection of chlamydial inclusions combining the use of cycloheximide-treated McCoy cells and immunofluorescence staining. Journal of Clinical Microbiology 6(3): 285–292

Thompson S, Lopez B, Wong K-H, Ramsey C, Thomas J, Reising G, Jenks B, Peacock W, Sanderson M, Goforth S, Zaidi A, Miller R, Klein L 1982 A prospective study of Chlamydia and Mycoplasma infections during pregnancy: relation to pregnancy outcome and maternal morbidity. In: Mardh P-A, Holmes K K, Oriel J D, Piot P, Schachter J (eds) Chlamydial infections, Elsevier Biomedical, Amsterdam p 155–158

Tipple M A, Beem M, Saxon E 1979 Clinical characteristics of the afebrile pneumonia associated with Chlamydia trachomatis infection in infants less than 6 months of age. Pediatrics 63: 192–197

Wager G P, Martin D H, Koutsky L, Eschenbach D A, Daling J R, Chiang W T, Alexander E R, Holmes K K 1980 Puerperal infectious morbidity: relationship to route of delivery and to antepartum Chlamydia trachomatis infection. American Journal of Obstetrics and Gynecology 138(7): 1028–1033

Wang S-P, Grayston J T 1970 Immunologic relationship between genital TRIC, lymphogranuloma venereum, and related organisms in a new microtiter indirect microimmunofluorescence test. American Journal of Ophthalmology 70: 367–374

Wang S-P, Grayston J T 1982 Microimmunofluorescence antibody responses in Chlamydia trachomatis infection, A review. In: Mardh P-A, Holmes K K, Oriel J D, Piot P, Schachter J (eds) Chlamydial infections, Elsevier Biomedical, Amsterdam

Washington A E, Gove S, Schachter J, Sweet R L 1985 Oral contraceptives, Chlamydia trachomatis infection and pelvic inflammatory disease: Journal of the American Medical Association 253(15): 2246–2250

Westrom L, Mardh P-A 1982 Genital chlamydial infections in the female. In: Mardh P-A, Holmes K K, Oriel J D, Piot P, Schachter J (eds) Chlamydial infections, Elsevier Biomedical, Amsterdam p 121–139

Yoder B L, Stamm W E, Koester M C, Alexander R E 1981 Microtest procedure for isolation of Chlamydia trachomatis. Journal of Clinical Microbiology 13(6): 1036–1039

4. Laboratory diagnosis of *Haemophilus ducreyi* infections

Allan R. Ronald

HISTORY

Chancroid or the 'soft chancre' was first recognised as a genital ulcer disease distinct from syphilis in 1852 by Basereau in France. The etiologic agent was initially described by a Naplese physician Ducrey in 1889. He autoinoculated the forearm skin of three patients with purulent material from their genital ulcer and at weekly intervals inoculated a new site. Following five or more serial transfers of material from the most recent ulcer, he described a short chaining streptobacillary rod in the exudate. While Ducrey was unable to find the organism in pus from buboes and he could not culture the organism in vitro, he concluded that it was responsible for the 'soft chancre' and that others were incorrect in attributing a major role to 'common microorganisms of suppuration' (Ducrey, 1889).

Between 1888 and 1901, several microbiologists successfully cultured *H. ducreyi* (Bezancon et al, 1900). However, during the next threequarters of a century, controversy continued as to the significance of *H. ducreyi* as an etiologic agent in genital ulcer disease. *H. ducreyi* could not be reproducibly cultured from many patients with presumed chancroid. Most investigators used a variety of liquid media for primary isolation. Cultivation on solid media was unpredictable and the organism was rarely isolated in pure culture. In 1920, Teague & Diebert reported that clotted rabbit, or human blood heated to 55°C for five minutes, was a satisfactory medium. Following overnight incubation, the broth culture was stained and a search made for gram-negative rods in long 'parallel chains', or 'school of fish arrangements'. Unfortunately, several species of gram-negative rods, particularly anaerobes, are usually present in chancroidal exudate and the specificity, sensitivity and reproducibility of these techniques were never critically ascertained. As late as 1935, the US Public Health Service was still skeptical about the etiology of chancroid stating 'this is a local disease of the external generative organs in which a sore develops. The cause of this sore is believed to be an infection with a germ, although some physicians question the part which this germ plays' (Greenblatt & Sanderson, 1938).

Beeson (1946) made a series of important observations with regard to the culture of *H. ducreyi*. Growth was enhanced by increased humidity and CO_2 in the ambient environment; all strains required red cells and many required serum for growth on primary isolation. Unfortunately, these observations went largely unnoticed and were not incorporated into routine technology for culture of *H. ducreyi*. Microbiologists argued for years about the need to inactivate human or rabbit blood clots before inoculation of exudate pus from the ulcer. Deacon et al (1956) noted that virulent, freshly-isolated organisms grew equally well in both activated and inactivated clots, but that contaminants proliferated more readily when the clot was inactivated. Avirulent laboratory strains only grew in inactivated clot cultures. Recently Odumeru et al (1984) have shown that virulent isolates are resistant to killing by serum whereas isogenic avirulent isolates are killed rapidly by serum in the presence of complement. Presumably this explains the failure of laboratory stock isolates to grow in blood clot cultures unless complement is inactivated by heating.

Delayed cutaneous hypersensitivity to *H. ducreyi* antigens and serologic tests have been used to diagnose chancroid (Dienst & August, 1942). These tests were both insensitive and non-specific and are currently not in use.

Chancroid is epidemic in many countries in the developing world and is the second most frequently diagnosed sexually transmitted disease in some regions. In industrialised nations, chancroid has disappeared as an epidemic disease, occurring only sporadically as a result of periodic importation. However, clusters and limited epidemics of chancroid continue to occur with recent outbreaks in Winnipeg, Canada in 1975, in the Netherlands in 1979, and in California in 1981 (Hammond et al, 1980; Nayyar et al, 1979; Centers for Disease Control, 1982). Although investigators in Sheffield, England have reported that chancroid is endemic in this region, and that cultures from a variety of ulcers including clasical genital herpes are frequently positive for *H. ducreyi*, these observations have not been confirmed in other studies (Kinghorn et al, 1982; Diaz-Mitoma, in press).

TAXONOMY AND BIOCHEMICAL CHARACTERISATION

Winslow proposed in 1917 that Ducrey's bacillus be included in the genus Haemophilus (Winslow et al, 1921). Lwoff & Pirosky (1937) confirmed its requirement for hemin (X-factor). Kilian (1976) and more recently Hammond et al (1978) demonstrated the absence of enzyme activity by the use of the porphyrin test, which tests for the synthesis of porphyrin from delta aminoleavulinic acid. *H. ducreyi* lacks hemin synthethase which catalyses the insertion of iron into the protoporphyrin nucleus. It is the only human pathogen in the genus Haemophilus with a requirement for hemin, as determined by the porphyrin test (Kilian, 1976).

Kilian (1976) confirmed the gram negative character of the *H. ducreyi* cell wall by electron microscopy. He also determined that the guanosine-plus-cytosine content was 0.38 mole fraction. More recently, Albritton et al (1984) have investigated the DNA relatedness within the genus Haemophilus. They have shown that, although the organism shares some antigenic relationships with other members of the genus Haemophilus, DNA-DNA hybridisation indicates a distant relationship with relative DNA homology to *H. influenzae* of only 0.18. This was confirmed by the inefficient heterospecific transformation of streptomycin-resistance markers from *H. influenzae* to *H. ducreyi*.

H. ducreyi has few biochemical characteristics which permit specific identification. All *H. ducreyi* strains are H_2S and indol negative. Haemin (x-factor) requirement cannot be demonstrated by growth around a disc impregnated with hemin on trypticase agar owing to the failure of this medium to support the growth of *H. ducreyi*. However, the requirement for hemin can be shown on a gonococcal agar base supplemented with glucose (0.1%), glutamine (0.01%), and cysteine (0.05%) (Hammond et al, 1978). The porphyrin test described by Kilian can also be used to test for haemin requirement. The oxicase reaction is positive if NNNN-tetramethyl-p-phenylenediamine is used as a substrate but variable or negative when NN-dimethyl-p-phenylene-diamine is used (Sottnek et al, 1979). The catalase test has been consistently reported to be negative if H_2O_2 is dropped on colonies on the agar surface. However, Sturm & Zanen (1984) reported that the tube test was positive for all of their 29 isolates. All strains are alkaline phosphatase positive and the nitrate reductase reaction is positive for most isolates. Sturm & Zanen (1984) investigated enzymic activities of 29 *H. ducreyi* strains using a heavy suspension of bacterial cells. None of their strains were found to produce glycosidase, decarboxylase, gelatinase, urease, DNAase or hyaluronidase. However, all strains produced L-arginine aminopeptidase, alkaline phosphatase and valerate esterase. These investigators obtained variable results with the nitrate reductase and oxidase tests. They speculate that there may be different biotypes of *H. ducreyi*. Additional investigation is required to determine if these occur.

STAINING AND ISOLATION

a Staining

H. ducreyi stain faintly with safranin and crystal violet. Although, few gram negative organisms share the classical spatial description of *H. ducreyi*, ulcer exudate rarely demonstrates this characteristic appearance (Nsanze et al, 1981). Although some microbiologists have found the Gram stain to be specific and sensitive (Taylor et al, 1984), others have refuted this observation (Nsanze et al, 1981). As a result, the role of the Gram stain in the diagnosis of *H. ducreyi* infection in patients with genital ulcer remains controversial. Alternate techniques to immediately identify *H. ducreyi* in ulcer or buboe exudate are needed. Although immunofluoresence has been reported to be useful, no commercial preparation is yet available (Denys et al, 1978). Newer techniques, specifically monoclonal antibodies and DNA probes, should be investigated and may permit immediate diagnosis. Hansen & Loftus (1984) have recently described a monoclonal antibody that reacts with a variety of *H. ducreyi* isolates and is able to detect *H. ducreyi* in lesion material from rabbits.

b Specimen collection

Specimens for culture should be obtained from the purulent ulcer base. However, the ulcer does not require extensive cleaning. Whenever possible, a dark field examination and a virus culture for *H. simplex* should be obtained as part of the laboratory investigation. A variety of swabs, including both cotton and calcium alginate, have been used successfully for *H. ducreyi*. Transport systems have not been evaluated, and best results are obtained by direct immediate inoculation of the specimen onto the agar surface.

c Media

Suppurating inguinal lymph nodes should be aspirated and the pus cultured on media for *H. ducreyi* and blood agar. Buboe pus is usually sterile unless a draining sinus has developed. Occasionally, *S. aureus* or other potential pathogens are isolated from buboes. Their role as 'pathogens' is uncertain.

A variety of cultural media have been proposed for the primary isolation of *H. ducreyi*. A number of these tested and described since 1978, are summarised in Table 4.1.

Table 4.1   Solid media for primary *H. ducreyi* isolation

Results	Agar	Supplements	Primary culture results
Hammond et al (1978)	Gonococcal	Bovine hemo-globin (Difco) 1% IsoVitaleX (BBL) Vancomycin	7 of 16
Sottnek et al (1979)	Heart infusion	5% Defibri-nated rabbit blood, 10% fetal bovine serum, Vancomycin	16 of 17
Hafiz et al (1984)	Proteose Peptone #3	Rice starch, Gelatin Gluta-mine, Ferric nitrate, 5% equine blood, Vancomycin	9 of 10
Oberhofer & Back (1982)	Mueller Hinton (BBL)	5% Sheep Blood 1% IsoVitaleX (BBL) Vancomycin	33 positive cultures
Hannah & Greenwood (1982)	Chocolate agar (Clinical Standards)	Vancomycin	51 of 62
Nobre (1982)	Columbia agar base (Difco)	10% heated defibrinated equine blood, 1% Polyvitex, Vancomycin	42 of 74
Sturm & Zanen (1984)	Columbia (Difco)	30% hemolysed horse blood, 2.5% yeast dialysate, vancomycin	Not tested
Nzanse et al (1984)	(a) Meuller-Hinton (BBL)	5% chocolated horse blood, Vancomycin	122 of 163
	(b) Gonococcus (GIBCO)	2% bovine Hemoglobin, 5% fetal calf serum, 1% CVA (GIBCO) Vancomycin	143 of 163

In 1978, Hammond et al reported that *H. ducreyi* grew well on gonococcal agar base, supplemented with 1% bovine haemoglobin, and 1% IsoVitaleX. The incorporation of 3 mg/L of vancomycin prevented overgrowth of gram-positive cocci, while permitting the growth of all strains of *H. ducreyi*. The Winnipeg isolates did not require added serum for primary culture. However, glutamine and cystine each enhanced growth and some strains required these amino acids. In subsequent studies Hammond *et al* (1978) confirmed that *H. ducreyi* require haemin for growth. In contrast to *Haemophilus influenzae* and other haemin requiring strains that grow well with a haemin concentration of 1–10 mg/L of haemin, *H. ducreyi* strains grow optimally at levels of haemin between 25–50 mg/L. Excellent growth of laboratory strains can be obtained on a more defined agar medium containing peptides, glucose, glutamine, cysteine and haemin.

Subsequent studies have compared optimal growth for primary isolation on several media. Sottnek et al (1979) enriched media with a variety of animal and human sera. Of four sera tested, only fetal bovine sera supported a heavy growth of all four strains of *H. ducreyi* strains. Six agar bases were compared. Growth was heaviest on heart infusion agar, but Mueller-Hinton agar supported growth well. Columbia agar, Proteus peptone # 3 agar and GC base agar were all slightly less optimal growth media. Strains did not grow well on trypticase soy agar. Sottnek et al (1979) used 5% defibrinated rabbit blood as a source of haemin, and found that it was superior to bovine haemoglobin. Oberhofer & Back (1982) compared 5% sheep blood in Mueller-Hinton agar to human blood clot tubes. Isolates were obtained from 33 patients over an eight-year period consistently on Mueller-Hinton sheep agar. Hafiz et al (1984) described the Sheffield medium, which consists of Proteus peptone #3, rice starch, gelatin, and agar with an added supplement consisting of gutamine, glucose and ferric nitrate. Equine haemin (0.02%) and 5% defibrinated horse blood are added to provide hemin. They reported that this medium produced more luxurient growth than previously described media. However, in Kenya, the Sheffield medium has failed to support *H. ducreyi* on primary isolation (Piot et al, 1983). Nobre (1982) compared 20% defibrinated rabbit blood in Columbia blood agar base, with chocolate agar (10% defibrinated horse blood in Columbia agar base plus a vitamin supplement) and found that the chocolate agar with horse blood was superior and achieved an isolation rate of 56%. Sturm & Zanan (1984) reported that 'Beiling agar', a mixture of two parts Columbia agar base and one part haemolised horse blood supplemented with 2.5% yeast dialysate, gave excellent results. Taylor et al (1984) isolated *H. ducreyi* in Thailand on Mueller-Hinton agar base, supplemented with 5% chocolatised horse blood, 5% fetal calf serum, and 1% Iso-VitaleX. They compared this medium with heart infusion agar base with 5% rabbit blood, and 5% calf serum. Mueller-Hinton agar with equine blood was superior to heart infusion agar.

Unfortunately, none of these seven studies have determined the specific nutritional requirements for *H. ducreyi* or compared various culture media for primary isolation. In recent studies in Kenya, we prospectively compared gonococcal agar base supplemented with 1% bovine haemoglobin and 5% fetal calf serum with Mueller-Hinton agar base with 5% chocolated horse blood (Nsanze et al, 1984). Of 163 total isolates of *H. ducreyi*, 143 grew on gonococcal agar base with bovine haemoglobin and serum; 122 grew on Mueller-Hinton agar base supplemented with horse blood. However, 23 strains of *H. ducreyi* were isolated from Mueller-Hinton agar only; 41 from the GC agar only. Transfer of these isolates to the alternate medium generally demonstrated poor or no growth. Overall, with the use of both media, we were able to isolate *H. ducreyi* from 81% of 201 men with clinical chancroid.

In a subsequent study we found that a second culture obtained 48 hours after an initial negative culture yielded a positive growth for *H. ducreyi* in seven of 18 patients investigated (Dylewski et al in press). Patients who had an initial positive culture were confirmed by the second culture in 46 of 54 attempts. From this study we assume that the overall sensitivity of a single culture in patients who ultimately prove to have *H. ducreyi*-positive ulcers, is only about 76%. The reasons for this low cultural sensitivity were not apparent and require further investigation.

d Cultural environment

H. ducreyi have a number of unique requirements. All strains grow best between 30°C and 33°C, and many strains on primary isolation will not grow if the temperature is 36°C or higher. Many isolates, however, do grow at temperatures as low as 22°C (Sturm & Zanen, 1984). A proportion of isolates, particularly on primary isolation, are CO_2 dependent, and growth is enhanced in the presence of CO_2 (Nsanze et al, 1984). Increased humidity facilitates the growth of most *H. ducreyi* strains. All isolates will grow well anaerobically. *H. ducreyi* grows best at a neutral pH (Sturm & Zanen, 1984). In most situations, a candle extinction jar with a moistened paper towel, incubated at 33°C, provides an excellent environment for the culture of *H. ducreyi*. Conditions favourable for the culture of campylobacter have also been found to be suitable for *H. ducreyi* (Sturm & Zanen, 1984). Growth is scanty at 24 hours and the typical colonies are usually only apparent at 48–72 hours. Culture plates should not be discarded as negative until the fifth day.

e Colonial morphology and selection of H. ducreyi

Colonies of *H. ducreyi* are often difficult to distinguish from other fastidious organisms. Although slight alpha-haemolysis occurs on rabbit or sheep blood agar, this does not occur with blood from other species. As reported by Hafiz et al (1982), all colonies of *H. ducreyi* aggregate starch, and this has been found useful by several investigators. Otherwise, individual colonies have to be selected for Gram stain and subculture. Unfortunately, the cellular morphology on Gram stained smears on primary isolation plates is seldom characteristic. However, relatively pure cultures of *H. ducreyi* have a distinctive colonial morphology. The colonies vary in size, giving a polymorphic appearance. Often the variation in size and opacity give the impression of a mixed culture. Most colonies measure less than 1.0 mm in diameter. Characteristically they have a yellow-grey colour, are dome shaped, and are difficult to remove with an inoculating needle. The colonies are extremely cohesive and can be pushed intact across the agar surface. They are autoagglutinable in saline.

INDICATIONS FOR CULTURE AND PREDICTIVE VALUE OF A POSITIVE CULTURE

Genital ulceration due to any of the classic etiologic agents *T. pallidum*, *H. simplex* or *H. ducreyi* can be extremely variable in appearance in both men and women. In particular, chancroid can be readily confused with both primary syphilis or ulcerative herpetic lesions. Epidemiologic and therapeutic studies can only be carried out if the etiology of genital ulcer disease is proven by laboratory diagnosis.

In industrialised nations, cultures for *H. ducreyi* should be provided for patients with:

(a) a clinical syndrome compatible with chancroid.
(b) genital ulcers that are darkfield negative and culture negative for HSV.
(c) an epidemiologic history of contact with an individual from an endemic region
(d) a sex contact of a patient with chancroid.
(e) ulcers on the genitalia and possibly other contact sites presenting during an epidemic of chancroid.

Unfortunately, in developing countries, laboratory resources cannot be made available to permit routine culture for *H. ducreyi*. However, reference laboratories should be able to undertake periodic surveys of genital ulcers to confirm the proportion due to *H. ducreyi* and to collect strains for determination of antimicrobial susceptibility patterns. Cultures may also be required for unusual or complicated patients. New, rapid, simple and inexpensive technologies for the diagnosis of *H. ducreyi* are urgently needed in developing countries.

In both industrialised and developing countries, careful darkfield microscopy repeated on at least two occasions, and serology for syphilis are most important laboratory investigations to exclude syphilis. In Kenya, *T. pallidum* occurs concomitantly with *H. ducreyi* in about 5% of genital ulcers. Additional patients have incubating or latent syphilis. Mandatory treatment with benzathine penicillin is essential if laboratory resources cannot be provided to exclude absolutely syphilis in these patients.

A positive culture for *H. ducreyi*, as for *Neisseria gonorrhoeae*, defines an abnormal state. Although studies from Sheffield, England have suggested that *H. ducreyi* may commonly colonise the genital tract, this has not been confirmed by other workers in England, Winnipeg or Kenya (Kinghorn et al, 1982; Diaz-Mitoma in press; Mallard et al, 1983, Plummer et al, 1983). However, secondarily exposed female sex partners of males with chancroid may have asymptomatic infection of the cervix (Plummer et al, 1983a). The duration and outcome of the cervical carriage is unknown. Although asymptomatic infection of the smegma was described by Brams in 1924, this has not been confirmed with current technology and positive cultures in males have only been associated with genital ulcers (Plummer et al, 1983a).

In Nairobi, *H. ducreyi* can be isolated from about 80% of males with clinical chancroid. The clinical and epidemiologic features and the therapeutic response of patients who are *H. ducreyi* culture negative are similar to those who are culture positive (Plummer et al, 1983c). These patients may be infected with *H. ducreyi* with unique nutritional requirements not provided by the culture media. However, many culture negative ulcers heal without specific treatment and we have postulated that *H. ducreyi* in a proportion of these patients have already been eradicated from the ulcer, either spontaneously or by previous treatment. Alternately, these ulcers may have an entirely unique etiology. In Swasiland, Ursi et al (1982) cultured an unusual fastidious gram-negative rod from patients who were *H. ducreyi* culture negative. Attempts to culture this organism in Kenya and in Winnipeg have been unsuccessful. Clarification of the issue of *H. ducreyi* culture negative ulcers must await the development of non cultural techniques for the detection of *H. ducreyi*.

ANTIMICROBIAL PROFILE

For over 30 years, the sulfonamides were predictably effective therapy for chancroid. The tetracyclines, streptomycin, kanamycin, chloramphenicol, and even cephalothin have been shown to be effective alternative agents. Curiously, despite in vitro susceptibility of *H. ducreyi* to both penicillin and ampicillin, no prospective clinical studies were undertaken with these agents. During the Vietnam conflict, clinical failures with the sulfonamides and tetracyclines began to appear. Unfortunately, until improvements in culture technology permitted cultivation of *H. ducreyi*, reasons for therapeutic failures were not explored. However, in 1981, we demonstrated in studies in Kenya that failure of treatment with sulfonamides, tetracyclines, and ampicillin were directly related to in vitro resistance (Fast et al, 1983). If *H. ducreyi* persists in the ulcer following treatment, the organism is almost invariably resistant and the ulcer fails to heal. This correlation between clinical response and in vitro susceptibility also provided further evidence for the unique significance of *H. ducreyi* in the etiology of chancroid (Fast et al, 1982).

Antimicrobial susceptibility can be determined with the agar dilution technique on gonococcal medium base enriched with 1 g of haemoglobin per 100 ml and 1% IsoVitalex. Antimicrobial agents are incorporated into the agar at 50°C to yield final concentrations increasing in a log_2 dilution series from 0.005 to 128 mg/L. The sulfonamide and trimethoprim susceptibilities are performed on gonococcal medium enriched with 0.1% glucose, 0.01% glutamine, and 0.025% hemin with added 5% lysed horse blood. The agar is poured into a 90 ml petri dish to a depth of 4 ml and stored for up to one week at 4°C. Following inoculation with a Steer's replicator, the plates are incubated in 5% CO_2 at 33°C in an atmosphere saturated with water vapour. The plates are read after 48 hours of incubation (Hammond et al, 1978).

Antimicrobial susceptibility varies markedly from one geographic area to another. However, most *H. ducreyi* isolates throughout the world carry one of three beta-lactamase encoding plasmids. The smallest of these plasmids is identical to the smaller (West African) gonococcal beta-lactamase encoding plasmid (Anderson et al 1984, McNicol & Ronald, 1984). Although ampicillin or other penicillins are of limited use because of the prevalence of these plasmids, the beta-lactamase enzyme is inhibited by clavulanic acid and the combination of amoxicillin with clavulanic acid is an effective treatment regimen (Fast et al, 1982).

Sulphonamide resistance is also widely prevalent. In Thailand, all isolates studied are completely resistant to sulphonamide (Taylor, personal communication). In Kenya, high level sulphonamide resistance is due to a 4.9 Mdal plasmid which is similar to sulphonamide resistance plasmids present in enterobacteriaceae (Albritton et al, 1984). Moderate resistance to sulphonamides (20–80 mg/L) occurs in about one-third of strains from Kenya and is not plasmid mediated (Plummer et al, 1983b). Although all *H. ducreyi* in Kenya have remained uniformly susceptible to trimethoprim, in vitro resistance to trimethoprim is occurring in South East Asia. Sulfonamide-trimethoprim combinations continue to be quite effective in East Africa but are no longer a satisfactory treatment regimen in Thailand (Taylor personal communication). Most strains are resistant to tetracycline; resistance can be mediated by a large conjugative plasmid (Albritton et al, 1984). Chloramphenicol resistance is also widely prevalent in strains from Thailand (Taylor personal communication).

Fortunately, erythromycin continues to be uniformly active against *H. ducreyi*. The third generation cephalosporins, ceftriaxone and cefotaxime are also very active in vitro and have been used successfully to treat chancroid (Plummer et al, 1984). The oxyquinolone agents rosoxacin, enoxacin, and ciprofloxacin are also very effecitve in vitro and have given an excellent clinical response in early therapeutic trials. Table 4.2 summaries the antimicrobial susceptibility of *H. ducreyi* to antimicrobial agents.

Continuing worldwide surveillance of the antimicrobial susceptibility of *H. ducreyi* and periodic screening for plasmids is necessary. A proportion of the isolates in Kenya have a 21.7 Mdal cryptic plasmid which has been found to be conjugative and able to mobilise the smaller non-conjugative plasmids into other *H. ducreyi* and other

Table 4.2 Antimicrobial resistance of *Haemophilus ducreyi*

	Range of MIC mg/L	% Resistant	Mechanism of Resistance
sulfonamides	2.0–640	high level $\gg$ 15% (21) moderate > 30%	plasmid-mediated unknown
trimethoprim	0.125–32	> 10% (5,21)	unknown
tetracycline	0.25–32	> 50% (19)	some plasmid-mediated
erythromycin	0.0005–0.06	none known (20)	—
ampicillin	0.5–> 128	> 90% (5,20)	plasmid-mediated β-lactamase
streptomycin	0.5–10	unknown	—
cefotaxime	0.001–0.06	none known	—
ceftriaxone	0.001–0.03	none known	—
rosoxacin	0.001–0.008	none known	—
chloramphenicol	0.3–16	< 1%	plasmid-mediated chloramphenicol acyltransferase
enoxacin	0.008–0.03	none known	—
rifampin	0.0001–1.0	only noted in in laboratory strains	unknown
spectinomycin	1–12	none known	—
kanamycin	1–8	variable	unknown
vancomycin	8–> 128	all virulent strains (20) tested resistant to > 8 mg/L	unknown
polymyxin	32–128	all virulent strains (20) tested	unknown

species of Haemophilus (Deneer et al, 1982). The continuing epidemiology and evolution of antimicrobial resistance of the organism and its plasmids will provide opportunities for further study.

REFERENCES

Albritton W L, Brunton J L, Slaney L, Maclean I W 1984 Plasmid mediated sulfonamide resistance in *Haemophilus ducreyi*. Antimicrob Agents Chemother 24: 187–189

Albritton W L, Maclean I W, Slaney L A, Ronald A R, Deneer H 1984 Plasmid-mediated tetracycline resistance in *Haemophilus ducreyi*. Antimicrob Agents Chemother 24: 187–189

Albritton W L, Setlow J K, Thomas M, Sottnek F, Steigerwalt A G 1984 Heterospecific transformation in the genus *Haemophilus*. Mol Gen Genet 193: 358–363

Anderson B, Albritton W L, Biddle J, Johnson S R 1984 Common β-lactamase-specifying plasmid in *Haemophilus ducreyi* and *Neisseria gonorrhoeae*. Antimicrob Agents Chemother 24: 296–297

Beeson P B 1946 Studies on chancroid IV. The ducrey bacillus; growth requirements and inhibition by antibotic agents. Proc. Soc Exp Biol Med 6: 81–85

Bezancon F, Griffon V, Le Sourd L 1900 Culture du bacille du chancre mou. DR Seances Soc Biol Paris 52: 1048–1051

Brams J 1924 Isolation of ducrey bacillus from the smegma of thirty men. Journal of the American Medical Association 82: 1166–1167

Centers for Disease Control 1982 Chancroid — California, Morbid Mortal Weekly Rep 31: 173–175

Deacon W E, Albritton D C, Obusky S, Kaplan W 1956 VDRL chancroid study. I. A simple procedure for the isolation and identification of *Haemophilus ducreyi*. Journal of Investigative Dermatology 26: 399–406

Deneer H, Slaney L, Maclean I W, Albritton W L 1982 Mobilization of nonconjugative antibiotic resistance plasmids in *Haemophilus ducreyi*. J Bact 149: 726–732

Denys G A, Chapel T A, Jeffries C D 1978 An indirect fluorescent antibody technique for *Haemophilus ducreyi*. Health Lab Sci 15: 128–132

Diaz-Mitoma F, Benningen G, Slutchuk M, Ronald A R, Brunham R C Etiology of non-vesicular ulcers in Winnipeg. Sexually Transmitted Diseases (Submitted)

Dienst R B, August G A 1942 A new preparation of antigen for intracutaneous diagnosis of chancroidal infection. American Journal of Syph Gonorrhea Vener Dis 26: 201–203

Ducrey A 1889 Experimental untersurchungel uber den Ansteekungsstoff des weichen Schaukers und uber die Bubonas. Monatsh Prakt Dermatol 9: 387–405

Dylewski J, Nsanze H, Maitha G, Ronald A R Laboratory diagnosis of *Haemophilus ducreyi*: sensitivity of culture media. Diagnos Micro and Infect Dis (in press)

Fast M V, Nsanze H, D'Costa L J, et al 1983 Antimicrobial therapy of chancroid: an evaluation of five treatment regimens correlated with in vitro sensitivity. Sexually Transmitted Diseases 10: 1–6

Fast M V, Nsanze H, D'Costa L J, Plummer Fa, Karasira P, Maclean I W, Ronald A R 1982 Treatment of chancroid by clavulanic acid with amoxycillin in patients with β-lactamase-positive *Haemophilus ducreyi* infection. Lancet ii: 509–511

Greenblatt R B, Sanderson E S 1938 The intradermal chancroid bacillary antigen test as an aid in the differential diagnosis of the venereal bubo. American Journal of Surgery 41: 384

Hafiz S, Kinghorn G R, McEntegart M G 1982 Starch aggregation as a presumptive test for *Haemophilus ducreyi*. Lancet ii: 872

Hafiz S, McEntegart M G, Kinghorn G R 1984 Sheffield medium for cultivation of *Haemophilus ducreyi*. British Journal of Venereal Diseases 60: 196–198

Hammond G W, Lian C J, Wilt J C, Albritton W L, Ronald A R 1978 Determination of the hemin requirement of *Haemophilus ducreyi*: evaluation of the porphyrin test and media used in the satellite growth test. Journal of Clinical Microbiology 7: 243–246

Hammond G W, Lian C J, Wilt J C, Ronald A R 1978 Antimicrobial susceptibility of *Haemophilus ducreyi*. Antimicrob Agents Chemother 13: 608–612

Hammond G W, Lian C J, Wilt J C, Ronald A R 1978 Comparison of specimen collection and laboratory techniques for isolation of *Haemophilus ducreyi*. Journal of Clinical Microbiology 7: 39–43

Hammond G W, Slutchuk M, Scatliff J, Sherman E, Wilt J C, Ronald A R 1980 Epidemiologic, clinical, laboratory and therapeutic features of an urban outbreak of chancroid in North America. Review of Infectious Diseases 2: 867–879

Hannah H, Greenwood J R 1982 Isolation and rapid identification of *Haemophilus ducreyi*. Journal of Clinical Microbiology 16: 861–864

Hansen E J, Loftus T A 1984 Monoclonal antibodies reactive with all strains of *Haemophillus ducreyi*. Infectious Immun 44(1): 196–198

Kilian M 1976 A taxonomic study of the genus *Haemophilus*, with the proposal of a new species. Journal of Gen Microbiology 93: 9–62

Kinghorn G R, Hafiz S, McEntegart M G 1982 Pathogenic microbial flora of genital ulcers in Sheffield with particular reference to herpes simplex and Haemophilus ducreyi. British Journal of Venereal Diseases 58: 377–380

Lwoff A, Pirosky I 1937 Determination du facteur de crossance pour *Haemophilus ducreyi*. CR Seances Soc Biol (Paris) 124: 1169

Mallard R H, Macaulay M E, Riordan T, Choudhary F H, Chandiok S, Bhattacharyya 1983 *Haemophilus ducreyi* infection in Manchester. Lancet 2: 283

McNicol P J, Ronald A R 1984 The plasmids of *Haemophilus ducreyi*. J Antimicro Chemother 14: 561–573

Nayyar K C, Stolz E, Michel M F 1979 Rising incidence of chancroid in Rotterdam. British Journal of Venereal Diseases 55: 439–441

Nobre G N 1982 Identification of *Haemophilus ducreyi* in the clinical laboratory. Journal of Medical Microbiology 15: 243–245

Nsanze H, Fast M V, D'Costa L J, Tukei P, Curran J, Ronald A R 1981 Genital ulcers in Kenya. British Journal of Venereal Diseases 57: 378–381

Nsanze H, Plummer F A, Maggwa A B N, Maitha G, Dylewski J, Piot P, Ronald A R 1984 Comparison of media for the primary isolation of *Haemophilus ducreyi*. Sexually Transmitted Diseases 11: 6–9

Oberhofer T R, Back A E 1982 Isolation and cultivation of *Haemophilus ducreyi*. Journal of Clinical Microbiology 15: 625–629

Odumeru J A, Wiseman G M, Ronald A R 1984 Vurulence factors of *Haemophilus ducreyi*. Infect Immun 43: 607–611

Piot P, Slottmans L, Nsanze H, Ronald A R 1983 Isolating Haemophilus ducreyi. Lancet 2: 909–910

Plummer F A, D'Costa L J, Nsanze H, Dylewski J, Karasira P, Ronald A R 1983a Epidemiology of chancroid and *Haemophilus ducreyi* in Nairobi. Lancet 2: 1293–1295

Plummer F A, Nsanze H, D'Costa L J, Karasira P, Maclean I W, Ellison R H, Ronald A R 1983b Single-dose therapy of chancroid with trimethoprim-sufametrole. New England Journal of Medicine 309: 67–71

Plummer F A, Nsanze H, D'Costa L J, Maggwa N, Girouard Y, Karasira P, Albritton W, Ronald A R 1983c Short course of single dose antimicrobial therapy of chancroid in Kenya: reports of studies with Rifampin-Trimethoprim and Rifampin alone. Review of Infectious Diseases 5: S565

Plummer F A, Maggwa A B N, D'Costa L J, Nsanze H, Karasira P, Maclean I W, Ronald A R 1984 Cefotaxime treatment of *Haemophilus ducreyi* infection in Kenya. Sexually Transmitted Diseases 11: 304–307

Sottnek F O, Biddle J W, Kraus S J, Weaver R E, Stewart J A 1979 Isolation and identification of *Haemophilus ducreyi* in a clinical study. Journal of Clinical Microbiology 12: 170–174

Sturm A W, Zanen H C 1984 Characteristics of *Haemophilus ducreyi* in culture. Journal of Clinical Microbiology 19(5): 672–674

Sturm A W, Zanen H C 1984 Enzymic activity of *Haemophilus ducreyi*. Journal of Medical Microbiology 18: 181–187

Taylor D N, Duangmani C, Suvongse C, O'Connor R, Pitarangsi C, Panikabutra K, Echeverria P 1984 The role of *Haemophilus ducreyi* in penile ulcers in Bangkok, Thailand. Sexually Transmitted Diseases 11: 148–151

Taylor D N Personal communications

Teague O, Diebert O 1920 The value of the cultural method in the diagnosis of chancroid. Journal of Urology 4: 543–546

Ursi J P, VanDyck E, Ballard R C, Jacob W, Piot P, Meheus A Z 1982 Characterization of an unusual bacterium isolated from genital ulcers. Journal of Medical Microbiology 15: 97–103

Winslow C E A, Broadhurst J, Buchanan R E, Krumweide C, Rogers L A, Smith G H 1921 The families and genera of the bacteria. Preliminary report of the Committee of the Society of American Bacteriologists on characterization and classification of bacterial types. Journal of Bacteriology 2: 505–566

5. Genital herpes simplex virus infections: natural history and therapy

Lawrence Corey

INTRODUCTION

Genital herpes simplex virus (HSV) infections have represented, to many, the prototype disease of the 'new' era in genitourinary medicine. However, while the prevalence of genital herpes has increased in most western industrialised nations in the last 15 years, the disease was a well described entity in the early 18th century.

HISTORY

The French physician John Astruc described genital herpes in 1736, and the first English translation appeared in his 'Treatus of Venereal Disease' in 1754 (Astruc 1736). In 1893, genital herpes was diagnosed in 9.1% of 846 prostitutes visiting an infirmary (Hutfield, 1966), and in 1886, Diday & Doyon published the monograph 'Les Herpes Genitaux' in which they observed that genital herpes often appeared after a venereal infection such as syphilis, chancroid, or gonorrhea. These authors also described cases of recurrent genital herpes and proposed that the eruptions were related to nervous 'trigger mechanisms' acting by way of the sacral plexus.

Fluid from oral-labial infection was shown to be infectious to other humans in the late nineteenth century. The disease was successfully transferred to rabbits in 1920, and HSV was grown in vitro in 1925 (Baum, 1920; Cruter, 1924; Parker, 1925). In the 1920s Lipshutz inoculated material from genital herpetic lesions into the skin of humans, eliciting clinical infection within 48–72 hours in six persons and 24 days in one case. In other experiments, he observed that protection in rabbits from corneal infection with specimens from genital herpes occurred only with strains originating from the genital sites and not from oral-labial sites (Lipshutz, 1921). From these and other experiments, he surmised that there were epidemiological and clinical differences between oral and genital herpes. However, most workers felt that the viruses of genital and labial herpes were identical. In the early 1960s, Schneweis, Dowdle & Nahmias reported that HSV could be divided by neutralisation tests into two antigenic types, and that there was an association between the antigenic type and the site of viral recovery (Schneweis, 1962; Dowdle et al, 1967; Nahmias & Dowdle, 1968). These observations led to the benchmark studies on the epidemiology of genital herpes in the late 1960s and early 1970s.

EPIDEMIOLOGY OF GENITAL HERPES

Prevalence of genital HSV infections

The reported prevalence of genital herpes appears to depend upon the demographic and clinical characteristics of the patient population studied and whether clinical and/or laboratory techniques are used for diagnosis. In the United Kingdom in 1981, genital herpes accounted for 3.73% of all diagnoses in genitourinary medicine clinics (Chief Medical Officer, 1984) Nationwide reporting of statistics for genital herpes is not available in the United States. However, it appears that the frequency of genital HSV varies greatly between clinics. In Seattle, genital HSV infection was diagnosed in 5.6% of all persons attending the sexually transmitted disease (STD) clinics in King County, Washington in 1982 and 4.2% in 1984. Whether the slight fall in prevalence is due to a true decrease in the disease, less referral to the STD clinic because of the availability in the private sector of an approved form of treatment, or shift in demographic population of persons attending the clinic is uncertain (Table 5.1).

Table 5.1   Reported prevalence of genital HSV infections in King County, Washington, Sexually Transmitted Disease Clinics 1976–1982

Year	1976	1977	1978	1979	1980	1981	1982	1983	1984
No. Cases HSV	1014	1011	1146	1251	1525	1686	1922	1349	1223
First episode	NA	NA	NA	NA	NA	NA	942	680	628
Recurrent episode	NA	NA	NA	NA	NA	NA	980	669	595
% HSV cases caucasian	94%	92%	89%	87%	88%	87%	NA	NA	NA
No. cases of N. gonorrhoeae	4834	4501	4664	4266	3789	2883	2526	2110	1759
Total No. STD clinic visits	39 803	38 722	39 440	35 890	35 207	33 313	34 209	30 554	28 722
% STD visits due to HSV	2.5%	2.6%	2.9%	3.5%	4.3%	5.1%	5.6%	4.41%	4.26%
Ratio N. gonorrhoeae to HSV	4.8:1	4.5:1	4.1:1	3.4:1	2.5:1	1.7:1	1.3:1	1.6:1	1.4:1

(NA = not available)

HSV has been isolated from 0.3–5.4% of males and 1.6–8% of females attending STD clinics (Wentworth et al, 1973; Jeansson & Molin, 1970; Jeansson & Molin, 1974). In non-VD clinic patient populations, HSV has been isolated from the genital tract in from 0.25% to 4.0% of patients (Rauh, et al, 1977; Taintivanich & Tharavawij, 1980; Knox et al, 1979; Vesterinen et al, 1977). Many of these patients are asymptomatic. Asymptomatic infection of the genital tract at or near term in women attending OB-GYN clinics has ranged from 0.24–4% of attendees (Vontver et al, 1982; Bolognese et al, 1976; Harger et al, 1983; Tejani, et al, 1979; Scher et al, 1982).

The prevalence of clinically diagnosed genital herpes is greater in caucasian than non-caucasian populations (Table 5.1). In STD clinics seeing a high proportion of non-caucasians, genital herpes is reported only one tenth as frequently as *Neisseria gonorrhoea* infection (STD Fact Sheet). However, student health centres seeing middle and upper class young adults, in whom the prevalence of gonococcal infection is very low, report that genital HSV infections are 7–10 times more common than gonorrhoea (Sumaya et al, 1980). In addition, genital HSV infections appear to be more frequently diagnosed in heterosexual than homosexual men (Judson et al, 1980; Mann et al, 1984)

Increasing prevalence of infection

In many populations, genital HSV infections appear to have increased in prevalence in the last decade. Consultations for genital herpes with private practitioners increased in the US from 3.4 per 100 000 patient consultations in 1966 to 29.2 per 100 000 consultations in 1979 (Becker et al, 1985). in Rochester, Minnesota, a population based epidemiologic study indicated that the incidence of genital HSV increased from 12.5 cases per 100 000 population in the years 1965 through 1970 to 48.1 in the years 1970 through 1975 and then to 82.3 cases per 100 000 population in the years 1975 through 1980 (Chuang et al, 1983). The shift in the spectrum of STDs during the late 1970s and 1980s in the US is illustrated by the change in the ratio of *N. gonorrhoeae* to genital herpes cases seen in STD clinics in King County, Washington. In 1976 this rate was 4.8 to 1 while in 1982–1984 it averaged 1.4 to 1, a result of both a decrease in *N. gonorrhoeae* and an increase in genital HSV infections. In the United Kingdom, the rate of genital HSV in STD clinics has increased from 14.97 cases in 1976 to 21.61 cases per 100 000 population in 1980; an average increase of 9% per year (Chief Medical Officer, 1984).

While the prevalence of genital HSV infections has markedly increased over the last 10 years in many populations throughout the world, in other population groups no evidence of an increasing prevalence of genital HSV infection has been noted. For example, the high prevalence of cytologically detected genital HSV infections noted in the predominantly black lower socioeconomic status populations studied in Atlanta, Georgia in the 1960s, has remained relatively constant over the decade of the 1970s (Nahmias et al, 1966; Nahmias et al, 1969a; Nahmias 1983; Rawls et al, 1971; Josey et al, 1972). These data suggest that genital herpes may be increasing in frequency in some population groups, especially those with a previously low prevalence of genital herpes, e.g., middle class caucasion population. Whether these apparent increases reflect a true increase in the prevalence of genital herpes or an increasing recognition and use of diagnostic facilities to confirm the diagnosis is uncertain. The increased incidence of neonatal HSV infection recently demonstrated in King County, Washington, indicates that at least part of the observed increase is probably related to a real increase in the incidence of infection (Sullivan-Bolyai et al, 1983).

Prevalance of HSV antibody

The prevalence of antibody to HSV increases with age and varies with socioeconomic status (Nahmias & Roizman 1973; Nahmias et al, 1970a; Wentworth & Alexander, 1971; Holzel et al, 1953). Studies of the seroepidemiology of HSV-2 infections are affected by the difficulty of distinguishing the human immune response between HSV-1 and HSV-2 infections. Some serologic tests such as the standard complement fixation antibody assay do not distinguish the antibody response between the two HSV types (Rawls et al, 1979). Several serologic tests (neutralisation, indirect immunofluorescence, passive haemagglutination, indirect haemagglutination, ELISA and RIA) have been developed which will distinguish between antibody to HSV-1 and to HSV-2 (Rawls et al, 1970; Plummer et al, 1970; Prakash & Seth, 1979; Lerner et al, 1974). Nethertheless, serologic cross reactions between the two HSV types are common. For example, in persons with prior HSV-1 infections, much of the antibody response to a new HSV-2 infection appears to be directed at common rather than type-specific antigenic determinants (Yeo et al, 1981). In addition, it may be difficult to detect the presence of HSV-2 antibody in the presence of high titers of HSV-1 antibody (McClung et al, 1976). Because of this, many of the currently available serologic techniques tend to underestimate the true prevalence of HSV-2 infection. The development of new diagnostic reagents using type-specific antigens and/or antibody systems will hopefully improve the specificity and sensitivity of seroepidemiologic surveys of HSV-2 infection (Eberle & Courtney, 1981; Pereira et al, 1982).

Serologic studies of western industrialised populations in the post World War II era found that 80–100% of middle aged adults of lower socioeconomic status possessed antibodies to HSV, as compared to 30–50% of adults of higher socioeconomic groups (Nahmias et al, 1970a). In the US in the early 1960s, HSV antibody was detected in 40% of 8–14 year-olds seen in a private paediatric group compared to 80% of those of a similar age attending outpatient clinics at an urban public hospital (Porter et al, 1969). The higher prevalence of antibody to HSV in lower socioeconomic class persons was due to an increased frequency of both HSV-1 and HSV-2 infections (Nahmias et al, 1970a; Nahmias & Roizman 1973).

Antibodies to HSV-2 are not routinely detected in sera until puberty, and antibody prevalence rates correlate with past sexual activity. HSV-2 antibodies were detected in 80% of female prostitutes, up to 60% of adults of lower socioeconomic status, 10% of higher socioeconomic groups, and 3% of nuns (Duenas et al, 1972). In the 1970s, the anti-HSV-2 prevalence rate was 7–20% in male and female volunteer blood donors in England compared to 60% in volunteer blood donors from prison populations (Roome et al, 1975). In Ibaden, Nigeria, HSV-2 antibodies were detected in 20% of volunteer blood donors and in 27% of women attending family planning clinics (Montefiore et al, 1980). A small population of young children in tropical areas have HSV-2 antibodies, suggesting that non-sexual transmission may occasionally occur in this population and climate (Montefiore et al, 1980; Johnson et al, 1981). In the late 1970s, HSV-2 antibodies were detected by an ELISA technique in 50% of men and women reporting to an outpatient medical dispensary in Scandinavia (Vestergaard & Rune, 1980; Grauballe & Vestergaard, 1977). Recently a randomised survey of caucasian middle class adults in metropolitan Toronto (North America) indicated a prevalence rate of HSV-2 antibody in 17.8% of women and 12.1% of men; only 20% of men and 13% of women gave a history of having had symptomatic genital lesions (Stavraky et al, 1983).

Few serosurveys are available in similar population groups comparing antibody prevalence rates to HSV-1 and HSV-2 over a period of time. However, separate studies of the prevalence of HSV antibody in the United Kingdom indicated that in 1953, 85% of caucasian children between three and 15 years of age possessed CF antibody to HSV-1 as compared to only 41% in 1965. In the 1965 survey, antibody to HSV was detected in 35% of 14–19 year olds and 69% of 15–19 year olds (Smith et al, 1967).

Several important epidemiologic questions remain to be answered before one can adequately assess the prevalence and incidence of genital HSV infections. There appears to be a substantial difference between the prevalence of HSV antibody and the prevalence of disease. Whereas the prevalence of HSV-2 antibody is greatest in persons of lower socioeconomic status, the prevalence of recognised genital herpes even in STD clinics is greater in middle class caucasian persons. It is intriguing to speculate that the increase in clinically recognized genital HSV infection is occurring in those areas and population groups where the age specific prevalence of oral-labial HSV-1 infection is decreasing. These data suggest that prior HSV-1 infection may play a role in partially protecting against the acquisition of clinically symptomatic infections (see below).

CLINICAL MANIFESTATIONS OF GENITAL HERPES

First episodes of genital herpes

The clinical manifestations and recurrence rate of genital herpes are influenced both by host factors, past exposure to HSV-1, previous episodes of genital herpes, gender and viral type (Corey et al, 1983a). First episodes of genital herpes are often associated with systemic symptoms, involve multiple genital and extragenital sites, and have a prolonged duration of viral shedding and lesions (Adams et al, 1976; Vontver et al, 1979; Kaufman et al, 1973). Patients with first episodes of genital herpes who have clinical or serologic evidence of prior HSV infection tend to have a milder illness than those experiencing true primary infection, i..e. experiencing their first infection with either HSV-1 or HSV-2 (Corey et al, 1981). About 60% of persons who attend our genital HSV clinic with their first episode of symptomatic genital herpes had primary infection with either HSV-1 or HSV-2. Most persons with non-primary first episodes of genital HSV infection have serologic evidence of past HSV-1 infection. However, 10–30% of persons with first episodes of disease have serologic evidence of past HSV-2 in acute phase sera, indicative of past asymptomatic acquisition of HSV-2 (Corey et al, 1978a; Corey et al, 1982a; Bernstein et al 1984).

Past oral-labial HSV-1 infection may decrease the acquisition of genital HSV-1 infections (Reeves et al, 1981). Genital HSV-1 infections have been reported in 5–50% of persons experiencing first episodes of infection (Kalinyak et al, 1977; Kawana et al, 1976; Barton et al, 1981). In Seattle, in the years 1975–1980, HSV-1 was isolated from genital lesions in 21 (7%) of 286 persons with first episodes of genital herpes. Between the years 1980–1983, 14% of first episodes of genital herpes have been due to HSV-1. Ninety-five per cent of the patients with first episode HSV-1 infection have lacked anti-HSV in acute phase sera, i.e. had true primary infection, suggesting that prior HSV-1 infection protects against the acquisition of genital HSV-1 disease.

Prior HSV-1 infection also ameliorates the severity of first episodes of genital herpes. For example, only 16% of persons with first episode non-primary genital HSV-2 infection demonstrate systemic symptoms during the course of illness as compared to 62% and 68% of patients with primary HSV-2 or primary genital HSV-1 infections. The severity or local pain (8.7 days) duration of viral shedding from lesions, (6.8 days) and duration of lesions (15.5 days) are also less than patients with primary HSV-2 disease (11.8, 11.4 and 18.6 days respectively) (Fig. 5.1). The duration of symptoms and lesions are similar between patients with primary HSV-1 and primary HSV-2 infections (Reeves et al, 1981; Corey et al, 1983a).

Primary genital herpes

Symptoms

Primary genital HSV infection is characterized by a high frequency and prolonged duration of systemic and local symptoms. Fever, headache, malaise, and myalgias are reported in nearly 40% of men and 70% of women with primary HSV-2 disease ($p < 0.05$) (Table 5.2). Systemic symptoms appear early in the course of the disease, usually reaching a peak within the first 3–4 days after onset of lesions, and gradually recede over the subsequent 3–4 days.

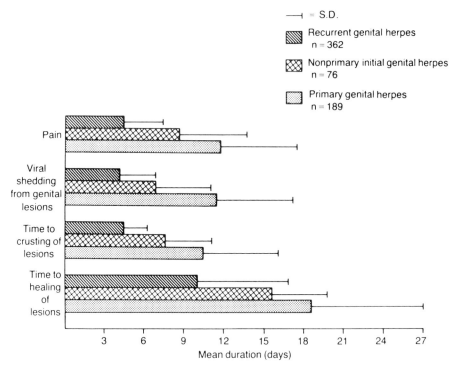

Fig. 5.1 Clinical course of untreated genital HSV Infection: comparison of the duration of local pain, viral shedding, time to crusting of genital lesions and time to healing of genital lesions in patients with first episode primary, first episode non-primary and recurrent genital herpes. The mean difference in the duration of each of the listed signs between each of these 3 stages of disease is significant ($p < 0.01$ for each comparison). SD = standard deviation.

Table 5.2   Clinical symptoms and signs of primary genital HSV-2

	Men	Women
% With constitutional symptoms*	39%	68%
Mean duration (days) local pain	10.9	11.9
% with dysuria*	44%	83%
Mean duration (days) dysuria*	7.2	11.9
Mean area (mm²) of lesions	427	550
Mean duration viral shedding from lesion (days)	10.5	11.8
Mean duration lesions (days)*	16.5	19.7

* $p < 0.05$ by Chi Square

Pain, itching, dysuria, vaginal or urethral discharge, and tender inguinal adenopathy are the predominant local symptoms of disease. Painful lesions are reported in 95% of men (mean duration 10.9 days) and 99% of women (mean duration 12.2 days) with primary HSV infection. Dysuria, both external and internal, appears more frequently in women (83%) than men (44%). HSV has been isolated from the urethra and urine of both men and women with primary genital herpes, suggesting that HSV urethritis and/or cystitis, in addition to external dysuria resulting from urine touching active genital HSV lesions, may account for the high frequency and long duration of dysuria in women (Corey et al, 1983a; Corey et al, 1983c; Person et al, 1973).

Urethral discharge and dysuria is noted in about one third of men with primary HSV-2 infection of the external genitalia. HSV can be isolated from a urethral swab or first voided urine of these men. The urethral discharge is usually clear and mucoid, and the severity of dysuria is often out of proportion to the amount of urethral discharge elicited on genital examination. Gram stain of the urethral discharge usually reveals between five and fifteen polymorphonuclear leukocytes per oil immersion field. Occasionally a mononuclear cell response is seen.

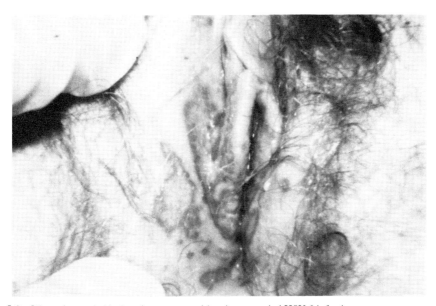

Fig. 5.2   Ulcerative genital lesions in a woman with primary genital HSV-2 infection.

The clinical symptoms of pain and irritation from lesions gradually increase over the first 6–7 days of illness, reaching their maximum intensity between 7 and 11 days of disease, and gradually recede over the second week of illness. Tender inguinal adenopathy usually appears during the second and third week of disease and is often the last symptom to resolve. Inguinal and femoral lymph nodes are generally firm, non-fluctuant and tender when palpated. Suppurative lymphadenopathy is a very uncommon manifestation of genital herpes.

Signs
In both men and women with primary genital HSV infection, widely spaced bilateral pustular or ulcerative lesions on the external genitalia are the most frequent presenting sign. Lesions are characteristically described as starting as papules or vesicles which rapidly spread over the genital area. At the time of the first clinic visit, multiple small pustular lesions which coalesce into large areas of ulceration are usually present (Fig. 5.2). The size and shape of the ulcerative lesions vary greatly between patients. These ulcerative lesions persist from between four and fifteen days until crusting and/or reepithelialisation occurs. In general, lesions in the penile and mons areas

crust over before complete reepithelialisation ensues. Crusting does not occur on mucosal surfaces. Residual scarring from lesions is uncommon. New lesion formation (the development of new areas of vesication or ulceration during the course of infection) occurs in over 75% of patients with primary genial herpes. New lesions usually form between days 4 and 10 of disease.

The median duration of time from which HSV can be isolated from lesions as defined from the onset of lesions to the last positive culture is 12 days. The mean time (about 10.5 days) from the onset of vesicles to the appearance of the crust stage correlates well with the duration of viral shedding (Fig. 5.1). However, since there is considerable overlap between the duration of viral shedding and the duration of crusting and since mucosal lesions do not crust, patients should be advised not to resume sexual activity until lesions have completely reepithelialised. The mean time from the onset of lesions to complete reepithelialisation of all lesions appears slightly longer in women (19.5 days) than in men (16.5 days).

Concomitant vulvar and cervical HSV infection
Ninety per cent of women with primary genital HSV-2 infection, 70% of women with primary genital HSV-1 infection, and 70% of women with non-primary genital HSV-2 infection have concomitant HSV cervicitis (Adams et al, 1976; Corey et al, 1983a; Barton et al, 1981). The high rate of isolation of HSV from the cervix in first episodes contrasts sharply with the 12–20% isolation rate in women who present with recurrent external genital lesions (Adams et al, 1976; Guinan et al, 1981; Corey et al, 1983a). Primary genital HSV cervicitis may be symptomatic (causing a purulent vaginal discharge) or asymptomatic (Josey et al, 1966). In most cases of primary HSV cervicitis the cervix appears abnormal to inspection (Fig. 5.3). The appearance may include areas of diffuse or focal friability and redness, extensive ulcerative lesions of the exocervix, or severe necrotic cervicitis. The cervical gram stain will reveal a neutrophilic reaction ($\geq$20 polymorphonuclear cells per oil immersion field). First episode HSV infection of the cervix usually involves the squamous epithelium of the exocervix as well as endocervical cells. The clinical differentiation between HSV and mucopurulent cervicitis due to *C. trachomatis* and/or *N. gonorrhoeae* infection may be difficult.

In women with primary genital herpes, the mean duration of viral shedding from the cervix (11.4 days) is similar to that from lesions of the external genitalia, and there is a close correlation between the duration of cervical viral excretion and the duration of viral shedding from external genital lesions.

Pharyngeal infection
HSV of the pharynx is commonly seen in association with primary genital herpes and may be the presenting complaint. Both HSV-1 and HSV-2 may cause pharyngitis and almost all patients report oral-genital exposure (Embil et al, 1981; Corey et al, 1983a). We have isolated HSV from the pharynx of 11% of patients with primary HSV-2 infection, 20% of patients with primary HSV-1 infection, 1% of patients with non-primary initial genital herpes, and 1% of persons with recurrent genital herpes. HSV was isolated from the pharynx in 70% of persons with primary genital herpes who complained of sore throat during the acute episode of disease. HSV is infrequently isolated from patients attending an STD clinic without pharyngitis. Clini-

cal signs of HSV pharyngitis may vary from mild erythema to a diffuse ulcerative pharyngitis (Evans & Dick, 1964; Glezen et al, 1975). The inflammatory response to these large areas of ulceration may produce a whitish exudate; when this is wiped away the extensive ulceration may be visualised. In rare cases severe swelling of the posterior pharynx resulting in obstruction of the airway may occur (Tustin & Kaiser, 1979). Extension of the ulcerative posterior pharyngeal lesions into the anterior gingival area may occur in about 50% of patients. Most patients with HSV pharyngitis have tender cervical nodes, and constitutional symptoms, such as fever, malaise, myalgia

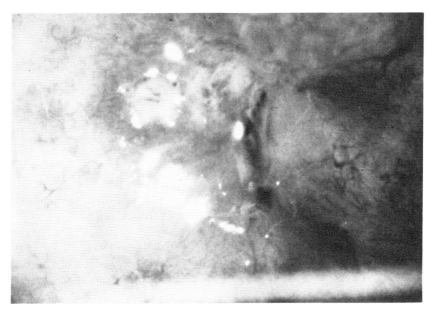

Fig. 5.3 Lesions of HSV cervicitis.

and headache are common. Many are misdiagnosed as having streptococcal pharyngitis. Recently, Lafferty et al (1985) have reported that HSV-2 pharyngitis may cause more frequent fever and constitutional symptoms than HSV-1 pharyngitis. While pharyngeal HSV-1 infection may result in the subsequent development of recurrent oral-labial HSV-1 infection, recurrent oral-labial HSV-2 infections are very uncommon (Lafferty et al, 1985).

Complications of genital herpes
The complications of first episodes of genital herpes are related both to local extension and spread of virus to extragenital sites. The most frequent complication is the development of lesions at extragenital sites (Table 5.3). Central nervous system involvement and fungal superinfection are also frequently encountered. Complications of primary genital herpes occur more frequently in women than in men (Corey et al, 1983a).

CENTRAL NERVOUS SYSTEM COMPLICATIONS
Central nervous system involvement may occur in several forms, including aseptic meningitis, transverse myelitis, or what has been called the sacral radiculopathy syn-

Table 5.3 Complications of primary genital HSV-2 infection

	Approximate frequency
I. Central Nervous System Complications	
% With stiff neck, headache and photophobia	28%
% Hospitalised with aseptic meningitis	5%
Sacral autonomic nervous system radiculopathy†	1%
Transverse myelitis	rare
II. HSV Pharygitis	10%
III. Development of Extragenital Lesions	21%
Lip	3%
Buttock, groin	9%
Breast	2%
Finger	6%
Eye	1%
Disseminated cutaneous infection	very rare
IV. Direct Extension of Disease	
Pelvic inflammatory disease syndrome (including endometritis)	1%
Pelvic cellulitis	rare
Suppurative lymphadenitis	rare
V. Fungal Superinfection	
Yeast vaginitis	14%

* All three symptoms present on two consecutive examinations
† Constipation, urinary retention, and sacral anesthesia

drome (Ross & Stevenson, 1961; Klastensky et al, 1972; Caplan et al, 1977). In patients with primary genital HSV-2 infection seen at the University of Washington Genital Herpes Clinic, meningeal irritation (defined as the presence of stiff neck, headache and photophobia on two consecutive examinations) was reported in 36% of women and 13% of men (p < 0.001). Hospitalisation was required for clinically overt aseptic meningitis in 6.4% of women and 1.6% of men with primary HSV-2 infections. All of the hospitalised patients were febrile, had Kernig's and Brudzinski's signs on physical examination and had a CSF pleocytosis. Routine lumbar puncture was not performed on all non-hospitalised patients. However, a study of primary genital herpes in the early 1900s reported a high frequency of CSF pleocytosis in patients without overt clinical evidence of meningeal irritation, suggesting that meningeal involvement may be a frequent occurrence with primary genital herpes (Ravaut & Darre, 1904).

Both HSV-1 and HSV-2 have been isolated from cerebrospinal fluid. HSV has been isolated from 0.5 to 3.0% of patients presenting to hospital with aseptic meningitis (Skoldenberg et al, 1975; Bayer & Gear, 1955). HSV aseptic meningitis appears to be more frequently associated with genital than oral-labial infection (Wolontis & Jeannson, 1977; Craig & Nahmias 1973). Fever, headache, vomiting, photophobia and nuchal rigidity are the predominant symptoms of HSV aseptic meningitis. Meningeal symptoms usually start from 3–12 days after onset of genital lesions. Symptoms generally reach a maximum 2–4 days into the illness and gradually recede over 36–72 hours. The cerebrospinal fluid in HSV aseptic meningitis is usually clear or slightly cloudy, and the opening pressure may be elevated. White blood cell counts in CSF may range from ten to over a thousand per mm^3 (mean 550). The pleocytosis is predominantly lymphocytic in adults, although early in the course of the disease and in neonates a predominantly polymorphonuclear response may be seen. The CSF glucose is usually more than 50% of the blood glucose, although hypoglycorrhachia has been reported; the CSF protein is slightly elevated (Brenton, 1980). If cultures are obtained within 24 hours of the onset of headache and photophobia HSV may be grown from the CSF. The differential diagnosis of HSV aseptic meningitis includes diseases which result in neurologic involvement and genital ulcerations: sacral herpes zoster, Behçet's syndrome, collagen vascuclar disease, inflammatory bowel disease, porphyria, and benign recurrent aseptic meningitis (Mollaret's syndrome).

Craig & Nahmias (1973) reported the isolation of HSV-2 from buffy coat collected in adults with HSV-2 meningitis. These investigators hypothesised hematogenous spread of virus into the central nervous system. In animal models, HSV appears to travel from involved mucocutaneous sites through peripheral nerves into the central nervous system (Overall et al, 1975; Renis et al, 1976; Kristensson et al, 1978). This form of neurotropic spread is often associated with the development of paralysis and/or death due to encephalitis, which rarely occur in human cases of aseptic meningitis associated with genital herpes. The pathogenesis of HSV meningitis is unclear. We have been unable to isolate HSV from buffy coat in patients with primary genital herpes (Corey, 1983c). Whether hematogenous, neurotropic, or a combination of both, the means by which virus reaches the CNS requires further study.

Aseptic meningitis associated with genital herpes appears to be a benign albeit uncomfortable disease in immunocompetent persons. Signs and symptoms of encephalitis are unusual, and neurologic sequelae are rare. Risk factors associated with the development of aseptic meningitis are not well understood. Whether antiviral chemotherapy will shorten the course or prevent the development of HSV-2 aseptic meningitis is currently unknown.

Both transverse myelitis and autonomic nervous system dysfunction have been described in association with genital HSV infection (Klastensky et al, 1972; Caplan et al, 1977;; Craig & Nahmias, 1973). Symptoms of sacral nervous system dysfunction include hyperaesthesia or anaesthesia of the perineal, lower back and anal regions; difficulty in urinating and constipation. Physical examination reveals a large bladder, decreased sacral sensation and poor rectal and perineal sphincter tone. In men, a history of impotence and absent bulbocavernous reflexes may be present. CSF pleocytosis may be present in some cases. Electromyography usually reveals slowed nerve conduction velocities and fibrillation potentials in the affected area, and urinary cystometric examination shows a large atonic bladder. Most cases gradually resolve over 4–8 weeks. In cases of transverse myelitis decreased deep tendon reflexes and muscle strength in the lower extremities, as well as the sacral neurologic dysfunction described above, are present. In one reported case, significant residual dysfunction was present years later (Craig & Nahmias, 1973).

Whether these neurologic abnormalities result from viral invasion of the central nervous system or an unusual immunologic response to infection is unknown. Paraesthesias, urinary retention and/or impotence have been noted in approximately 50% of men who present with HSV proctitis (Goodell et al, 1983). We have observed these symptoms in only 2 of 123 heterosexual women and 0 of 63 heterosexual men who presented with HSV infection of the penile or scrotal area. Of interest was the fact that both of the women who presented with sacral neurologic dysfunction also had anal HSV lesions. The mechanism for the more frequent association between HSV proctitis and these symptoms is unclear. Involvement of the dorsal nerve root ganglia (ganglionitis) has been postulated as one potential mechanism. Patients with these neurologic symptoms have been noted to have CSF pleocytosis. However, pleocytosis is common in primary genital herpes and is not specific for ganglionitis. To date, our group has studied six women and two men with these symptoms. In four women sacral nerve conduction studies revealed slowed nerve condition and the presence of bladder dysfunction, usually motor and/or mixed sensory/motor involvement. In both men, studies revealed no evidence of sacral nerve dysfunction, but both had severe perineal pain associated with inability fully to relax the perineal musculature. Thus, the pathogenesis of these complications may be varied. Controlled clinical trials of the use of antivirals or anti-inflammatory medications in these sacral neurologic syndromes have not been performed.

EXTRAGENITAL LESIONS
Extragenital lesions appear during the course of infection in as many as 15% of persons with primary first episodes, 10% with non-primary first episodes and 4% with recurrent genital herpes. Extragenital lesions occur 2–3 times more frequently in females than in males and extragenital lesions are most frequently found in the buttock, groin or thigh area. Occasionally HSV infections of the finger and eye can occur. Extragenital lesions characteristically develop during the second week of disease. The distribution of the lesions and their occurrence well into the course of disease suggest that the majority of extragenital lesions develop by autoinoculation of virus rather than viremic spread. Anatomic differences, especially contact with infected cervical-vaginal secretions, are the most likely explanation for the apparent increased risk of extragenital lesions in women.

DISSEMINATED INFECTION
Blood-borne dissemination, evidenced by the appearance of multiple vesicles over widespread areas of the thorax and extremities, rarely occurs (<0.5%) in persons with primary mucocutaneous herpes (Nahmias, 1970b; Ruchman & Dodd, 1950). Occasionally concomitant esophagitis, hepatitis, monoarticular arthritis (Friedman et al, 1980); (Joseph & Vogt, 1974; Flewett et al, 1969), thrombocytopenia (Whittaker & Hardson, 1978), and myoglobinuria (Schlesinger et al, 1978) may occur. Severe mucocutaneous and occasionally visceral dissemination of disease may occur in patients with atopic eczema and during pregnancy (Wheeler & Abele, 1966; Koberman et al, 1980; Peacock & Sarubbi, 1983; Young et al, 1976). In immunosuppressed patients, especially those with impaired cellular immune responses, reactivation of genital HSV infection can be associated with viremic spread of virus to multiple organs (Linnemann et al, 1976; Sutton et al, 1974; Ramsey et al, 1982; Meyers et al, 1980). These patients may develop interstitial pneumonia, hepatitis, and pneumonitis, similar to the manifestations of disseminated infection of the neonate (Nahmias & Dowdle, 1969b). Disseminated visceral infection in the immunosuppressed and pregnant patient is a disease of potentially high mortality. Systemic antiviral chemotherapy should be considered.

LOCAL EXTENSION OF DISEASE
Extension of HSV infection into the uterine cavity may occasionally occur (Abraham, 1978; Barton et al, 1982; Schneider et al, 1982). HSV has been isolated from the endometrium and occasionally from the fallopian tubes of women undergoing laparo-

scopy for pelvic inflammatory disease. Most studies suggest this is infrequent and that HSV is a very uncommon cause of pelvic inflammatory disease.

SUPERINFECTION

Bacterial superinfection of genital herpes in non-immunosuppressed patients is uncommon. In rare cases, pelvic cellulitis presenting as an advancing erythema and swelling of the perineal area is encountered. In this instance systemic antimicrobial therapy should be administered. Fungal superinfection may, however, be encountered during the course of first episodes of genital herpes. Characteristically, monilial infection develops during the second week of disease, is associated with a change in character of the vaginal discharge and reemergence of local symptoms such as vulvar itching and irritation. Typical hyphal yeast forms can be demonstrated on microscopy of vaginal secretions.

Recurrent genital herpes

Symptoms and signs

In contrast to first episodes of genital infection, the symptoms, signs and anatomic sites of infection of recurrent genital herpes are localised to the genital region (Adams et al, 1976; Guinan et al, 1981; Corey et al, 1983a). Local symptoms such as pain and itching are mild compared to first episodes of genital infection and the duration of the episode usually ranges from 8–12 days (Fig. 5.1). Approximately 50% of persons with recurrent genital herpes develop symptoms in the prodromal phase of illness, i.e. prior to the appearance of lesions. Prodromal symptoms vary from a mild tingling sensation, occurring $\frac{1}{2}$ to 48 hours prior to the eruption, to shooting pains in the buttocks, legs or hips 1–5 days prior to the episode. In many patients these symptoms of sacral neuralgia are often the most bothersome part of the episode. Sacks (1984) has reported that in many patients these prodromal symptoms may occur without the subsequent development of lesions. Whether this is associated with reactivation of virus and an abortive lesion due to an active host response is unknown.

Symptoms of recurrent genital herpes tend to be more severe in women. In the 362 patients with untreated recurrent genital herpes followed at the Genital Herpes Clinic at the University of Washington pain associated with lesions was a complaint of 88% of women (mean duration 5.9 days), as compared to 67% of men (mean duration 3.9 days). In addition, pain was more severe in women. Dysuria was reported in only 27% of women with recurrent disease. Most reported only external dysuria and isolation of HSV from the urethra was uncommon in both sexes (3–9%).

Lesions of recurrent genital HSV are usually confined to one side, with an area of involvement approximately one-tenth that of primary genital infection (Figures 5.4a and 5.4b). The average duration of time that HSV can be isolated from lesions is about 4 days; and the mean time from the onset of lesions to crusting of lesions averaged between 4 and 5 days for both men and women. The mean time from onset of vesicles to complete reepithelialisation of lesions was about 10 days. Although symptoms of recurrent genital disease tend to be more severe in females, objective signs of disease are similar in the two sexes.

Considerable overlap in the severity and duration of disease exists between patients (Fig. 5.1— note standard deviation for lesions, pain). In addition, the severity of

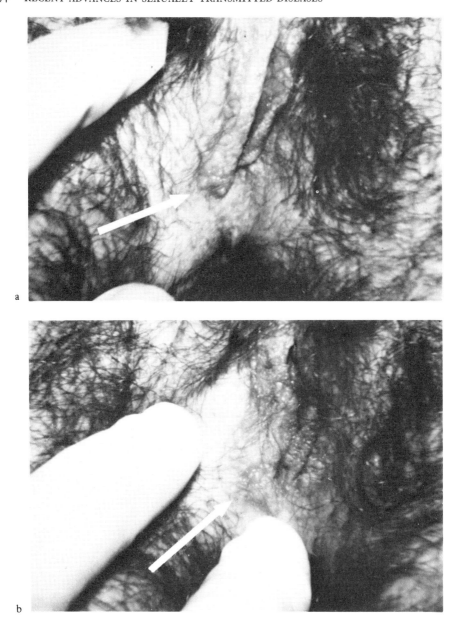

Fig. 5.4 (a) Group of unilateral vesicular lesions in a woman with recurrent genital herpes.
(b) Same lesions 24 hours later, small vesicles have formed coalescent painful ulcer.

any one individual episode of disease in any one patient may vary greatly during the course of disease. Some patients with recurrences have only 1–2 lesions lasting 6–7 days, while others may have 15–20 lesions lasting 12–16 days. Factors which are related to these variations in clinical expression are largely unexplored. This variability makes clinical assessment of the response to therapy difficult to assess.

Other clinical syndromes associated with genital HSV infection

HSV cervicitis
Herpes simplex virus may involve the cervix alone, without involvement of the external genitalia (Josey et al, 1966). Cervical HSV infection may be asymptomatic or may present as a symptomatic cervicitis. It is currently unknown what percentage of women who contract first episode genital HSV infection develop cervicitis alone compared with those with both vulvar and cervical disease.

Asymptomatic excretion of virus from the cervix may occur concomitant with episodes of vulvar lesions as well as between episodes of recurrent vulvar disease (Rattray et al, 1980; Vontver et al, 1982). The frequency of detection of HSV infection of the cervix varies according to the frequency with which patients are sampled. Rattray et al (1978) followed six women with recurrent vulvar genital herpes with twice weekly viral cultures of the cervical and vulvar area. Twenty-three clinical and virological recurrences of HSV were recorded in these women during 190 weeks of follow-up. Three recurrences were associated with asymptomatic excretion of virus; one with a small vulvar lesion noted only by the examiner, from which HSV was isolated; one with no external lesions, although HSV was isolated from a vulvar skin culture; and one in which HSV was isolated from the cervix. Thus in this small group of women with recurrent genital herpes, asymptomatic HSV infection of the cervix accounted for one of 23 clinical and virological recurrences of genital herpes. Adam et al (1979) also demonstrated transient asymptomatic excretion of HSV from the cervix in three women who were sampled regularly over three months. Brown et al (in press) followed pregnant women with first and recurrent genital herpes with weekly cultures during the course of gestation. Asymptomatic cervical infection was detected from 5% of cervical cultures among women with first as compared with 1.4% in those with recurrent disease. These data suggest asymptomatic cervical infection may occur more frequently early in the long-term natural history of genital herpes.

Isolation of HSV from the vulvar area without clinical signs and symptoms of infection has also been described, and may be even more frequent than cervical viral shedding. Vontver et al (1982) described asymptomatic vulvar shedding in 0.75% and asymptomatic cervical excretion in 0.66% of cultures in a cohort of pregnant women with known genital herpes.

Herpes simplex virus antigen has been demonstrated in cervical-vaginal secretions when HSV culture was negative (Adam et al, 1979; Moseley et al, 1981; Goldstein et al, 1983). It is currently unknown whether this is a reflection of short but frequent periods of viral shedding in which infectious virus is quickly inactivated by local immune mechanisms, or defective viral replication. These studies do, however, indicate that viral shedding from the cervix is intermittent, resembling the intermittent appearance of external genital lesions (August et al, 1979).

HSV urethritis
As discussed earlier, among patients with primary genital herpes who present with external genital lesions, HSV has been isolated from the urethra in 28% of men and 82% of women. This urethritis is usually symptomatic. HSV urethritis may also occur as the sole symptomatic manifestation of genital herpes. In a recent study

of women with the urethral syndrome (dysuria-frequency syndrome), HSV was iso-lated from the urethra or cervix in 5% (Stamm et al, 1980). HSV has been isolated from the urine of both men and women with dysuria or haematuria, and cystoscopy has in some of these cases revealed mucosal ulcerations. It is likely that HSV cystitis occasionally occurs as a result of ascending infection from the urethra into the bladder.

Herpes simplex proctitis
HSV has been isolated from rectal mucosal and rectal biopsies in men and women with symptoms of rectal pain and discharge (Goodell et al, 1983; Quinn et al, 1983; Waugh, 1976). In a prospective study of 100 consecutive homosexual men who pre-sented to an STD clinic with symptoms of rectal discharge and pain, HSV was isolated from rectal swabs and/or rectal biopsies in 23% and was the most frequent cause of nongonoccal proctitis in homosexual men (Goodell et al, 1983). Patients with HSV proctitis usually present with the acute onset of rectal pain, discharge, tenesmus, constipation, and bloody and/or mucoid rectal discharge. Fever, malaise, and myalgia are common, and urinary retention, dysesthesia of the perineal region, and impotence may be reported. External perianal lesions are seen in about one-half the cases. Anos-copy and/or sigmoidoscopy generally reveal a diffuse, friable rectal mucosa, although occasionally discrete ulcers of the rectal mucosa may be present. In most cases the pathology is limited to the lower ten centimeters of the rectum. Rectal biopsies of involved mucosa generally reveal diffuse ulceration and lymphocytic infiltration. If multiple histologic sections are performed, intranuclear inclusions may be demon-strated in rectal biopsies in about 50% of cases.

Both HSV-1 and HSV-2 have been isolated from patients with HSV proctitis (Levine & Saeed, 1979; Goodell et al, 1983). Recurrences of this disease have been described and may be mild and/or asymptomatic. Recent controlled trials suggest that oral acyclovir therapy may reduce the duration of HSV proctitis (Rompalo et al, 1985).

Genital ulceration
HSV infection causes 40–60% of genital ulcers in patients presenting to gynaecological practices or STD clinics in western industrialised countries (Chapel et al, 1978; Kinghorn et al, 1982). In underdeveloped nations, however, genital HSV infection is an infrequent cause of genital ulceration (Plummer et al, 1983; Meheus et al, 1982). The varied size, symptoms, and appearance of genital HSV lesions may make clinical diagnosis of genital ulceration, especially single ulcers, difficult. HSV may be isolated from many lesions attributed by patients to 'trauma' or irritation. In addition clinical differentiation of genital ulceration due to HSV, *Treponema pallidum* and *Hemophilus ducreyi* may be difficult. For this reason, laboratory confirmation of the diagnosis in patients who present with genital ulceration should be sought. Occasionally patients may have concomitant *T. pallidum* and HSV infections (Chapel et al, 1979).

Chronicity of genital HSV infections
There are still large gaps in our knowledge concerning the natural history and chroni-city of genital herpes. Long-term prospective studies of the subsequent rate of recur-rence of persons who acquire symptomatic primary infection are unavailable. Many basic questions such as, does the frequency of disease change over time, remain un-answered.

Prospective studies of patients who present with symptomatic primary genital herpes infection have shown that after one year of follow-up 55% of those with HSV-1 genital infections will develop recurrences, compared with >90% of those with primary HSV-2 infection. The median time to first recurrence was 42.5 days in patients with primary HSV-2 infections compared to 115 days in patients with primary HSV-1 infections. The mean rate of recurrences over time was also significantly less in patients with HSV-1 as compared to patients with primary HSV-2 infections, (0.10 recurrences per month in patients with primary HSV-1 infections versus 0.32 in patients with genital HSV-2 infection ($p < 0.001$)). Conversely, oral-labial HSV infections recur more frequently than oral-labial HSV-2 infection. These differences in recurrence rate between the two viruses at these anatomic sites help explain the well-known anatomic predilection for HSV-2 infections to be 'below the waist' and HSV-1 'above the waist'. The mechanisms behind this behaviour are unknown. The factors influencing recurrence of disease after primary infection are poorly understood. Among patients followed after first episode primary HSV-2 infection 40% experienced >6 recurrences in the first year of follow-up (Gold et al, 1985). The frequency of recurrences did not correlate with severity of the primary episode nor subsequent antibody response. The first year recurrence rate among those with primary and non-primary HSV-2 infection appear similar. A large questionnaire survey of over 6000 persons with symptomatic recurrent genital herpes conducted in the US indicated that the median number of yearly clinical recurrences of genital herpes was between five and eight (Knox et al, 1982). Recurrences of genital herpes do not follow a uniform pattern. The time of onset of disease and the number of recurrences over time which an individual experiences may vary greatly between patients and over time in any individual patient. For example, we have recently followed a cohort of patients with frequently recurring genital herpes over an 8 month period. In this population which averaged 1.17 recurrences per month, only 28 of 92 patients exhibited less than a 30% change in their clinical recurrence rate in the first as compared to second 4 months of observation. Twenty-three of the 92 patients had at least a 50% increase and 25 of 92 a 50% decrease in their recurrence rates in the first as compared to subsequent 4 month periods. These observations again indicate the difficulty in assessing response to therapy using anecdotal observations.

Current dogma suggests that the recurrence rate of genital herpes decreases over time. However, little data supports this. Our 3 year prospective follow-up of patients who presented with first episode disease has shown no significant drop in recurrence rates with time (Table 5.4). This is, however, a short time in the long-term natural history of this disease and further long-term evaluations are needed.

Table 5.4   Mean no. recurrences of genital herpes by 6 month intervals in patients who presented with symptomatic first episode disease and followed >24 months

	Patients with primary HSV-1 n = 6	Patients with primary HSV-2 n = 47	Non-primary HSV-2 n = 16
First 6 months	0.5 ± 0.6	2.32 ± 2.30	3.5 ± 2.74
Second 6 months	0.17 ± 0.7	1.57 ± 2.13	3.69 ± 3.11
Third 6 months	0.17 ± 0.7	2.76 ± 2.57	3.13 ± 2.49
Fourth 6 months	0.17 ± 0.7	2.28 ± 2.23	2.50 ± 2.10

'Trigger' mechanisms associated with recurrent genital herpes are also largely unknown. Guinan et al (1981) found a clustering of genital HSV episodes during the menstrual period. Others have shown no relationship between the onset of lesions and menstrual cycle or frequency of sexual activity (Vontver et al, 1979; Rattray et al, 1978). Anecdotal observations have suggested that such diverse phenomena as emotional stress, heat, moisture, climate change, pregnancy, oral contraceptive use, anaesthesia and trauma might be 'trigger' factors associated with recrudesences of HSV. However, objective data are lacking. Reinfection with different strains of HSV may occasionally occur (Buchman et al, 1979). Recent studies have, however, indicated that exogenous reinfection with new strains of HSV-2 appear in heterosexual populations to be a very infrequent cause of recurrent genital herpes (Schmidt et al, 1984). Infection with multiple strains of the same virus type may, however, be a more common occurrence in more promiscuous and/or immunosuppressed populations (Heller et al, 1982).

SEXUAL TRANSMISSION OF GENITAL HSV

Knowledge of the sexual transmission of genital herpes is scanty. The risk of acquiring disease from a sex partner during symptomatic or asymptomatic periods is unknown. Mertz et al (1985) recently evaluated the source contacts of 63 patients who presented with first episodes of genital herpes. The median time from first sexual exposure to the source contact and development of disease in the index patient was 4 months. Two-thirds of the source contacts had an obvious clinical history of genital HSV infection. However only one-third of the source contacts were aware of the diagnosis at the time of presumed transmission. These data suggest that educating patients regarding the high transmissibility of infection during periods when mildly symptomatic lesions are present might decrease transmission of HSV disease.

Transmission of genital herpes by sexual contact with an asymptomatic excretor of virus occurs and appears to be an important source of infection. Asymptomatic excretion of HSV has been demonstrated in saliva, cervical and seminal secretions. Douglas & Couch (1970) demonstrated asymptomatic excretion of HSV in saliva in 2% of adults, and there are reports of transmission of genital HSV-1 infection from oral-genital sex during periods of asymptomatic salivary excretion of virus (Embil et al, 1981). Asymptomatic cervical viral shedding has been shown to result in transmission to sexual contacts or infants (Whitly et al, 1980a). In the few studies in which virus has been titred from cervical secretions during asymptomatic episodes, the titre of HSV is 2–3 logs less than that recovered from lesions (Guinan et al, 1980; Merriman et al, 1984; Brown et al, 1979). However, whether the frequency of transmission from asymptomatic shedding is less than from symptomatic lesions is unknown.

HOST IMMUNE RESPONSES TO INFECTION

A large series of clinical and experimental observations indicate that host responses to infection influence the acquisition of disease, severity of infection, resistance to development of latency, maintenance of latency and frequency of HSV recurrences (Lopez, 1985). However, detailed analysis of the aspects of the host immune response which are most closely correlated with disease expression, and experimental evidence to determine which specific manifestations of the response are correlated with the subsequent clinical course of disease, are lacking. Some aspects of experimental recurrent herpes virus infection, e.g. stromal opacities associated with herpetic keratitis, appear to be related more to the host immune response than to virus induced damage (Pavan-Langston, 1979). Immunocompromised patients, especially those receiving immunosuppressive medication, and patients with T cell dysfunction, experience severe genital and oral HSV infections (Sutton et al, 1974; Linnemann et al, 1976; Meyers et al, 1980). As noted earlier, prior HSV-1 infection as evidenced by the presence of antibody in acute phase sera, ameliorates the signs and symptoms of first episodes of genital disease. These clinical observations and experimental animal studies indicate that both the humoral and cellular immune systems play a role in affecting the frequency and severity of mucocutaneous HSV infection (Kirchner, 1982).

Humoral immune responses
Numerous antibodies appear to be made in response to HSV infections. In primary HSV infection, complement fixing, neutralising, cytotoxic, precipitating and non-precipitating antibodies have been demonstrated (Norilld, 1985). Complement enhanced neutralising antibody and antibody-dependent cellular cytotoxicity (ADCC) antibody appear early in the course of disease (Shore et al, 1976). These antibodies persist at high levels throughout illness, and recrudescent infection appears to occur in the face of high levels of neutralising antibody (Reeves et al, 1981; Douglas & Couch, 1970).

In most animal systems, passive transfer of antibody to HSV will ameliorate infection, especially if the antibody is given in high titre (Worthington et al, 1980). In animals, Stevens & Cook (1974) noted that the passive instillation of anti-HSV immune serum globulin was important to the maintenance of latent infection. Evidence that high levels of neutralising antibody are present in humans with recurrent disease suggests that 'non-neutralising' antibodies may fluctuate in the course of disease. However, fluctuations in serum antibodies to viral specified polypeptides prior to the reactivation of disease have not to date been identified (Zweerink & Corey, 1982; Ashley & Corey, 1984b). Recently monoclonal antibodies to a variety of the viral surface glycoproteins have been shown in animal models to protect against subsequent viral challenge. Thus, although passive transfer experiments in animals suggest that humoral antibodies may modify and/or attenuate the severity of HSV infection. The role of the humoral immune system in reactivation disease is currently unclear.

Cellular immune response
While humoral immune responses appear to stay at high levels throughout the course of infection, many studies have shown that in vitro cellular immune responses to HSV antigens appear to fluctuate throughout the course of disease (Corey et al, 1978a; Shillitoe et al, 1978; O'Reilly et al, 1977). An association between the development of disseminated HSV infection and a markedly reduced in vitro 'natural killer' cell activity against HSV infected fibroblasts has been reported (Ching & Lopez, 1979).

Other studies evaluating macrophage and lymphocyte populations, including cytotoxic T cells, natural killer cells, lymphoproliferative responses, and T suppressor cell responses indicate that all of these cell populations play a role in host defense mechanisms to HSV infection (Ennis, 1973a & b; Morahan et al, 1977; Hirsch et al, 1970; Kohl & Loo, 1982). For example, newborns who have decreased macrophage activity suffer from severe HSV infections (Hirsch et al, 1970; Mintz et al, 1980). Newborn animals administered activated macrophages from adult animals and subsequently inoculated with HSV experience a lower mortality rate. In addition, substances which activate macrophages, e.g. *Corynybacterium parvum*, increase the resistance of animals to HSV infection, while depletion of animals' macrophages with silica increases the mortality and death rate from HSV infection (Zismann et al, 1970; Morahan et al, 1977).

Patients with HSV infections generally have normal in vitro responses to mitogens such as pokeweed, phytohemagglutinin and concanavalin A as well as to heterologous antigens such as candida and SK-SD. These responses do not appear to vary during the course of illness. However, fluctuations in HSV antigen specified cellular immune responses do occur (Corey et al, 1978a; Shillitoe et al, 1978; O'Reilly et al, 1977; Rasmussen et al, 1974). For example, patients who had localised primary genital herpes made high amounts of an HSV antigen specified lymphokine, lymphocyte derived chemotactic factor (LDCF), early in the course of disease. In contrast, those patients who experienced systemic symptoms with primary genital infection did not make high levels of this lymphokine antigen (Rattray et al, 1980). Similarly, an inverse correlation between the mean peak lymphoproliferative response to HSV antigen and the time course of this response has been shown in patients with primary genital herpes (Corey et al, 1978a). These studies, and those mentioned earlier in immunosuppressed patients, indicate that cellular immune host factors are important factors influencing the severity of primary HSV episodes.

The role of the cellular immune response in reactivation infection is less clear. O'Reilly et al (1977) noted a decrease in lymphocytotoxin prior to the onset of recurrent HSV infection. However, many investigators have not found significant alterations in cellular immune responses prior to reactivation of genital HSV infection (Rasmussen et al, 1974). Recent studies have reported changes in the ratio of T cell subsets $(T_4:T_8)$ early in the course of reactivation infection (Sheridan et al, 1982), and the duration and level of circulating gamma interferon has also been correlated with the time between recurrences of oral-labial HSV (Cunningham & Merigan, 1983).

THERAPY OF GENITAL HERPES

Concepts and goals

Goals for the therapy of genital herpes include: 1. prevention of infection and/or 2. shortening the clinical course of disease, including the frequency of complications of primary infection such as aseptic meningitis and urinary retention; 3. preventing the development of latency and subsequent clinical recurrences after initial genital infection; 4. preventing subsequent recurrences of disease in those with established latency; 5. decreasing the transmission of disease; and 6. eradicating established latent infection.

It is likely that one therapeutic entity will not be effective in accomplishing all the above goals for HSV infection. For example, an antiviral drug may be the most effective way of speeding the rate of healing and resolution of symptoms. However, an HSV vaccine appears to be the most logical approach for preventing infection. Likewise, it is unlikely that a herpes vaccine will affect the clinical course and subsequent recurrence rate in someone with already established latent infection. Conversely, if fluctuations in the cellular immune response is an important factor in recrudescent infection, a specific immune modulator may prevent recurrences of disease in those with established latency. This form of therapy may not, however, have any effect on the rate of healing or resolution of symptoms. As first episode genital HSV infection affects multiple anatomic areas, systemic therapy appears to be the best approach for shortening the duration of systemic complications. An oral antiviral medication that is safe in pregnancy and can be given for a short time period may be useful for the prevention of transmission of disease to the neonate. While recurrent genital herpes is usually localised to the external genitalia and amenable to topical antiviral therapy, there is no direct clinical or experimental evidence to suggest that shortening the course of recurrent episodes will affect the subsequent recurrence rate of disease. The short duration of symptoms and signs of recurrent genital herpes suggests that early application of a medication, especially during the prodromal period, may be necessary in order to have clinical utility.

Chemotherapy of genital herpes

Current status
Chemotherapeutic approaches to the treatment of genital HSV infection can be categorised into five areas: 1. antiviral compounds, 2. topical surfactants or detergents, 3. photodynamic dyes, 4. immune modulators, and 5. vaccines (Table 5.5). Many of the listed compounds which inhibit HSV in vitro have been studied only in vitro or in animal models of primary infection, and only a few have been subjected to rigorous randomised controlled clinical evaluations (Corey & Holmes, 1983b).

Acyclovir
A series of clinical trials conducted over the last few years have shown that the antiviral acyclovir (ACV) is clinically useful in the therapy of some aspects of genital HSV infections. Acyclovir is a nucleoside analogue that is a substrate for HSV specified thymidine kinase. Acyclovir is selectively phosphorylated in HSV-infected cells by this viral enzyme to ACV-monophosphate (ACV-MP). Cellular enzymes then phosphorylate ACV-MP to ACV-triphosphate, a competitive inhibitor and chain terminator of viral DNA polymerase (Elion et al, 1977) (Fig. 5.5).

ACV has potent in vitro activity against both HSV-1 and HSV-2 (Crumpacker et al, 1982). In animal models topical or systemic ACV markedly reduces the severity of mucocutaneous HSV infections, and if administered within 96 hours after inoculation of virus prevented ganglionic latency (Klein et al, 1979a, b; Field et al, 1979). Studies of first episode genital herpes have indicated that intravenous, oral and topical acyclovir are effective in shortening the clinical course of first episode primary genital herpes (Corey et al, 1982a; Corey et al, 1983d; Mindel et al, 1982; Bryson et al, 1983; Nilson et al, 1982; Mertz et al, 1984). Systemic therapy has the advantage of shortening the duration of constitutional symptoms and signs of HSV cervicitis and urethritis. For this reason, in first episodes of genital herpes systemic therapy

Table 5.5   Results of controlled therapeutic trials of mucocutaneous HSV infections in immunocompetent patients

Compound	Type of HSV infection	Dose and route of administration	Result
Antivirals:			
Acyclovir	Genital	5% ointment in polyethylene glycol (PEG) 4–6 times daily	Shortened local symptoms and lesions of first infection — decreased viral shedding in recurrent infections.
		5% cream (polyethylene glycol 6 times daily)	Shortened local symptoms and lesions of first episode, shortened lesions and viral shedding in recurrent genital episodes.
		5 mg/kg IV every 8 hours	Shortened local and systemic symptoms and signs of severe primary herpes
		200 mg po 5 × daily	Shortened local and systemic symptoms and signs of primary genital herpes. Shortened lesions and viral shedding of recurrent genital herpes, patient initiated better results than physician initiated
	Recurrent oral-labial	5% ointment in PEG 4 times daily	Decreased viral titer, no clinical effect
		5% cream 6 × daily	Same shortening of lesion duration inpatient initiated study
Ara-A	Genital and oral	3% cream	Ineffective in primary or recurrent genital infection
(vidarabine)			
Ara-AMP	Recurrent oral	10% cream	Ineffective
2-Deoxy-d-glucose	Genital	0.19% gel in 20% miconazole nitrate cream	Ineffective in animals, efficacy in humans claimed
IUdR	Oral and genital	0.1%–2% cream	Ineffective
	Oral and genital	5 and 20% solution in DMSO 3 times daily	Shortens viral shedding and lesions
	Genital	30% solution in DMSO 4 times daily	Reduced viral shedding, no clinical effect, toxic
L-Lysine	Oral	500 mg twice daily	Ineffective in shortening course of reducing frequency of recurrences
Ribavirin	Genital	800 mg per day orally	Reduction in disease severity (?) confirmation required
Phosphonoformate	Oral-labial	3% cream 6 times daily 4 days	Shortened time of papular and vesicular stages of disease
	Genital	3% cream for 7 days	Shortening of lesions and duration of vesicular and ulcerative lesions
Topical Surfactants			
Ether	Genital	4 times daily	Toxic, ineffective
	Oral-labial	6 times daily	Ineffective
Chloroform	Oral		Ineffective
Nonoxynol 9	Genital	4 times daily	Ineffective
Photodynamic Inactivation:			
Neutral red	Oral	3–6 times over 2 days	Ineffective
Proflavine	Genital	3 times over 1 day	Ineffective

Table 5.5   (*contd*)

Compound	Type of HSV infection	Dose and route of administration	Result
Vaccinations:			
Smallpox	Oral-labial	Intradermal	Ineffective, toxic
BCG	Genital	Intradermal	Ineffective
Polio	Oral-labial	Oral vaccine	Ineffective
Influenza	Oral-labial and genital	Subcutaneous	No controlled trials
Interferons: Leukocyte interferon	Oral-labial	70 000 units/kg per day IM for 5 days	Decreases frequency of reactivation and lesions when given prophylactically
Recombinant alpha interferon	Genital	Subcutaneous 3–10 millions units daily × 3–5 days	Ineffective in decreasing duration of lesion; headache and side effects

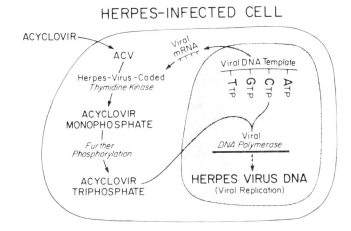

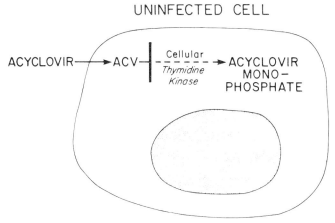

Fig. 5.5   Mechanism of action of the antiviral drug acyclovir.

is preferred to topical treatment (Corey et al, 1983d). In addition, as almost all patients can be treated as outpatients, oral acyclovir is preferable to intravenous treatment for first episode genital herpes. None of the acyclovir formulations when used as a therapy for first episode disease have been shown to decrease the subsequent rate of recurrence of disease (Mertz et al, 1984; Corey et al, 1985).

The use of acyclovir in recurrent genital herpes is less clear cut. Clinical studies of 5% acyclovir in polyethylene glycol ointment have shown minimal efficacy in shortening the course of recurrent genital herpes (Corey et al, 1982a; Reichman et al, 1984; Luby et al, 1984). Recent studies of 5% acyclovir in propylene glycol, however, have shown efficacy of this preparation in shortening the case of recurrent genital lesions. In these studies, the duration of viral shedding is reduced by about 50% (3 days to 1.5 days) and lesions by about 30% i.e. from 8–10 days to 5–7 days (Fiddian et al, 1983). In animal models, the cream preparation of acyclovir appears to have better penetration of the drug into skin and enhanced healing. Oral acyclovir tablets (200 mg 5 times daily for 5 days) taken within 36 hours of onset of lesions have also been shown to shorten the course of viral shedding of men and women with recurrent genital herpes. Initiating therapy even earlier, i.e., before onset of lesions, enhances the clinical efficacy (Reichman et al, 1984).

Recent studies have shown that oral acyclovir tablets taken daily can effectively decrease (but not completely abrogate) the subsequent development of clinical episodes of disease (Douglas et al, 1985; Straus et al, 1984; Mindel et al, 1984). In a series of studies in which persons with frequent (6–12 episodes of recurrences per year) were given two, three, or five 200 mg acyclovir tablets daily for 4–6 months, over 95% of persons had a marked decrease in their clinical recurrence rate. While breakthrough recurrences occur in about 30% of persons, the frequency of the episodes even in those who recurred was reduced to about one every 3 months. Daily therapy has been well tolerated. To date, most authorities recommend discontinuing suppressive therapy at 6–9 months after initiation. Reassessment of the patient's recurrence rate to determine if continued therapy is indicated should be performed. At present, data regarding the frequency of asymptomatic HSV infection on acyclovir is not available. Similarly whether the frequency of breakthroughs increases with use, and the long-term toxicities and effects of therapy on transmission of disease are not understood. Thus, daily suppressive therapy should be used judiciously. Studies of the efficacy and toxicity of oral acyclovir in pregnancy are unavailable.

Balancing these studies of clinical efficacy is the in vitro and in vivo description of acyclovir resistant mutants (Crumpacker et al, 1982; Field et al, 1980; Sibrack et al, 1982; Burns et al, 1982). Little information is yet available on repeated use of acyclovir preparations in immunocompetent patients with genital herpes. Whether frequent intermittent therapy will enhance the development of acyclovir resistant viruses and whether the transmission of acyclovir resistent viruses becomes clinically important (hence reducing the efficacy of acyclovir in first episode disease) is unknown. One time use of the agent does not appear to result in the emergence of clinically significant resistance (McLaren et al, 1983). Until these questions are answered, definite recommendations as to how to use acyclovir in patients with recurrent genital herpes cannot be made. At present, we do not recommend routine use of the medication for the treatment of all recurrences. Judicious use, especially of suppressive therapy, can benefit persons with frequent recurrences.

Other antivirals

Because of the interest in therapy of genital herpes, numerous other compounds have been investigated. A brief overview of the controlled clinical investigations of other antivirals in genital HSV infections is presented below.

Vidarabine (adenine arabinoside, ARA-A) is an antiviral compound which selectively inhibits HSV DNA polymerase. Intravenous ARA-A is effective in decreasing the mortality of HSV encephalitis and neonatal herpes (Whitley et al, 1980b; Whitley et al, 1981). However, topically applied 3% ARA-A cream and a 10% cream made from the more soluble monophosphate derivative, ARA-AMP, are ineffective in shortening the course of initial or recurrent genital and oral-labial infections (Adams et al, 1976; Spruance et al, 1979a). Reevaluation of the use of topical ARA-AMP in recurrent genital herpes is underway.

Topical application of idoxuridine (IDU) (Stoxil) has also been shown to be ineffective in shortening the course of oral or genital herpes (Burnette & Katz, 1962). In 1966, MacCallum & Juel-Jensen used the organic solvent dimethylsulfoxide (DMSO) to increase the penetration of IDU into skin. They demonstrated that a 5% IDU-DMSO mixture compared to DMSO hastened healing of oral-labial HSV. Davidson-Parker (1977) compared topical treatment of recurrent genital herpes with 20% IDU-DMSO, 5% IDU-DMSO, and 100% DMSO alone. In this study, the mean time to healing from onset of therapy was 3.9 days in the 20% IDU group, 5.7 days in the 5% IDU group, and 6.3 days in the DMSO treated group ($p < 0.05$), and the duration of viral shedding was 2.1, 2.9, and 4.1 days respectively. Silvestri et al (1982) compared 30% IDU-DMSO with 100% DMSO alone and with normal saline in initial and recurrent genital herpes. While the 30% IDU-DMSO mixture shortened viral shedding in both initial and recurrent genital herpes, no effect was noted on the duration of symptoms, rate of healing or subsequent recurrence rate of disease. In addition, toxicity associated with prolonged ulceration of genital lesions was seen with a 40% IDU-DMSO mixture.

One study purported to show the efficacy of topical 2-deoxy-D-glucose dissolved in a miconazole cream in reducing the severity and frequency of initial and recurrent genital herpes (Blough & Giuntoli, 1979). However, in animal models of genital HSV infections, 2-deoxy-D-glucose has proven ineffective in the therapy of genital herpes (Kern et al, 1982). Further studies of 2-deoxy-D-glucose in genital HSV infections are needed (Corey & Holmes, 1980).

Two published controlled studies of L-lysine therapy have shown no efficacy of this substance in ameliorating the effects or reducing the rate of recurrence of oral-labial HSV infection (Milman et al, 1978; Scheibel & Jesson, 1979). Topical trifluorothymidine is licensed for therapy of herpetic keratitis, but no studies in mucocutaneous HSV infection have been conducted. The medication has been shown to have fetal toxicity in animals.

There are only a few controlled trials in the English literature on the use of ribavirin in mucocutaneous HSV infections. One recent study purported to show clinical efficacy of this compound in a double blind placebo controlled trial in recurrent genital HSV infection. Unfortunately, no virological data to assess the results on the duration of viral shedding from lesions were performed. In addition, clinical responses seemed to diminish with subsequent episodes (Bierman et al, 1981). Recent studies have indicated about 10% of recipients develop a mild hyperbilirubinemia with this medication. Rarely this may be associated with a hemolytic anaemia (Smith et al, 1980). Further investigations of ribavirin in genital HSV investigations are needed.

Phosphonoformate (PFA) and its related compound phosphonoacetic acid (PAA) are potent inhibitors of the DNA polymerase of herpes simplex virus (Kern et al, 1978). In recurrent oral-labial disease, topical preparations of phosphonoformate appear to speed the rate of healing and decrease the duration of viral shedding (Wallin et al, 1981). In one study, topical application to recurrent genital lesions also appeared to shorten the duration of lesions (Wallin et al, 1983). Studies as to whether in vitro resistance of clinical HSV isolates to PFA occur have not yet been published. Absorption of this drug into bone limits the systemic use of this medication and may be a concern with repeated topical application.

In summary, the recent development of effective antivirals for herpes simplex virus have opened up promise for the therapy of genital HSV infection. This is especially true in those patients with first episodes of genital herpes in whom early therapy may alleviate the morbidity of this infection. In recurrent genital disease, antiviral therapy with acyclovir or phosphonofomate may shorten the course of illness but does not reduce subsequent recrudescences of disease. Oral acyclovir capsules taken daily can be an effective suppressive of the disease, especially with six monthly use. The longer term safety of chronic acyclovir therapy has not yet been fully evaluated. While the emergence of resistance may be a concern, the development of other antiviral compounds may allow the physician more flexibility in his approach to therapy of recurrent episodes of genital herpes.

Topical surfactants/antiseptics
HSV is a lipid enveloped virus and dissolution of the envelope reduces infectivity. However, to date all double-blind placebo controlled investigations of topical surfactants such as ether and chloroform have shown these medications to be ineffective in shortening the course or duration of initial or recurrent genital or oral-labial HSV infections (Corey et al, 1978b; Guinan et al, 1980; Taylor et al, 1977). While anecodotal data are available concerning the in vitro effects of betadine, silver and zinc compounds on HSV, well controlled double blind investigations of these preparations in human genital herpes have not been conducted (Friedrich & Masukawa, 1975).

Photodynamic inactivation
Double-blind placebo controlled trials of photodynamic inactivation using neutral red and/or proflavine dyes showed them to be ineffective in shortening the course of recurrent genital or oral infection (Felbee et al, 1973; Myers et al, 1975). HSV treated with these agents is still, however, capable of causing cell transformation in vitro. Because of the lack of clinical benefit and potential toxicity these medications should not be used in mucocutaneous HSV infection.

Non-specific immune modulators
Immune modulators such as levamisol and transfer factor have received some attention for the therapy of genital HSV infection. Controlled clinical trials of levamisol in primary genital herpes have not been conducted. Levamisol had no effect in recurrent mucocutaneous infection (Chang & Fiumara, 1978; Spruance et al, 1979b; Jose & Minty, 1980; Bierman, 1978; Russell et al, 1978). Similarly, well controlled clinical

trials enrolling adequate numbers of patients with genital herpes of the immune poten-
tiator isoprinosine have not been conducted.

Few studies of transfer factor in mucocutaneous HSV infection have been reported.
In a small study conducted at Emory University in Atlanta, Georgia, transfer factor
offered no clinical benefit in preventing recurrences of genital herpes (Starr, 1977).
Recently, transfer factor has been shown to be effective in decreasing the acquisition
of varicella in immunosuppressed children (Steele et al, 1980). The fluctuations in
in vitro cellular immune responses to HSV antigens appear more marked and more
frequent than in varicella-zoster infection and may make preparation of an effective
transfer factor more difficult. No studies have been performed of transfer factor in
prevention of primary genital herpes.

Interferon has been used in herpetic keratitis as well as for prophylaxis of recurrent
oral-labial disease after facial nerve decompression (Jones et al, 1976; Pazin et al,
1978). Low doses of interferon have given equivocal results in treatment of mucocutaneous HSV infection, but routine administration of interferon immediately prior
to and after surgery for trigeminal neuralgia was partially effective in prevention of
subsequent oral-labial HSV infection (Pazin et al, 1978). In addition, interferon recipients also had less tendency to develop recrudescences of infection after operation.
In renal transplant patients, interferon did not reduce the frequency of HSV infections
(Cheeseman et al, 1979). Studies of the use of interferon for the prophylaxis and
therapy of genital herpes are currently underway. To date, subcutaneous or intramuscular administration of 3–10 million units of recombinant alpha interferon within
the first 24–36 hours after onset has not reduced the severity of recurrent genital
herpes (Gnann et al, 1984). Whether more chronic administration and higher doses
will be clinically beneficial and well tolerated will require further study.

Heterologous vaccines
Many heterologous vaccines such as smallpox, BCG, influenza, and polio vaccines
have been used as therapies for genital HSV infection. A controlled study of smallpox
vaccine in recurrent oral-labial herpes indicated that this vaccine was ineffective in
reducing the recurrence rate of disease (Kern & Schiff, 1959). Deaths from disseminated vaccinia infection have occurred, and this potentially dangerous form of therapy
should be actively discouraged (Anonymous, 1979).

Controlled evaluations of BCG vaccine have shown no effect on the recurrence
rate of genital HSV infection (Bierman, 1976; Douglas et al, 1985). No immunologic
or virologic rationale has emerged to suggest that either influenza or polio vaccine
should ameliorate the course of genital HSV infections. A recent controlled evaluation
of polio vaccine has shown no efficacy (Tager, 1974).

Prophylaxis of infection
Currently no proven effective means of prophylaxis of HSV has been established.
Barrier forms of contraception, especially condoms, may decrease transmission of
disease. Transmission of disease when lesions were present despite the use of a condom
may still occur. Spermicides contain the topical surfactant nonoxynol-9, which inacti-
vates HSV in vitro. Nonoxynol-9 has been shown to be ineffective in the treatment
of established genital HSV infection (Vontver et al, 1979). No data are, however,
available to determine if it would be effective in decreasing transmission of disease.

Similarly, it is unknown whether oral contraceptive use increases the relative risk of acquiring HSV infection. Because of the intermittent nature of excretion and subsequent exposure to the virus and the long term 'risk' of acquiring infection from a chronically infected partner, an effective HSV vaccine appears to offer much more convenient, safe and potentially efficacious way of preventing acquisition of infection than chronic or 'prophylactic' antiviral chemotherapy.

HSV vaccines
Experimental evidence in animals indicate that HSV vaccines can protect against the acquisition of infection and development of latency (Scriba, 1978; Kitces et al, 1978; Cappel et al, 1980; Hilleman et al, 1981). There is, however, no experimental or theoretical data yet generated to suggest that vaccine given to someone with established latent infection and/or disease will subsequently modify the clinical course of their HSV infection. Inactivated herpes virus vaccines are available in Europe (Lupidon G and H). Well-controlled evaluations of these preparations either in reducing the risk of acquiring disease or recurrence rate of disease have not been performed. Because of the potential oncogenicity of HSV-2 in animals, most authorities feel that any potential HSV vaccine should be free of all viral genetic material (Allen & Rapp, 1982). These concerns have provided the impetus to develop purified HSV subunit vaccines. However, an essential piece of information is missing from our current knowledge of the pathogenesis and natural history of genital HSV infections; this is an understanding of what are the important virological and host factors associated with resolution of disease. What antigen(s) are required to protect one from acquiring disease and/or are associated with resolution of clinically symptomatic disease? Are there immune responses to specific viral polypetides which can maintain latency? If so, theses antigens could be incorporated into a vaccine preparation.

At present, the best candidate vaccines have been inactivated vaccines from which viral DNA has been removed (Skinner et al, 1982; Hilleman et al, 1981). One approach has been to develop subunit vaccines to the viral surface glycoproteins. The viral glycoproteins have been shown to be involved in neutralisation and cytotoxicity responses to the virus (Dix et al, 1981; Balachandran et al, 1982; Carter et al, 1981). Recombinant DNA techniques have provided the tools to produce large quantities of highly immunogenic protein. In addition, use of novel vectors such as smallpox vaccine have been proposed by some. Early trials indicate the vaccines are immunogenic and protective in animals. Immunogenicity and clinical trials of these HSV vaccines are currently underway.

SUMMARY

Genital herpes simplex virus infection is a disease of major public health importance. In the last 10 years, genital herpes has increased in prevalence in some population groups, especially white middle class caucasian men and women between the ages of 15 and 35 years. First episodes of genital HSV infection involve multiple anatomic sites, lasts 3–4 weeks, and have a high rate of complications. In contrast, episodes of recurrent genital disease are of much milder intensity and duration. The major morbidity of recurrent genital herpes is its frequency of recurrence, its chronicity, and its effects on the patients' personal relationships and sexuality. A possibility of increased risk of subsequent cervical carcinoma and the potential transmission of the disease to the neonate are major concerns to women. Studies in the last few years with new antiviral compounds such as acyclovir suggest that these substances may reduce the severity and duration of acute episodes of genital herpes. The effects of these substances on reducing the transmission of disease and subsequent recurrence rate of disease are, however, unknown. The development of effective forms of immuno-prophylaxis of HSV infection offers several new potential approaches in the management of HSV infections; especially in reducing the acquisition of disease. Further investigations on the mechanism of recurrence and risk factors associated with recurrence will hopefully provide the understanding to design effective forms of immunoprophylaxis. As animal models of recurrent genital HSV infection are not analagous to human infection, well controlled clinical evaluations of humans are essential if we are to further our understanding of the pathogenesis of human HSV infections. Fortunately, genital HSV patients are one of the most cooperative and rewarding patient populations in which to conduct long-term studies of the natural history of disease. These controlled studies of the natural history of disease are critical in order to direct laboratory research into new diagnostic and therapeutic uses, as well as to generate the information necessary to design appropriate clinical trials evaluating new therapies and/or vaccines. In the meantime, knowledge of the natural history of the disease is also of direct vital importance to the physician in providing the patient with the information necessary to understand this complex entity, and to identify risk factors which will decrease the transmission of disease to sexual partners and neonates.

REFERENCES

Abraham A A 1978 Herpesvirus hominis endometritis in a young woman wearing an intrauterine device. American Journal of Obstetrics and Gynecology 131: 340–343

Adam E, Kaufman R H, Mirkovic R R, Melnick J L 1979 Persistence of virus shedding in asymptomatic women after recovery from herpes genitalis. Obstetrics and Gynecology 54: 171–173

Adams H G, Benson E A, Alexander E R, Vontver L A Remington M A, Holmes K K 1976 Genital herpetic infection in men and women: clinical course and effect of topical application of adenine arabinoside. Journal of Infectious Diseases 133: A151–A159

Allen W P, Rapp F 1982 Concept review of genital herpes vaccines: NIAID workshop. Journal of Infectious Diseases 145: 413–421

Ashley R L, Corey L 1984a Effect of acyclovir treatment of primary genital herpes on the antibody response to herpes simplex virus. Journal of Clinical Investigation 73(3): 681–688

Ashley R, Corey L 1984b Association of herpes simplex virus polypeptide specific antibodies and the natural history of genital herpes infections. Herpesvirus. Alan R. Liss, New York, NY 21: 37–54

Astruc J De Morbis Venereis Libri Sex. Paris, 1736

August M J, Nordlund J J, Hsiung G D 1979 Persistence of herpes simplex virus types 1 and 2 in infected individuals. Archives of Dermatology 115: 309–10

Anonymous 1979 Adverse reactions to smallpox vaccinations — 1978. Morbidity and Mortality Weekly Report 28: 265–267

Balachandran N, Bacchetti S, Rawls W E 1982 Protection against lethal challenge of BAIB/c mice by passive transfer of monoclonal antibodies to five glycoproteins of herpes simplex virus type 2. Infection and Immunity 37(3): 1132–1137

Barton I G, Kinghorn G R, Walker M J, Al-Omer L S, Potter C W, Gunner E B 1981 Association of HSV-1 with cervical infection. Lancet 2: 1108

Barton I G, Kinghorn G R, Najem S, Al-Omar L S, Potter C W 1982 Incidence of herpes simplex virus types 1 and 2 isolated in patients with herpes genitalis in Sheffield. British Journal of Venereal Disease 58: 44–47

Barton I G, Najem S N, Walker M J, Potter C W 1982 Isolation and characterization of two strains of herpesvirus hominis type 1 from fallopian tubes. Medical Microbiology 15: 62–71

Baum O 1920 Uber die ubentragbarkeit des herpes simplex auf die kaninchen hourhaut. Derm Wosch; 70:105

Bayer P, Gear J 1955 Virus meningo-encephalitis in South Africa. South African Journal of Laboratory and Clinical Medicine 1:22

Becker T M, Blount J H, Guinan M E 1985 Genital herpes infections in private practice in the United States, 1966 to 1981. Journal of the American Medical Association 253: 1601–1603

Bernstein D I, Lovett M A, Bryson Y J 1984 Serologic analysis of first episode nonprimary genital herpes simplex virus infection. The American Journal of Medicine 77: 1055–1059

Bierman S M 1976 BCG immunoprophylaxis of recurrent herpes progenitalis. Archives of Dermatology 112: 1410–1415

Bierman S M 1978 Double-blind crossover study of levamisole as immunoprophylaxis for recurrent herpes progenitalis. Cutis 21: 352–354

Bierman S M, Kirkpatrick W, Fernandez H 1981 Clinical efficacy of ribavirin in the treatment of genital herpes simplex virus infection. Chemotherapy 27: 139–145

Blough H A, Giuntoli R L 1979 Successful treatment of human genital herpes infections with 2-deoxy-D-glucose. Journal of the American Medical Association 241: 2798–2801

Bolognese R J, Corson S L, Fuccillo D A, Traub R, Moder F, Sever J L 1976 Herpes-virus hominis type II infections in asymptomatic pregnant women. Obstetrics and Gynecology 48: 507–510

Brenton D W 1980 Hypoglycorrhachia in herpes simplex type 2 meningitis. Archives of Neurology 37: 317

Brown Z A, Kern E R, Spruance S L, Overall J C Jr 1979 Clinical and virologic course of herpes simplex genitalis (Medical Progress). Western Journal of Medicine 130: 414

Brown Z A, Vontver L A, Benedetti J, Critchlow C W, Hickok D E, Sells C J, Berry S, Corey L Recurrent genital herpes in pregnancy: variation of recurrence rates by trimester and risk factors associated with asymptomatic viral shedding. American Journal of Obstetrics and Gynecology (in press)

Bryson Y J, Dillon M, Lovett M et al 1983 Treatment of first episodes of genital herpes simplex virus infection with oral acyclovir. A randomized double-blind controlled trial in normal subjects. New England Journal of Medicine 308: 916–921

Buchman T G, Roizman B, Nahmias A J 1979 Demonstration of exogenous genital reinfection with herpes simplex virus type 2 by restriction endonuclease fingerprinting of viral DNA. Journal of Infectious Diseases 140: 295–304

Burnette J W, Katz S L 1962 A study of the use of 5 iodo-2'-deoxyuridine in cutaneous herpes simplex. Journal of Investigative Dermatology 40: 7–8

Burns W H, Saral R, Santos G W, Laskin O L, Lietman P S, McLaren C, Barry D W 1982 Isolation and characterization of resistant herpes simplex virus after acyclovir therapy. Lancet 1: 421–423

Caplan L R, Kleman F J, Berg S 1977 Urinary retention probably secondary to herpes genitalis. New England Journal of Medicine 297: 920–921

Cappel R, DeCuyper F, Rickaert F 1980 Efficacy of a nucleic acid-free herpetic subunit vaccine. Archives of Virology 65: 15–23

Carter V C, Schaffer P A, Tevethia S S 1981 The involvement of herpes simplex virus type 1 gycoproteins in cell-mediated immunity. Journal of Immunology 126(5): 1655

Chang T, Fiumara N 1978 Treatment with levamisole of recurrent herpes genitalis. Antimicrobial Agents and Chemotherapy 13: 809–12

Chapel T, Brown W J, Jeffres C, Stewart J A 1978 Microbiological flora of penile ulcerations. Journal of Infectious Diseases 137: 50–57

Chapel T A, Jeffries C D, Brown W J 1979 Simultaneous infection with treponema pallidum and herpes simplex virus. Cutis 24: 1912

Cheeseman S H, Rubin R H, Stewart J A et al 1979 Controlled clinical trial of prophylactic human-leukocyte interferon in renal transplantation. New England Journal of Medicine 300: 1345–1349

Chief Medical Officer 1984 Sexually transmitted diseases. British Journal of Venereal Disease 60: 199–203

Ching C, Lopez C 1979 Natural killing of herpes simplex virus type 1-infected target cells: normal human responses and influence of antiviral antibody. Infection and Immunity 26: 49–56

Chuang T-Y, Daniel Su W P, Perry H O, Ilstrup D M, Kurland L T 1983 Incidence and trend of herpes progenitalis, a 15-year population study. Mayo Clinic Proceedings 58: 436–441

Corey L, Reeves W C, Holmes K K 1978a Cellular immune response in genital herpes simplex virus infection. New England Journal of Medicine 299: 986–991

Corey L, Reeves W C, Chiang W T, Vontver L A, Remington M, Winter C, Holmes K K 1978b Ineffectiveness of topical ether for the treatment of genital herpes simplex virus infection. New England Journal of Medicine 299: 237–239

Corey L, Holmes K K 1980 The use of 2-deoxy-D-glucose for genital herpes. Journal of the American Medical Association 243: 29

Corey L, Holmes K K, Benedetti J, Critchlow C 1981 Clinical course of genital herpes: implications for therapeutic trials. In: Nahmias A J, Dowdle W R, Schinazi K F (eds) The human herpesviruses. New York, Elsevier, 496–502

Corey L, Nahmias M E, Guinan M E, Guinan M E, Benedetti J K, Critchlow C W, Holmes K K 1982a A trial of topical acyclovir in genital herpes simplex virus infections. New England Journal of Medicine 306: 1313–1319

Corey L, Benedetti J K, Critchlow C, Remington M R, Winter C A, Fahnlander A L, Smith K Y, Salter D L, Keeney R E, Davis L G, Hintz M A, Connor J D, Holmes K K, 1982b Double blind controlled trial of topical acyclovir in genital herpes simplex virus infections: the Seattle experience. American Journal of Medicine 73(1A): 326–334

Corey L, Adams H G, Brown Z A, Holmes K K 1983a Genital herpes simplex virus infection: Clinical manifestations, course and complications. Annals of Internal medicine 98· 958–972

Corey L, Holmes K K 1983b. Genital herpes simplex virus infection: current concepts in diagnosis, therepy and prevention. Annals of Internal Medicine 98: 973–978

Corey L, Fife K H, Benedetti J K, Winter C, Fahnlander A, Connor J D, Hintz M A, Holmes K K 1983c Intravenous acyclovir for the treatment of primary genital herpes. Annals of Internal Medicine 98: 914–921

Corey L, Benedetti J, Critchlow C, Mertz G, Douglas J, Fife K, Fahnlander A, Remington M L, Winter C, Dragavon J 1983d Treatment of primary first episode genital HSV infections with acyclovir: results of topical, intravenous and oral therapy. Journal of Antimicrobial Chemotherapy 12: 3093–3094

Corey L, Mindel A, Fife K H, Suthereland S, Benedetti J, Adler M W Risk of recurrence after treatment of first episode genital herpes with intravenous acyclovir. Sexually Transmitted Diseases, (in press)

Craig C, Nahmias A, 1973. Different patterns of neurologic involvement with herpes simplex virus types 1 and 2: isolation of herpes simplex virus from the buffy coat of two adults with meningitis. Journal of Infectious Diseases 127: 365–372

Crumpacker C S, Schnipper L E, Marlowe S I, Kowalsky P N, Hershey B J, Levin M J 1982 Resistance to antiviral drugs of herpes simplex virus isolated from a patient treated with a cyclovir. New England Journal of Medicine 306: 343–348

Cruter W 1924 Das herpesvirus seine aetiologische und klinische bedeutung. Munch Med Wsch; 71: 1058–1060

Cunningham A, Merigan T C 1983 Alpha interferon production appears to predict time of recurrence of herpes labialis. Journal of Immunology 130: 2397–2400

Davidson-Parker J D 1977 A double blind trial of idoxuridine in recurrent genital herpes. Journal of Antimicrobial Chemotherapy 3: Suppl A: 131–139

Deture F A, Drylie D M, Kaufman H E, Centifanto Y M 1976 Herpes virus type 2 isolation from seminal vesicle and testes. Urology 7: 541

Diday P, Doyon A 1886. Les Herpes Genitaux. Paris, Masson et Cie

Dix R D, Pereirea L, Baringer R J 1981 Use of monoclonal antibody directed against herpes simplex virus glycoproteins to protect mice against acute virus-induced neurological disease. Infection and Immunity 34(1): 192–199

Douglas J M, Vontver L A, Reeves W C, Benedetti J, Critchlow C, Holmes K K, Corey L. 1985 Ineffectiveness and toxicity of BCG vaccine for the prevention of recurrent genital herpes. Antimicrobial Agents and Chemotherapy 27: 203–206

Douglas RG Jr, Couch RB 1970 A prospective study of chronic herpes simplex virus infection and recurrent herpes labialis in humans. Journal of Immunology 104: 289–295

Dowdle W R, Nahmias A J, Harwell R W et al 1967 Association of antigenic type of herpesvirus hominis with site of viral recovery. Journal of Immunology (99): 974–980

Duenas A, Adam E, Melnick J L, Rawls W E 1972 Herpesvirus type 2 in a prostititue population. American Journal of Epidemiology 95: 483

Eberle R, Courtney R J 1981 Assay of type-specific and type-common antibodies to herpes simplex virus types 1 and 2 in human sera. Infection and Immunity 31: 1062–1070

Elion G B, Furman P A, Fyfe J A, de Miranda P, Beauchamp L, Schaeffer H J 1977 Selectivity of action of an antiherpetic agent, 9-(2-hydroxyethoxymethy) guanine. Proceedings of the National Academy of Science USA 74: 5716–5720

Embil J A, Manuel F R, McFarlane S 1981 Concurrent oral and genital infection with an identical strain of herpes simplex virus type 1. Sexually Transmitted Diseases 8: 70–73

Ennis F A 1973a Host defense mechanisms against herpes simplex virus. I. Control of infection in vitro by sensitized spleen cells and antibody. Infection and Immunity 7: 898–904

Ennis F A 1973b Host defense mechanisms against herpes simplex virus. II. Protection conferred by sensitized spleen cells. Journal of Infectious Diseases 127: 632–638

Evans A S, Dick E C 1964 Acute pharyngitis and tonsilitis in University of Wisconsin students. Journal of the American Medical Association 190: 699–708

Eron L J, Toy C, Santo Mauro D, Puretz D M Interferon therapy of recurrences of genital herpes.

Abstract No. 1242, 24th Interscience Conference on Antiviral Agents and Chemotherapy. October 810, 1984, Washington DC

Felbee T D, Smith E B, Knox J M, Wallis C, Melnick J L 1973 Photodynamic inactivation of herpes simplex. Journal of the American Medical Association 223: 289–292

Fiddian A P, Goldmeier D, Kinghorn G R, deLoning G A S, Thinj R N Successful treatment of recurrent genital herpes with topical acyclovir: comparison with oral therapy. Abstract 180, International Society for STD Research 5th International Meeting, August 1983, Seattle, Washington

Field H J, Bell S E, Elion G P, Nash A A, Wildy P 1979 Effect of acycloguanosine treatment on acute and latent herpes simplex infections in mice. Antimicrobial Agents and Chemotherapy 15: 554–61

Field H J, Darby G 1980 Pathogenicity in mice of strains of herpes simplex virus which are resistant to acyclovir in vitro and in vivo. Antimicrobial Agents and Chemotherapy 17: 209–216

Fife K H, Schmidt O, Remington M, Corey L 1983 Primary and recurrent concomitant genital infection with herpes simplex virus types 1 and 2. Journal of Infectious Diseases 147: 163

Flewett T H, Parker R G F, Philip W M 1969 Acute hepatitis due to Herpes simplex in an adult. Journal of Clinical Pathology 22: 60–61

Friedman H M, Pincus T, Gibilisco P et al 1980 Acute monoarticular arthritis caused by herpes simplex virus and cytomegalovirus. American Journal of Medicine 69: 241–247

Friedrich E G Jr, Masukawa T 1975 Effect of povidone-iodine on herpes genitalis. Obstetrics and Gynecology 45: 337–339

Glezen W P, Fernald G W, Lohr J A 1975 Acute respiratory disease of university students with special reference to the etiologic role of herpesvirus hominis. American Journal of Epidemiology 101: 111–120

Gnann J, Whitely R, Reichman R, Wolinsky S, Nahmias A, Keyserling H Controlled trial of parenteral interferon alpha-2 in the treatment of recurrent genital herpes. Abstract 1024, 24th Interscience Conference on Antimicrobial Agents and Chemotherapy, October 8–10, 1984, Washington, DC

Gold D, Benedetti J A, Critchlow C, Remington M, Winter C, Fahnlander A, Corey L Recurrence rate of symptomatic genital HSV-2 infection. Abstract, American Federation for Clinical Research, May 3–6, 1985, Washington DC

Goldstein L C, Corey L, McDougall J, Tollentino E, Spear P, Nowinski R C 1983 Monoclonal antibodies to herpes simplex viruses: use in antigenic typing and rapid diagnosis. Journal of Infectious Diseases 147: 829–37

Goodell S E, Quinn T C, Mkritchian E E, Schuffler M D, Corey L, Holmes K K 1983 Herpes simplex virus: an important cause of acute proctitis in homosexual men. New England Journal of Medicine 308: 868–871

Grauballe P C, Vestergaard B F 1977 ELISA for herpes simplex virus type 2 antibodies. Lancet 2: 1038–1039

Guinan M E, MacCalman J, Kern E R, Overall J C, Spruance S L 1980 Topical ether and herpes simplex labialis. Journal of the American Medical Association 243: 1059–1061

Guinan M E, MacCalman J, Kern E R, Overall J C, Spruance S L 1981 Course of an untreated episode of recurrent genital herpes simplex infection in 27 women. New England Journal of Medicine 304: 759–763

Harger J H, Pazin G J, Armstrong J A, Breinig M C, Ho M 1983 Characteristics and management of pregnancy in women with genital herpes simplex virus infection. American Journal of Obstetrics and Gynecology 145: 784

Heller M, Dix Rd, Baringer J R, Schachter J, Cante J E 1982 Herpetic proctitis and meningitis: recovery of two strains of herpes simplex virus type 1 from cerebrospinal fluid. Journal of Infectious Diseases 146: 1–6

Hilleman M R, Larson V M, Lehman E D et al 1981 Subunit herpes simplex 2 vaccine. In: Nahmias A J, Dowdle W R, Schinazi R D, (eds) The human herpesviruses: an interdisciplinary perspective. Elsevier, New York, 503–506

Hirsch M S, Zisman B, Allison A C 1970 Macrophages and age-dependent resistance to herpes simplex virus in mice. Journal of Immunology 104: 1140–1165

Holzel, A, Feldman G V, Tobin J O, Harper J 1953 Herpes simplex: a study of complement fixing antibodies at different ages. Acta Paediatr; Scand 42: 206–14

Hutfield DC 1966 History of herpes genitalis. British Journal of Venereal Disease 42: 263–268

Jeansson S, Molin L 1970 Genital herpesvirus hominis infection: a venereal disease. Lancet 1: 1064

Jeansson S, Molin L 1974 On the occurrence of genital herpes simplex virus infection. Acta Dermatologica Venereologica 54: 479–85

Johnson A O, Salimonu L S, Osunkoya B O 1981 Antibodies to herpesvirus hominis types 1 and 2 in malnourished Nigerian children.
Archives of Diseases in Children 56: 45–48

Jones B R, Coster D J, Falcon M G, Cantell K 1976 Topical therapy of ulcerative herpetic keratitis with human interferon. Lancet 2: 128

Jose D G, Minty C C J 1980 Levamisole in patients with recurrent herpes infection. Medical Journal of Australia; 2: 390–394

Joseph T J, Vogt R J 1974 Disseminated herpes with hepatoadrenal necrosis in an adult. American Journal of Medicine 56: 735–739

Josey W E, Nahmias A J, Naib Z M, Utley D M, McKenzie W J, Coleman M T 1966 Genital herpes simplex infection in the fermale. American Journal of Obstetrics and Gynecology 96: 493–501

Josey W, Nahmias A, Naib Z 1972 The epidemiology of type 2 (genital) herpes simplex virus infection. Obstetric and Gynecology Survey 27: 295–302

Judson F N, Penley K A, Robinson M E, Smith J K 1980 Comparative prevalence rates of sexually transmitted diseases in heterosexual and homosexual men. American Journal of Epidemiology 112: 836–843

Kalinyak J E, Fleagle G, Docherty J J 1977 Incidence and distribution of herpes simplex virus types 1 and 2 from genital lesions in college women. Journal of Medical Virology 1: 175–181

Kaufman R H, Gardner H L, Rawls W E, Dixon R E, Young R L 1973 Clinical features of herpes genitalis. Cancer Research 33: 1446–1451

Kawana T, Kawaguchi T, Sakamoto S 1976 Clinical and virological studies on genital herpes (letter). Lancet 2: 964

Kern A B, Schiff B L, 1959 Smallpox vaccinations in the management of recurrent herpes simplex: a controlled evaluation. Journal of Investigative Dermatology 33: 99–102

Kern E R, et al 1978 Treatment of experimental herpesvirus infections with phosphonoformate and some comparison with phosphonoacetate. Antimicrobial Agents and Chemotherapy 14: 817

Kern E R, Glasgow L A, Klein R J, Friedman-Kien A E 1982 Failure of 2-deoxy-D-glucose in treatment of experimental cutaneous and genital herpes simplex virus (HSV) infections. Journal of Infectious Diseases 146 (2): 159–166

Kinghorn G R, Hafiz S, McEntegart M G 1982 Pathogenic microbial flora of genital ulcers in Sheffield with particular reference to herpes simplex virus and Haemophilus ducreyi. British Journal of Venereal Disease 58: 377–80

Kirchner H 1982 Immunology of infection with herpes simplex virus. In: Melnick J L, (ed) Houston, Texas

Kitces E N, Morahan P S, Tew J G, Murray B K 1978 Herpes simplex virus vaccine: protection from stomatitis, ganglionitis, encephalitis and latency. IARC Science Publication 24 (part 2) 1027–1032

Klastensky J, Cappel R, Snoeck J M, Flament J, Thiry L 1972 Ascending myelitis in association with Herpes simplex virus. New England Journal of Medicine 287: 182–184

Klein R J, Friedman-Kien A E, DeStefano E 1979a Latent herpes simplex virus infections in sensory ganglia of hairless mice prevented by acycloguanosine. Antimicrobial Agents and Chemotherapy 15: 723–729

Klein R J, Friedman-Kien A E, Yellin P B 1979b Orofacial herpes simplex virus infection in hairless mice: latent virus in trigeminal ganglia after topical antiviral treatment. Infection and Immunity 20: 130–135

Knox G E, Pass R F, Reynolds D W, Stagno S, Alford C A 1979 Comparative prevalence of subclinical cytomegalovirus and herpes simplex virus in the genital and urinary tracts of low-income urban women. Journal of Infectious Diseases 140: 419–422

Knox S R, Corey L, Blough H A, Lerner A M 1982 Historical findings in subjects from a high socioeconomic group who have genital infections with herpes simplex virus. Sexually Transmitted Diseases 9: 15–20

Koberman T, Clark L, Griffin W T 1980. Maternal death secondary to disseminated herpesvirus hominis. American Journal of Obstetrics and Gynecology 137: 742–743

Kohl S, Loo L S 1982 Protection of neonatal mice against herpes simplex virus infection: probable in vivo antibody dependent cellular cytotoxicity. Journal of Immunology 129: 370–376

Kristensson K, Vahlne A, Person L A, Lycke E 1978 Neural spread of herpes simplex virus type 1 and 2 in mice after corneal or subcutaneous (footpad) inoculation. Journal of Neurological Sciences 45: 331–340

Lafferty W, Remington R, Winter C, Fahnlander A, Corey L Natural history of concomitant pharyngeal and genital HSV infection: influence of viral type and anatomic site on recurrence rates. Abstract, American Federation for Clinical Research, May 3–6, 1985. Washington, DC

Lerner A M, Shippey M J, Crane L R 1974 Serological responses to herpes simplex virus in rabbits: Complement requiring neutralizing, conventional neutralizing, and passive hemmagglutinating antibodies. Journal of Infectious Diseases 129: 623–636

Levine J B, Saeed M 1979 Herpesvirus hominis (type 1) proctitis. Journal of Clinical Gastroenterology 1: 225–227

Linnemann C C, First M R, Alvira M M, Alexander J W, Schiff G M 1976 Herpesvirus hominis type 2 meningoencephalitis following renal transplantation. American Journal of Medicine 61: 703–708

Lipschutz B 1921 Untersuchungen uber die aetiologic der krankheiten der Herpesgrupbpe (Herpes zoster, herpes genetalis, Herpes februlis). Archives of Dermatology, Syph Birl; 136: 428–482

Lopez C 1985 Natural resistance mechanisms in herpes simplex virus infection. 1985 Roizman B and Lopez C (eds) In: The herpesviruses, Plenum Press, New York, vol. 4, p 37–60

Lopez C, Ryshke R, Bennett M 1980 Marrow-dependent cells depleted by 89 Sr mediate resistance to herpes simplex virus type 1 infection in mice. Infection and Immunity 28: 1028–1032

Luby J P, Gnann J W, Alexander W J, Hatcher V A, Freidman-Kein A E, Klein R J, Keyserling H, Nahmias A, Mills J, Schachter J, Douglas J M, Corey L, Sacks S L 1984 A collaborative study of patient-initiated treatment of recurrent genital herpes with topical aclycovir or placebo. Journal of Infectious Diseases 150: 1–6

MacCallum F O, Juel-Jensen B E 1966 Treatment of Herpes simplex virus skin infection with IDU in dimethylsulfoxide. Results of double-blind controlled trial. British Medical Journal 2: 805–807

Mann S L, Meyers J D, Holmes K K, Corey L 1984 Prevalence and incidence of herpesvirus infections among homosexually active men. Journal of Infectious Diseases 149: 1026–1027

McClung H, Seth P, Rawls W E, 1976 Relative concentration in human sera of antibodies to cross reacting and specific antigens of HSV virus types 1 and 2. American Journal of Epidemiology 104: 192–201

McLaren C, Corey L, Dekket C, Barry D W 1983 In vitro sensitivity to acyclovir in genital herpes simplex viruses isolated from acytclovir treated patients. Journal of Infectious Diseases 148: 868–875

Meheus A, VanDyck E, Ursi J P, Ballard R C, Piot P 1982 Etiology of genital ulcerations in Swaziland. American Venereal Disease Association 10: 33–35

Merriman H G, Woods S, Winter C, Fahnlander A, Corey L 1984 Secretory IgA antibody in cervicovaginal secretions in women with genital herpes simplex virus infection. Journal of Infectious Diseases 149(4): 505–510

Mertz G J, Schmidt O, Jourden J L, Guinan M E, Remington M L, Fahnlander A, Winter C, Holmes K K, Corey L 1985 Frequency of acquisition of first episode genital herpes simplex virus infection from symptomatic and asymptomatic source contacts. Sexually Transmitted Diseases 12: 33–39

Mertz G J, Critchlow C, Benedetti J, Reichman R C, Dolin R, Connor J, Redfield D C, Savoia M C, Richmann D D, Tyrrell D L, Miedzinski L, Portnoy J, Keeney R E, Corey L 1984 Double blind placebo-controlled trial of oral acyclovir in first episode genital herpes simplex virus infection. Journal of the American Medical Association 252: 1147–1151

Meyers J D, Flournoy N, Thomas E D 1980 Infection with herpes simplex virus and cell-mediated immunity after marrow transplant. Journal of Infectious Diseases 142: 338–346

Milman N, Scheible J, Jessen O 1978 Failure of lysine treatment in recurrent herpes simplex labialis. Lancet, 2: 942

Mindel A, Adler M W, Sutherland S, Fiddian A P 1982 Intravenous acyclovir treatment for primary genital herpes. Lancet 1: 697–700

Mindel A, Faherty A, Hindley D, Weller I V D, Sutherland S, Fiddian A P, Adler M W 1984 Prophylactic oral acyclovir in recurrent genital herpes. Lancet 57–59

Mintz L, Drew W L, Hoo R, Finley T N 1980 Age-dependent resistance of human alveolar macrophages to herpes simplex virus. Infection and Immunity 28: 417–420

Montefiore D, Sogbetun A O, Anong C N, 1980 Herpesvirus hominis type 2 infection in Ibadan: problem of non-venereal transmission. British Journal of Venereal Disease 56: 49–53

Morahan P S, Kern E R, Glasgow L A 1977. Immunomodulator-induced resistance against herpes simplex virus. Proceedings Social Experimental Biological Medicine 154: 615–620

Moseley, R, Corey L, Winter C, Benjamin D 1981 Comparison of the indirect immunoperoxidase and direct immunofluorescence techniques with viral isolation for the diagnosis of genital herpes simplex virus infection. Journal of Clinical Microbiology 13: 913–918

Myers M G, Oxman M N, Clark J E, Arndt K A 1975 Failure of neutral-red photo-dynamic inactivation in recurrent herpes simplex virus infections. New England Journal of Medicine 293: 945–949

Nahmias A J, Naib Z M, Josey W E, Clipper A C 1966 Genital herpes simplex infection virologic and cytologic studies. Obstetrics and Gynecology 29: 395–400

Nahmias A J, Dowdle W R 1968 Antigenic and biologic differences in herpesvirus hominis. Progress Medical Virology 10: 110–159

Nahmias A J, Dowdle W R, Naib Z M et al 1969a Genital infection with type 2 herpes virus hominis: a commonly occurring venereal disease. British Journal of Venereal Disease 45: 294–8

Nahmias A J, Dowdle W R, Josey W E et al 1969b Newborn infection with herpesvirus hominis types 1 and 2. Journal of Pediatrics 75: 1194–1203

Nahmias A J, Josey W E, Naib Z M, Luce C F, Duffey A 1970a Antibodies to herpesvirus hominis types 1 and 2 in humans. American Journal of Epidemiology 91: 539–546

Nahmias A J 1970b Disseminated herpes simplex virus infections. New England Journal of Medicine 282: 684–685

Nahmias A J, Roizman D 1973 Infection with herpes simplex virus 1 and 2. New England Journal of Medicine 299: 667–674, 719–725,781–789

Nahmias A J 1983 (Personal communication)

Nilson A E, Assen T, Halsos A M, Kinge B R, Tjotta E A L, Wikstrom K, Fiddian A P 1982 Efficacy of oral acyclovir in the treatment of initial and recurrent genital herpes. Lancet; Sep 11: 571–573

Norilld B 1985 Humoral immune response to herpes simplex virus infections. Roizman B, Lopez C, (eds) In: The herpesviruses, Plenum Press, New York, vol. 4, p 69–85

Notkins A L 1974 Immune mechanisms by which the spread of viral infections is stopped. Cellular Immunology 11: 478–483

O'Rcilly R J, Chibbaro A, Anger E et al 1977 Cell-mediated immune response in patients with recurrent herpes simplex virus infections. II. Infection-associated deficiency of lymphokine production in patients with recurrent herpes labialis or herpes progenitalis. Journal of Immunology 108: 1095–1102

Overall J C Jr, Kern E R, Schlitzer R L, Friedman S B, Glasgow L A, 1975 Genital herpesvirus hominis infection in mice I: development of an experimental model. Infection and Immunity 11: 476–480

Parker F, Nye R W 1925 Studies on filterable viruses II: cultivation of herpes virus. American Journal of Pathology (1): 337–340

Pavan-Langston D R 1979. Ocular Viral Diseases. In: Galasso G J, Merigan T C, Buchanan R A (eds): Antiviral Agents and Viral Diseases of Man. New York, Raven Press 253–303

Pazin G J, Armstrong J A, Lam M T, Tarr G C, Jannetta R J, Ho M 1978 Prevention of reactivated herpes simplex infection by human leukocyte interferon after operation on the trigeminal root. New England Journal of Medicine 301: 225–230

Peacock J E, Sarubbi F A 1983 Disseminated herpes simplex virus infection during pregnancy. Obstetrics and Gynecology 61: 135–137

Pereira L, Dondero D V, Gallo P, Devlin V, Woodie J D 1982 Serological analysis of herpes simplex virus types 1 and 2 with monoclonal antibodies. Infection and Immunity 363–367

Person D A, Kaufman R H, Gardner H L, Rawls W E 1973 Herpesvirus type 2 in genitourinary tract infection. American Journal of Obstetrics and Gynecology 116: 993–995

Plummer F A, Nsanze H, Costa L J, Karasira P, Maclean I W, Ellison R H, Ronald A R 1983 Single-dose therapy of chancroid with trimethoprim-sulfametrole. New England Journal of Medicine 309(2): 67–71

Plummer G, Waner J L, Phuangsab A et al 1970 Type 1 and 2 herpes simplex viruses: Serological and biological differences. Journal of Virology 5: 51–59

Porter D D, Wimberly I, Benyesh-Melnick M 1969 Prevalence of antibodies to EB virus and other herpesviruses. Journal of the American Medical Association 208: 1675–1679

Prakash S S, Seth P 1979 Evaluation of indirect hemagglutination and its inhibition in the differentiation between antibodies to Herepes simplex virus types 1 and 2 for seroepidemiologic studies: Use of a II/I index threshold of 85 and an assay of type-specific antibodies. Journal of Infectious Diseases 139: 524–528

Quinn T C, Stamm W E, Goodell S E, Mkrtichian E, Benedetti J, Corey L, Schuffler M D, Holmes K K 1983 The polymicrobial origin of intestinal infections in homosexual men. New England Journal of Medicine 309: 576–582

Ramsey P G, Fife, K, Hackman R, Meyers J D, Corey L 1982 Herpes simplex virus pneumonia; clinical presentation and pathogenesis. Annals of Internal Medicine 97: 813–820

Rasmussen L E, Jordan G W, Stevens D A, Merigan T C 1974 Lymphocyte interferon production and transformation after herpes simplex infections in humans. Journal of Immunology 112: 728–736

Rattray M C, Corey L, Reeves W C, Vontver L A, Holmes K K 1978 Recurrent genital herpes among women: symptomatic versus asymptomatic viral shedding. British Journal of Venereal Disease 54: 262–265

Rattray M C, Peterman G M, Altman L C, Corey L, Holmes K K 1980 Lymphocyte-derived chemotactic factor synthesis in initial genital herpesvirus infections: correlation with lymphocyte transformation. Infection and Immunity 30: 110–116

Rauh J L, Brookman R R, Schiff G M 1977 Genital surveillance among sexually active adolescent girls. Journal of Pediatrics 90: 844

Ravaut P, Darre M, 1904 Les reactions nerveuses au cours des herpes genitaux. Ann Dermato Syphil (Paris), 5: 481–496

Rawls W E, Iwamoto K, Adam E, Melnick J L 1970 Measurement of antibodies to herpesvirus types 1 and 2 in human sera. Journal of Immunology 104: 599–606

Rawls W E, Gardner H L, Flunders R W, Lawry S P, Kaufman R H, Melnick J L 1971 Genital herpes in 2 social groups. American Journal of Obstetrics and Gynecology 110: 682–689

Rawls W E 1979 Herpes simplex viruses type 1 and 2, in Lennette E H, Schmidt N J: Diagnostic procedures for viral, rickettsial and chlamydial infections, 5th ed. Washington, DC, American Public Health Association; 309–354

Reeves W C, Corey L, Adams H G, Vontver L A, Holmes K K 1981 Risk of recurrence after first episodes of genital herpes: Relation to HSV type and antibody response. New England Journal of Medicine 305: 315–319

Reichman R C et al 1984 Orally administered acyclovir in the therapy of recurrent herpes simplex genitalis: a controlled trial. Journal of the American Medical Association 251(16): 2103–2108

Renis H E, Eidson E E, Mathews J, Gray J E 1976 Pathogenesis of herpes simplex virus types 1 and 2 in mice after various routes of inoculation. Infection and Immunity 14: 571–578

Rompalo A M, Mertz G J, Mkrtichian E E, Price C B, Stamm W E, Corey L 1985 Oral acyclovir versus placebo for the treatment of herpes simplex virus proctitis. Abstract, American Federation for Clinical Research, Carmel California, February 5–8, 1985

Roome A P C H, Montefiore D, Waller D, 1975 Incidence of Herpesvirus hominis antibodies among blood donor populations. British Journal of Venereal Disease 51: 324–328

Ross C A C, Stevenson J 1961 Herpes simplex meningoencephalitis. Lancet 2: 682–685

Ruchman I, Dodd K, 1950 Recovery of herpes simplex virus from the blood of a patient with herpetic rhinitis. Journal of Laboratory and Clinical Medicine 35: 434–439

Russell A S, Brisson E, Grace M 1978 A double-blind, controlled trial of levamisole in the treatment of recurrent herpes labialis. Journal of Infectious Diseases 137: 597–600

Sacks S L 1984 Frequency and duration of patient-observed recurrent genital HSV infections: characterization of the non-lesionsal prodrome. Journal of Infectious Diseases 150: 873–877

Scheibel M, Jesson O 1979 Lysine prophylaxis in recurrent herpes simplex labialis: a double-blind controlled cross over study. Acta Dermatologica Venereologica (Stockholm); 60: 85–87

Scher J, Bottone E, Desmond E, Simons W 1982 The incidence and outcome of asymptomatic herpes simplex genitealis in an obstetric population. American Journal of Obstetrics and Gynecology 144: 906–907

Schlesinger J J, Gandara D, Bensch K G 1978 Myoglobinuria associated with herpes-group viral infections. Archives of Internal Medicine 138: 422–424

Schmidt O W, Fife K H, Corey L 1984 Reinfection is an uncommon occurrence in patients with symptomatic recurrent genital herpes. Journal of Infectious Diseases 149(4): 645–646

Schneider V, Behm F G, Mumaw V R 1982 Ascending herpetic endometritis. Obstetrics and Gynecology 59: 259–262

Schneweis K E 1962 Z um antigenen aufbau des herpes simplex virus. Z Immunitaetsforsch 124: 173

Scriba M, 1978 Protection of guinea pigs against primary and recurrent genital herpes infections by immunication with live heterologous or homologous herpes simplex virus: implications for herpes virus vaccine. Medical Microbiology and Immunology 166: 63–69

Sheridan J F, Donnenberg A D, Aurelian L, Elpern D J 1982 Immunity to herpes simplex virus type 2. Journal of Immunology 129: 326–333

Shillitoe E J, Wilton J M A, Lehner T 1978 Sequential changes in cell-mediated immune response to Herpes simplex virus following primary herpetic infection in man. In: de The G, Henle W, Rapp F (eds) Oncogenesis and herpesviruses Part 2: Cell-virus Interactions, Host Response to Herpesvirus Infection and Associated Tumors, Role of Co-Factors. Lyon, France, International Agency for Research on Cancer

Shore S L, Black C M, Melewicz F M, Wood P A, Nahmias A J 1976 Antibody-dependent cell-mediated cytotoxicity to target cells infected with type 1 and type 2 herpes simplex virus. Journal of Immunology 116: 194–201

Shore S L, Milgrom H, Wood P A and Nahmias A J 1977 Antibody dependent cellular cytotoxicity to target cells infected with herpes simplex virus: functional adequacy in the neonate. Pediatrics 59: 22–28

Sibrack C D, Gutman L T, Wilfert C M, McLaren C, Barry D W 1982 Altered pathogenicity of acyclovir resistant herpes simplex virus type 1 from an immunodeficient child. Journal of Infectious Diseases 146 (5): 673–682

Silvestri D L, Corey L, Holmes K K 1982 Ineffectiveness of topical idoxuridine in dimethylsulfoxide for therapy of genital herpes. Journal of the American Medical Association 248: 953–959

Skinner G R B, Woodman C B J, Hartley C E, Buchan A, Fuller A, Durham J, Synnott M, Clay J C, Melling J, Wiblin C, Wilkins J 1982 Preparation and immunogenicity of vaccine Ac NFU, (S-) MRC towards the prevention of herpes genitalis. British Journal of Venereal Disease 58: 381–386

Skoldenberg B, Jeansson S, Wolontis S 1975 Herpes simplex virus 2 and acute aseptic meningitis. Scandinavian Journal of Infectious Disease 7: 227–232

Smith C B, Charette R P, Fox J P, Cooney M K, Hall C E 1980 Double-blind evaluation of ribavirin in naturally occurring influenza. In: Smith R A, Kirkpatrick W (eds) Ribavirin: a broad spectrum antiviral agent. New York, Academic Press, p 147–164

Smith I W, Pleutherer J F 1967 The incidence of herpesvirus hominis antibody in the population. Journal of Hygiene 65: 395–408

Spruance S L, Crumpacker C S, Haines H et al 1979a Ineffectiveness of topical adenine arabinoside

5'-monophosphate in the treatment of recurrent herpes simplex labialis. New England Journal of Medicine 300: 1180–1184

Spruance S L, Krueger G G, MacCalman J, Overall J C, Klauber M R 1979b Treatment of recurrent herpes simplex labialis with levamisole. Antimicrobial Agents and Chemotherapy 15: 662–665

Stamm W E, Wagner K F, Amsel R, Alexander E R, Turck M, Counts G W, Holmes K K 1980 Causes of the acute urethral syndrome in women. New England Journal of Medicine 303: 409–415

Starr S E 1977 Immunotherapy for recurrent herpetic infections. Cutis; 20: 596

Stavraky K M, Rawls W E, Chiavetta J, Donner A P, Wanklin J M 1983 Sexual and socioeconomic factors affecting the risk of past infections with herpes simplex virus type 2. American Journal of Epidemiology 118: 109–121

STD Fact Sheet, Edition 35. U.S. Department of Health and Human Services, Public Health Service, Centers for Disease Control. Atlanta, Georgia, 5–12

Steele R W, Myers M G, Vincent M M 1980 Transfer factor for the prevention of varicella-zoster infection in childhood leukemia. New England Journal of Medicine 303: 355–359

Straus S E, Takiff H E, Seidlin M, Bachrach S, Lininger L, DiGiovanna J J, Western K A, Smith H A et al 1984 Suppression of frequently recurring genital herpes; a placebo-controlled double-blind trial of oral acyclovir. New England Journal of Medicine 310: 1545–1550

Stevens J G, Cook M L 1974 Maintenance of latent herpetic infection: an apparent role for anti-viral IgG. Journal of Immunology 113: 1685–1693

Sullivan-Bolyai J, Hull H F, Wilson C, Corey L 1983 Neonatal herpes simplex virus infection in King County, Washington: Increasing incidence and epidemiologic correlates. Journal of the American Medical Association 250: 3059–3062

Sumaya C V, Marx J, Ullis K 1980 Genital infections with herpes simplex virus in a university student population. Sexually Transmitted Diseases 7: 16–20.

Sutton A L, Smithwick E M, Seligman S J, Kim D S 1974 Fatal disseminated herpesvirus hominis type 2 infection in an adult with associated thymic dysplasia. American Journal of Medicine 56: 545–553

Tager A 1974 Preliminary report on the treatment on recurrent herpes simplex with poliomyelitis vaccine (Sabin's). Dermatologica 149: 253–255

Taintivanich S, Tharavawij V 1980 Prevalence of genital herpes virus infection in Thai women. Southeast Asian Journal of Tropical Medicine Public Health; 11: 127–130

Taniguchi S, Yoshino K 1965 Studies on the neutralization of herpes simplex virus II. Analysis of complement as the antibody-potentiating factor. Virology; 26: 54–60

Taylor C A, Hendley S O, Greer K E, Gwaltney J M 1977 Topical treatment of herpes labialis with chloroform. Archives of Dermatology 113: 1150

Tejani N, Klein S W, Kaplan M 1979 Subclinical herpes simplex genitalis infections in the perinatal period. American Journal of Obstetrics and Gynecology 135: 547

Tustin A W, Kaiser A B 1979 Life threatening pharyngitis caused by herpes simplex virus type 2. Sexually Transmitted Diseases 6: 23–24

Vestergaard B F, Rune S J 1980 Type-specific herpes simplex virus antibodies in patients with recurrent duodenal ulcer. Lancet 1: 1273–1274

Vesterinen E, Purola E, Sadsela E et al 1977 Clinical and virological findings in patients with cytologically diagnosed gynecologic herpes simplex infection. Acta Cytology 21: 199–205

Vontver L A, Reeves W C, Rattray M et al 1979 Clinical course and diagnosis of genital herpes simplex virus infection and evaluation of topical surfactant therapy. American Journal of Obstetrics and Gynecology 133: 548–554

Vontver L A, Hickok D E, Brown Z, Reid L, Corey L 1982 Recurrent genital herpes simplex virus infection in pregnancy: infant outcome and frequency of asymptomatic recurrences. American Journal of Obstetrics and Gynecology 142: 75

Wallin J, Lernestedt J-O, Lycke E et al 1981 Therapeutic efficacy of trisodium phosphonoformate in treatment of recurrent herpes labialis (abstract) In: Nahmias A J, Dowdle W R, Schinazi R F (eds) The human herpesviruses, New York, Elsevier, 503: 5

Wallin J, Lernestedt J-O, Lycke E, Ogenstad S 1983 Topical treatment of recurrent genital herpes with foscarnet: a double blind placebo controlled study. Abstract No. 181, 5th International Society Meeting for STD Research, August 1–3, 1983, Seattle, Washington

Waugh M A 1976 Anorectal herpesvirus hominis infection in man. Journal of the American Venereal Disease Association 3:68

Wentworth B B, Alexander E R 1971 Seroepidemiology of infections due to member of the herpesvirus group. American Journal of Epidemiology 94: 496–507

Wentworth B B, Bonin P, Holmes K K, Alexander E R 1973 Isolation of viruses, bacteria and other organisms from venereal disease clinic patients: methodology and problems associated with multiple isolations. Health Lab Science 10: 75–81

Wheeler C E Jr, Abele D C 1966. Eczema herpeticum, primary and recurrent. Archives of Dermatology 93: 162–173

Whitley R J, Nahmias A J, Visintine A M, Fleming C L, Alford C A 1980a The natural history of herpes simplex virus infection of mother and newborn. Pediatrics 66: 489–494

Whitley R J, Nahmias A J, Soong S J, Galasso G G, Flemming C L, Alford C A 1980b Vidarabine therapy of neonatal herpes simplex virus infection. Pediatrics 66: 495–501

Whitley R J, et al 1981 Herpes simplex encephalitis vidarabine therapy and diagnostic problem. New England Journal of Medicine 304: 313

Whittaker J A, Hardson M D 1978 Severe thrombocytopenia after generalized HSV-2 infection. Southern Medical Journal 71: 864–866

Wolontis S, Jeannson S 1977 Correlations of herpes simplex virus types 1 and 2 with clinical features of infection. Journal of Infectious Diseases 135: 28–33

Worthington M. Conliffe M A, Baron S 1980 Mechanism of recovery from systemic herpes simplex virus infection. II. Effectiveness of antibody reconstitution of nude and neonatally thymectomized mice. Proceedings of the Society for Experimental Biology and Medicine 165: 462–468

Yeo J, Killington R A, Watson D H, Powell K L 1981 Studies on cross reactive antigens in herpes viruses. Virology 108: 256–266

Young E J, Killam A P, Greene J F 1976 Disseminated herpesvirus infection association with primary genital herpes in pregnancy. Journal of the American Medical Association 235: 2731–2733

Zisman B, Hirsch M S, Allison A C 1970 Selective effects of anti-macrophage serum, silica and anti-lymphocyte serum on pathogenesis of herpes virus infection of young adult mice. Journal of Immunology 104: 1155–1159

Zweerink H J and Corey L 1982 Virus-specific antibodies in sera from patients with genital herpes simplex virus infection. Infection and Immunity 37: 413–421

6. Genital papillomavirus infections: virology

D. J. McCance

INTRODUCTION

Papillomaviruses (papilla = nipple; oma = tumour) are a group of species specific viruses infecting a wide range of animals including such seemingly unlikely species as the chaffinch and African Gray Parrot (Jacobson et al, 1983; Osterhaus et al, 1983). The viruses produce in their hosts benign skin tumours (papillomas) which contain a variable amount of infectious virus. Common hand warts and plantar warts are the commonest skin papillomas of man, and those papillomaviruses infecting the genital areas are now recognised to be associated with a variety of lesions. Until recently little interest was generated in these viruses mainly because they cannot be grown in tissue culture as other viruses, and they were not linked to any major disease process. Now that they have been linked with genital cancers interest has been stimulated, but the problem of in vitro replication of these viruses remains, so genetic manipulation techniques are used to detect viral DNA in tissues and to help broaden our knowledge of the molecular organisation of this virus group. This chapter deals with the properties of the papillomaviruses and with the serological and molecular diagnosis of the various genital papillomavirus infections, while subsequent chapters deal more specifically with the types of lesions associated with infection and with their treatment.

HUMAN PAPILLOMAVIRUS (HPV) TYPES

The human papillomaviruses (HPV) are a genus within the family Papovaviridae — another genus within the family is the Polyomavirus group whose type species is the polyoma virus of mice. This genus also contains species specific viruses of which at least two, BK and JC, infect humans.

There are at present 30 types of human papillomavirus. The types are not differentiated serologically (HPV 1–3 and 4 only have been shown to have serological differences) as with other virus groups because of the lack of antigen available to produce antibodies for testing, since as mentioned these viruses cannot be grown in vitro (see next section). Instead, the genus is divided into types depending on the homology (percentage cross-hybridisation) of their DNA molecules, i.e. how similar the sequence or nucleotide pairings of the DNA of one HPV is to that of another. An arbitrary figure of 50% is set, so if a new papillomavirus is isolated and has a DNA molecule which has 50% or greater homology with a virus already isolated it will be placed into that typing group. If the homology is less than 50% then it is placed in a new group. Within the papillomavirus group cross hybridisation is very heterogeneous, with some HPV types having no detectable sequence homology e.g. HPV1, 2, 4,

7 while other types may be grouped on the basis of variable cross hybridisation e.g. HPV3, 10, 28 show 25–35% homology while HPV5, 8, 12, 14, 19, 20–23 show 5–40% homology and HPV9, 15, 17 show 6–22% homology (Kremsdorf et al, 1983; Kremsdorf et al, 1984; Orth, personal communication). There are at present four genital HPVs; HPV6, 11, 16 and 18. Recently HPV6 and HPV11 have been shown to have homology of the order of 82%, so these two isolates may be moved into the same typing group.

Several of the types are subdivided because although they show extensive cross-hybridisation the number of restriction sites for an endonuclease may vary e.g. HPV6a has no sites for EcoR1 but HPV6b has one site. Table 6.1 shows the common types of HPVs and their associated lesions.

Table 6.1   Human papillomavirus types and associated lesions

HPV types	Associated lesions
HPV1a, b, c	Plantar warts
HPV2a-e	Common hand warts
HPV3a, b	Flat warts/juvenile warts
HPV4	Plantar warts
HPV5a, b	Macules in EV[1] patients
HPV6a–f	Condylomata acuminata/CIN[2]I–III/VIN[3]I–III/Laryngeal papillomas
HPV7	'Butchers' warts
HPV8	Macules in EV patients
HPV9	Warts and macules in EV patients
HPV10a, b	Flat warts
HPV11a, b	Condylomata acuminata/CIN I–III/Laryngeal papillomas
HPV12	Warts and macules in EV patients
HPV13	Hyperplastic lesions on the neck
HPV14a, b	EV patients
HPV15	EV patients
HPV16	Condylomata acuminata/CIN I–III/VIN I–III/Malignant carcinoma of cervix and penis
HPV17a, b	EV patients
HPV18	Malignant carcinoma of cervix and penis
HPV19–29	Various warty lesions in EV patients
HPV30	Laryngeal carcinoma

[1] EV — Epidermodysplasia Verruciformis
[2] CIN — Cervical intraepithelial neoplasia
[3] VIN — Vulvar intraepithelial neoplasia

PHYSICAL AND CHEMICAL PROPERTIES

1. Structure

The virion is the complete mature virus particle including the genome and capsid proteins (coat proteins). The papillomavirus virion is 50 nm–55 nm in diameter and the capsid, which has an icosahedral symmetry, is made up of 72 individual capsomeres (protein subunits) (Fig. 6.1). The complete particles show a density of 1.34 g/cm³ in Cscl gradients while empty particles (without DNA) band at 1.29 g/cm³.

2. The genome

The virion contains a double stranded DNA molecule of 5×10^6 daltons molecular weight. The DNA in the virion has a supercoiled circular form (Form I), but two other configurations, nicked circular (Form II) and linear (Form III) are found on extraction of the DNA (Fig. 6.2). These latter two forms are produced on extraction

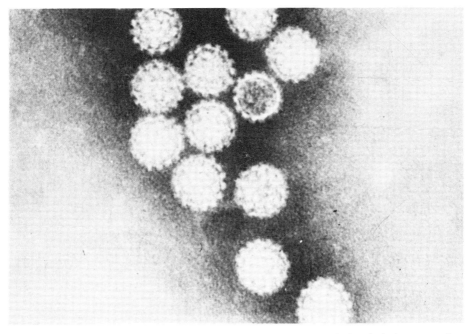

Fig. 6.1   An electromicrograph of human papillomavirus particles to show the icosahedral structure of the virion, with a diameter of 50–55 mm. Negative strain, X290,00 (courtesy of Dr J D Oriel).

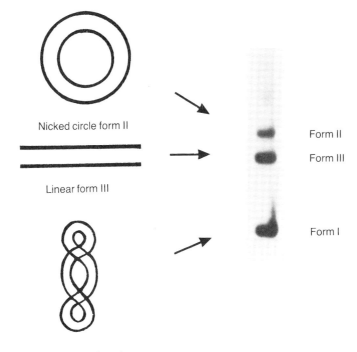

Fig. 6.2   Shows diagrammatically the three forms or configurations of the virion papillomavirus DNA and an autoradiograph of the relative positions after electrophoresis in an agarose gel.

of the DNA by the handling procedure and are also seen when extracting DNA from biopsy material (see later). The genomes of HPV type 1a (virus associated with plantar warts) and type 6b (genital warts) have been completely sequenced as has that of bovine papillomavirus type 1 (Chen et al, 1983; Danos et al, 1982; Schwarz et al, 1983). The organisation of the genomes (Fig. 6.3) is well conserved between types and can potentially code for 7–8 proteins although at present the precise number is unknown.

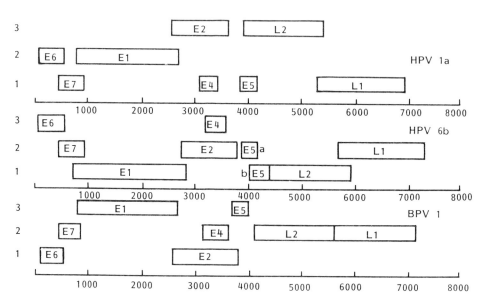

Fig. 6.3 Shows the possible open reading frames of HPV1a (top), HPV6b (middle) and BPV1 (bottom). Since DNA has three possible reading frames which are denoted on the left hand side, the boxes represent the possible mRNAs in each of these three frames. Reading frames designated L1 and L2 code for structural proteins. The function of products coded for by E frames is unknown although some are involved in the transformation of rodent cells in vitro by BPV1 (see later section).

3. Virus coded proteins

Figure 6.3 shows the theoretical open reading frames of the HPV types 1a and 6b. These open reading frames are regions of DNA bounded at the beginning and end with start and stop codons for the transcription of mRNA which when translated on ribosomes produces virally coded proteins. The L1 and L2 open reading frames probably code for the major capsid proteins (VP2 and 3). The only other information on the HPV coded capsid proteins is that there is a common structural antigen present in a masked form in the coat protein of the virion. This is exemplified when the coat protein is disrupted with detergent (sodium dodecyl sulphate, SDS) and then inoculated into an animal; the antibodies produced will cross react with all the human and animal papillomaviruses (Kurman et al, 1982). The antibodies raised only recognise disrupted papillomavirus particles and infected cells from papillomavirus induced lesions, since these cells contain the equivalent of disrupted particles as virions are being assembled during the replicative cycle There is a set of host cell coded histone proteins (H2a, H2b, H3 and H4) associated with the papillomavirus DNA also seen with the polyomavirus genus.

Serological differences between complete virions has been hampered by the difficulty of obtaining enough antigen from papillomavirus lesions, and the pooling of different warts may lead to erroneous results since there are by DNA-DNA hybridisation 30 different types of HPV many of which can produce lesions of similar clinical appearance. This has made serological data obtained in the past unreliable. It may be that when more is known about serological profiles of the HPV group 30 types can be accommodated in a much smaller number of serological groups.

REPLICATION OF PAPILLOMAVIRUSES

The replicative cycle of papillomaviruses appears to occur only in a differentiating squamous epithelium, with the full cycle producing infectious virus particles only completed in the most differentiated cells, i.e. the outer cells of the epithelium. Viral DNA may be detected in lower layers of the epithelium where no viral structural proteins are detected. The close alignment of papillomavirus replication with epithelial differentiation has constantly hampered attempts to replicate the viruses in vitro. Researchers using partially differentiating keratinocyte cultures in vitro have been successful in replicating papillomavirus DNA but no mature virus particles have been produced (La Porta & Taichman, 1982).

CELL TRANSFORMATION BY PAPILLOMAVIRUSES IN VITRO

Although papillomaviruses cannot be grown conventionally in tissue culture to produce infectious virus particles, insertion of the genome of bovine papillomavirus (BPV) into rodent fibroblasts has transformed these cells, and subsequent inoculation into nude mice produces tumours. The DNA is present as a free replicating episome in these cells so transformation can be achieved without detectable integration into the host cell chromosome (Law et al, 1981). There appear to be two regions of the genome important in this transformation process, but none of the proteins coded for by these areas have been characterised (Nakabaysahi et al, 1983). So far no HPV type has been shown to transform cells in vitro (Chesters & McCance 1985).

ONCOGENIC POTENTIAL OF HUMAN PAPILLOMAVIRUSES

Workers in the 1930s showed that the cottontail rabbit papillomavirus (CPRV) produced benign warts in its natural host the cottontail rabbit and that these benign tumours in 25% of cases would become malignant after 12 months (Rous & Beard, 1935; Syverton, 1952). Benign tumours produced in domestic rabbits would become malignant more frequently and within a shorter time. Also, application of hydrocarbons or tar produced in both animal species a higher and more rapid malignant conversion. The virus DNA was detected both in the benign and malignant lesions. These results suggested that the CRPV produced the benign lesions, but that other factors, genetic and environmental, may be necessary for production of malignant disease. More recently oesophageal, intestinal and bladder papillomas produced by bovine papillomavirus type 4 (BPV4) were shown to become malignant when cattle were fed on a diet of bracken (Jarrett et al, 1981). In this case the BPV4 DNA was only detected in the benign lesions and was not detectable after malignant conversion.

In humans, one third of patients with the rare autosomal recessive disease epidermo-dysplasia verruciformis (EV) develop squamous cell carcinomas, usually in areas exposed to sunlight. A percentage of these patients will have detectable HPV5 or 8 DNA sequences present in these lesions, and recently renal transplant patients who developed squamous cell carcinoma during their post operative immunosuppression were found to have HPV5 in these lesions. This suggests that given the right environmental or genetic conditions, benign lesions associated with HPV5 infection in particular, may develop into a carcinoma. Studies from Queensland in Australia, where squamous cell carcinoma is common amongst caucasians, show papillomavirus-like particles in hyperkeratotic lesions in sun damaged skin (Spradbrow et al, 1983). In Western Australia and Queensland BPV-like DNA sequences have been found in sheep and cattle with skin carcinomas of sun exposed areas around the nose and mouth and on the genitals (Vanselow & Spradbrow, 1982; Vanselow & Spradbrow, 1983).

The studies with animal papillomaviruses and EV patients show the association of these viruses with malignant conversion and sets a precedent when investigating the association of HPVs and genital cancers. Unfortunately there is no animal model for investigation of carcinoma of the cervix.

DETECTION OF PAPILLOMAVIRUS INFECTION

1. Culture methods

As already mentioned, no cell type has been found capable of replicating and producing infectious papillomavirus particles although several efforts have been made.

2. Immunochemical methods

As mentioned in the last section there have been difficulties in producing specific antibodies against single papillomavirus types. At the moment the antibody against the common antigen is used to detect HPV in lesions. This antibody can be raised against disrupted bovine papillomavirus extracted from bovine warts which are large and provide a plentiful supply of virions. The antibody can be used in two types of immunochemical staining technique. In all cases the principle of the test is the same. The tissue to be investigated can either be formalin fixed or snap frozen in liquid nitrogen. Sections cut from snap frozen blocks can then be fixed in methanol at $-20°C$ or acetone at room temperature after cryostat sectioning.

The specific anti-papillomavirus antibodies are interacted with the sections, the sections washed and then stained with anti-species antibodies which are tagged with a reagent which will visualise the specific antibody interactions. Anti-species antibodies are usually tagged with (a) a fluorescent dye e.g. fluorescein isothiocyanate or rhodamine (b) alkaline phosphatase or peroxidase. The latter two give the greater sensitivity and also make tissue definition much easier since fluorescent dyes are only seen against a dark background. Figure 6.4 shows a section from a cervical biopsy showing positively stained nuclei in the outer one third of the epithelium stained by the alkaline phosphatase method. Note that the positive cells are in the peripheral layers of the epithelium and these cells are producing structural antigens and mature virus particles. The staining is confined to the nucleus.

The detection rate of HPV antigens by this method in condylomata acuminata and cervical intraepithelial neoplasia (CIN) lesions is variable between studies, but 30–50% of biopsies exhibit positive staining with the antibody against the common structural antigen. There is a reduction in the percentage positive between CIN I and CIN III, probably due to the fact that mature particles are seen in the most

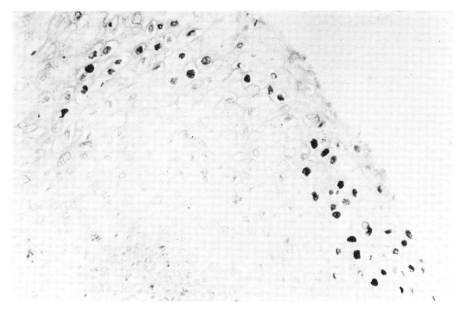

Fig. 6.4 Shows a section from a biopsy reacted with rabbit antipapillomavirus antiserum (containing antibodies against the papillomavirus common antigen) and subsequently stained with anti-rabbit antibodies tagged with alkaline phosphatase. A pink/red colour is developed using the appropriate enzyme substrate. The positive cell nuclei appear dark in this black and white plate and positive cells are found in the outer part of the epithelium (courtesy of Mr P G Walker).

differentiated cells of the epithelium and because in CIN III lesions there is complete disruption in polarity of the epithelium and few or no differentiated cells are seen in the outer cell layers of the epithelium.

3. DNA-DNA hybridisation

a Principle

It is possible to detect in a tissue a piece of viral DNA using an identical or partially identical viral DNA which has been previously isolated and purified. This latter DNA, called the probe, is usually labelled with a radio-isotope before mixing with the tissue DNA. Since both DNAs are double stranded, a denaturation step to produce single strands is carried out before mixing of the two sets of DNA (Fig. 6.5). A simple method of denaturation involves heating the DNA above its melting temperature (Tm), i.e. that temperature at which the two strands separate, and depends, if environment conditions are constant, on the deoxyguanosine + deoxycytidine triphosphate ratio (% G + C) of the DNA. The single strands are separated and when the single-stranded probe is mixed with the single-stranded total DNA from the tissue and the temperature dropped to below the Tm of the DNA, homologous single strands will re-anneal (Fig. 6.5). If any DNA in the tissue is homologous to the probe it can be detected since the probe strand is radio-labelled. This is the principle of all DNA-DNA hybridisation experiments, but in practice certain steps are taken to simplify the method and allow visualisation of re-annealed DNA by autoradiography.

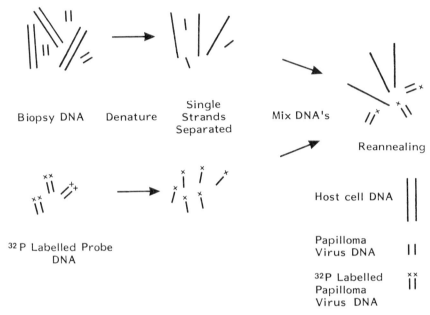

Fig. 6.5   Shows the principle of DNA-DNA hybridisation with the biopsy DNA containing both host chromosomal DNA (long lines) and papillomavirus DNA (short lines). The denaturation produces single stranded DNAs and each set of single strands can be separated and then the biopsy DNA and probe mixed and reannealing allowed to commence.

The following section introduces the method commonly used to detect papilloma virus DNA in biopsy material.

b Practice

(I) PREPARATION OF DNA FROM BIOPSY AND ELECTROPHORESIS

Total DNA is extracted from the biopsy by one of the standard techniques. This DNA when extracted carefully is very viscous, owing to the high molecular weight of cellular DNA. To make it easier to electrophorese the DNA is digested with restriction endonuclease enzymes which recognise small specific sequences of nucleotides, usually four or six base pairs in length, and digest or break each DNA strand at this site (Fig. 6.6). Most of the restriction endonucleases produce protruding complementary or 'sticky-ends' at the site of breakage which has the advantage that the piece of DNA can be joined to another fragment of DNA which is complementary due to digestion with the same enzyme. In this way DNA can be cloned into or joined to plasmid or phage DNA and replicated in bacterial cells to produce multiple copies of inserted DNA. This is a great advantage since papillomaviruses cannot be replicated in the conventional way, and it is used to produce sufficient viral probe DNA to carry out many hybridisation experiments.

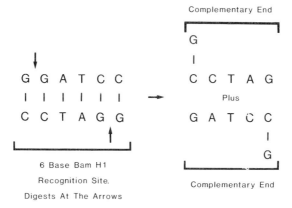

Fig. 6.6 Shows the nucleotide site of the restriction endonuclease *Bam* H1 and the complementary ends produced after digestion of DNA by the enzyme.

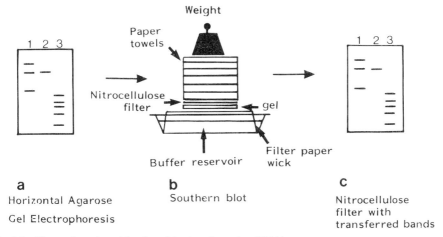

Fig. 6.7 Electrophoresis and Southern blotting of samples of DNA.
  (a) three wells (1, 2 and 3) in the horizontal contain DNA samples digested with different restriction enzymes producing different band patterns.
  (b) The transfer by Southern blotting of the bands in the gel to a nitrocellular filter, and
  (c) The resulting nitrocellulose filter containing the bands transferred from the gel. This filter can then be used for hybridisation studies.

The digested DNA from the biopsy is then electrophoresed through an agarose horizontal gel, which will separate out the total DNA into various sized fragments with the small ones moving fast and the larger ones running more slowly (Fig. 6.7a).

If the number of sites for a particular restriction endonuclease is known for HPV, e.g. *Bam*H1 has one site for HPV6a and 16 DNA, then by digesting with this enzyme a linear molecule will be produced (Fig. 6.2), and it will run a certain distance on the gel. After the gel has been run, usually for 10–15 hours at low voltage, the DNA fragments are denatured by alkali treatment which produces single-stranded molecules and then transferred to nitrocellulose paper by a process called Southern Blotting

(Southern, 1975; Fig. 6.7b). The capillary flow of the buffer from the reservoir through the gel and up through the paper towels, transfers the DNA through the thickness of the gel onto the nitrocellulose filter, where it is trapped. The result is the nitrocellulose filter becomes a image of what was on the gel and each band is transferred to the nitrocellulose in the same relationship to other bands as in the gel (Fig. 6.7c). To make sure the DNA is irreversibly stuck to the nitrocellulose the filter is baked at 80°C in a vacuum oven.

(II) RADIOLABELLING THE DNA PROBE
Searching for small amounts of viral DNA in the total DNA extracted needs probes which are labelled with a relatively high energy emitter at a high specific activity. This can be achieved using ^{32}P (phosphorus) labelled triphosphates (nucleotide triphosphates ATP, GTP, CTP, TTP) and by a process called nick translation (Rigby et al, 1977) the labelled triphosphates can replace the unlabelled nucleotides in the DNA probe. This is carried out by using a DNAase enzyme to nick or cut one strand of the DNA and then using a DNA polymerase to add on radiolabelled triphosphates at the site of the nick (Fig. 6.8). This produces a uniformly labelled piece of DNA as the DNAse activity is random along the DNA molecule.

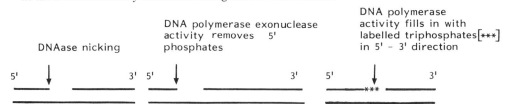

Fig. 6.8   Shows the process of nick translation to produce a radio-labelled DNA probe. Although only one site of activity is shown, the DNAase enzyme will nick the DNA randomly along its length resulting in radiolabelled areas throughout the DNA molecule.

(III) HYBRIDISATION
Before hybridisation can be carried out the probe is denatured by immersion in boiling water for 5 minutes to separate strands. It is then added to the hybridisation solution, which is placed with the nitrocellulose filters in a plastic bag, and hybridisation is carried out over a period of 15–48 hours depending on the concentration of the probe. After this period the filters are washed to remove the radiolabelled probe not hybridized to DNA on the filter. Hybridisation can be carried out in stringent or non-stringent conditions. This is controlled by the salt concentration and temperature of hybridisation, and stringent conditions are those which allow only identical or almost identical (80% or greater homology) DNA sequences to be detected while non-stringent conditions allow less closely related DNAs to be identified. If the salt concentration remains constant then the temperature controls stringency, and at stringent conditions the hybridisation and wash are usually carried out at temperatures of 10°–25°C below the melting temperature of DNA (Tm) whereas non-stringent would be 40°C below. A rough guide to how related the DNA detected is to the probe is that for every degree below the Tm 1% mismatch is detected so at 10°C below melting temperature DNA with 90% homology or greater is detected. Once hybridisation and washing are complete the filter is exposed to X-ray film for a varying period of time to visualise the viral bands that were in the original biopsy material. Figure 6.9a shows some

examples of HPV16 detected in biopsy material. The figure is the developed X-ray and shows viral DNA undigested and digested by the restriction endonuclease enzyme *Pst*1.

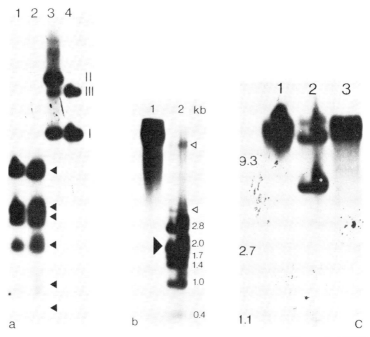

Fig. 6.9 Autoradiographs of papillomavirus bands after hybridisation with ^{32}P labelled HPV16 (a) and (b) and HPV18 (c).

(a) shows biopsy DNA digested with *Pst* 1 (lanes 1 and 2) and undigested (lanes 3 and 4). *Pst* 1 cuts HPV16 DNA into 6 pieces (arrow heads) while the undigested HPV16 shows three configurations of form I, II and III.

(b) shows biopsy DNA from a stage I malignant carcinoma of the cervix. Lane 1 shows the radioactive signal is confined to the high molecular weight host DNA and suggests that HPV16 is associated with host cell DNA in an integrated form. Lane 2 shows the band pattern after digestion with *Pst* 1. There are extra bands when compared to lanes 2, 3 of (a) marked with closed and open arrow heads. The two fainter bands (open arrow heads) may represent the HPV ends covalently linked to host DNA.

(c) Hela cell DNA undigested (lane 1), digested with *Bam* H1 (lane 2) and *Eco* R1 (lane 3), then hybridisation against HPV18. Again the undigested lane suggests HPV18 DNA is integrated within the host DNA and the unusual band pattern with the restriction enzymes confirms this. In (b) and (c) molecular weights are indicated in kilobases (kb).

TYPES OF HPV ASSOCIATED WITH DYSPLASIAS AND MALIGNANT DISEASE OF THE FEMALE LOWER GENITAL TRACT AND PENIS

Two groups of cytologists (Meisels & Fortin, 1976; Purola & Savia, 1979) first showed a possible association of wart virus infection and dysplasias of the cervix and vagina, and since that time these viruses have been associated with dysplasias and malignancies throughout the lower genital tract. Table 6.2 gives a summary of the type and site of genital lesions and the associated genital HPV types. HPV6 and 11 are most commonly seen in vulvar, perianal, cervical and penile condylomata acuminata but are also associated with cervical dysplasias or intraepithelial neoplasias type I through to the severe type III (CIN I–III) (Gissmann et al, 1982; Gissmann et al, 1983; McCance

Table 6.2   Genital HPV types[1] and the site of associated lesions

HPV type	Associated lesion	Site
HPVa-f	Condylomata acuminata	Vulva
		Vagina
		Cervix
		Penis — shaft
		— prepuce
		— urethral meatus
		Perianal
	CIN I–III	Cervix
	VIN I–III	Vulva
HPV11a, b	Condylomata acuminata	Vulva
		Cervix
		Perianal
	CIN I–III	Cervix
HPV16	Condylomata acuminata	Vulva, cervix and penis
	CIN I–III	Cervix
	VIN I–III	Vulva
	Bowenoid papulosis	Vulva and penis
	Malignant carcinoma	Cervix, vulva and penis
HPV18	Malignant carcinoma	Cervix and penis

[1] Apart from the types mentioned in the Table a few biopsies from malignant lesions have contained sequences similar to HPV10.

et al, 1983; Singer et al, 1984). These two types are also found in laryngeal warts in babies and young children, which suggests that they can be transmitted by aspiration during delivery if the woman is harbouring a papillomavirus infection, although accumulating evidence suggests that some adult laryngeal warts may be transmitted by oro-genital sexual practices (JAMA 1984). From the data on Table 6.2 it is striking that only two types of HPV16 and 18, are consistently associated with malignant carcinoma of the cervix. Work by Drs H. zur Hausen and L. Gissman in Germany has shown that 90% of all malignant carcinomas of the cervix have an HPV type detected in the lesion, with HPV16 accounting for some 60% (zur Hausen et al, 1984). HPV16 has also been found in CIN I–III and VIN I–III lesions, being more frequently detected in CIN III and vulvar intraepithelial neoplasias (VIN) grade III (Gissmann & zur Hausen, personal communication; McCance et al, 1985). One point that needs investigation is whether women who harbour HPV16 or 18 virus are at a greater risk of developing carcinoma of the cervix, while in women with lesions containing HPV6 or 11 the lesions either regress or at least do not progress to malignant

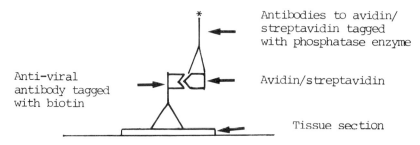

Fig. 6.10   Shows the detection of viral antigens in a tissue section using biotin labelled antibodies, followed by treatment with avidin or streptavidin which binds very efficiently with biotin. Following the addition of enzyme tagged anti-avidin/streptavidin to the section a colour reaction can be produced with the appropriate substrate and so visually indicate the presence of the viral antigens.

disease. This may also elucidate whether the association of HPV types with dysplastic and malignant lesions of the lower genital tract is casual or causal.

In the case of condylomata acuminata and CIN lesions the HPV DNA sequences are in a free form and not integrated into the genome (Fig. 6.9a), but in malignant lesions the majority have integrated sequences of either 16 or 18 (Fig. 6.9b). Hela cells, originally from a patient with squamous cell carcinoma, first cultured in the early 1950s, today show integrated sequences of HPV18 (Fig. 6.9c). More detailed information on the lesions associated with HPV infection will be given in the next chapter.

FUTURE DEVELOPMENTS IN DETECTION OF HPV TYPES

1. Detection by antibodies

With the increasing sophistication of genetic engineering it may be possible in the near future to produce specific HPV coded proteins which could be used to produce antibodies which may recognise antigens produced by individual or groups of HPV types. This may lead to easier detection methods, especially if antibodies were directed against early, non-structural proteins which would possibly be present in deeper layers of the lesion, rather than in the periphery of the lesion as are structural antigens. In addition antibodies labelled with biotin, which binds very tightly with avidin or streptavidin might be used. Addition of avidin/streptavidin which will then bind to any antibody on the section and the subsequent addition of anti-avidin/streptavidin antibodies tagged with alkaline phosphate/peroxidase enzymes (Fig. 6.10) would lead to the amplification of the initial specific antibody-antigen interaction.

2. Non-radiolabelled DNA probes for analysing DNA-DNA hybridisation

These DNA probes are in principle used in the same fashion as radiolabelled probes except that instead of incorporating ^{32}P/CTP, TTP, GTP, ATP, incorporation of biotin labelled UTP is accomplished by nick translation (Leavy et al, 1983). The hybridisation procedure is identical, but visualising DNA-DNA hybridisation on the nitrocellulose filter after washing involves adding avidin or streptavidin to the filter which will bind to any biotin containing probe. This interaction can be visualised by adding dye-labelled biotin or a dye-labelled anti-avidin/streptavidin antibody which will detect and visualise the initial hybridisation. The main advantage of these methods is that these probes do not contain radiolabel and do not decay (half-life of ^{32}P is 14 days) so they can be made and aliquots used for long periods. In addition they are safer to handle for laboratory personnel, but at the moment lack the sensitivity of ^{32}P labelled probes. This situation is changing and commercially available kits may be standard diagnostic reagents in the near future.

IMMUNE RESPONSES TO PAPILLOMAVIRUSES

Studies of the immune response to human papillomaviruses have been hampered by the lack of a virally infected target cell for a cytotoxic T cell assay, and of a type specific viral antigen for the measurement of the humoral response. Indications that the immune response is important in protecting and limiting lesions is obtained mostly from the studies with immunosuppressed patients. It has been observed that

42% of immunosuppressed patients will develop cutaneous warts after one year of immunosuppression (Spencer & Andersen, 1970; Spencer & Andersen, 1979). Patients with the rare autosomal recessive disease epidermodysplasia verruciformis (EV) appear to have a reduced cell-mediated response and develop multiple warts and flat macular lesions which contain a variety of HPV types, some found only in EV patients and not detected in the general population (Jablonska et al, 1982; Orth et al, 1978). One third of these patients develop squamous cell carcinoma usually in areas exposed to sunlight, with HPV types 5 and 8 commonly found in lesions. HPV5 has also been found in squamous cell carcinomas of renal allograft recipients (Lutzner et al, 1980; Lutzner et al, 1983). There have been reports of increased risk of condylomata acuminata and CIN as well as squamous cell carcinoma of the cervix amongst women immunosuppressed after renal transplantation, and of benign vulvar warts and cutaneous lesions developing into malignant lesions in women with a variety of lymphomas (Schneider et al, 1983; Shokri-Tabibzadek et al, 1981; Shelley & Wood, 1981). These fragmented but accumulating pieces of information suggest that the immune response is important in controlling wart virus infections, although little direct evidence of specific responses to wart virus infected cells or wart viruses themselves is available.

1. Humoral immunity

The HPV types 1–3 and HPV4 are the only human papillomaviruses to be grouped separately serologically (Pfister & zur Hausen, 1978). Several antibody studies using the complement fixation test and radioimmune assays have shown that there is an age distribution between these two groups with HPV 1–3 found mostly in 5–15 year olds while HPV4 is found most commonly in 20–25 year olds. Fifty percent of the 5–15 year olds have antibodies to HPV 1–3 but with increasing age this level falls (Pfister & zur Hausen 1978). Others have shown that anti-wart virus antibodies, of the IgM, IgG, and IgA classes, are detected in the serum of individuals with warts but that there is a difference between those with regressing and non-regressing warts. Most individuals with regressing warts had IgM (100%), IgG (97%) and IgA (80%) antibodies to wart virus antigens and 83% had IgM to wart virus infected cells while IgM was detected in 12% of those with non-regressing warts (Matthews & Shirodaria, 1973; Shirodaria & Matthews, 1975). There was a correlation between the patients with no detectable antibodies and the amount of viral antigens in their warts when stained with rabbit anti-HPV antibodies. In both these studies antibody tests were carried out either with virus antigens isolated from a single wart or by immunofluorescence with warts from the same patients, thus by-passing the problem with many studies of using pooled isolates which may contain many HPV types.

Antibodies against the genital wart viruses have not been studied, but genital lesions in particular contain small amounts of detectable viral antigen. In one study (Baird, 1983) antibodies to the common papillomavirus antigen was measured by Enzyme-Linked Immunosorbent Assay (ELISA) in a group of children (<5 years old) and normal women as controls, while women attending an STD clinic and women with anogenital warts, CIN or carcinoma of the cervix, were the test population. There were highly significant numbers with antibodies to the common antigen amongst women with anogenital warts, CIN and carcinoma of the cervix but in no other groups. This test measures antibodies to all HPV types, and it was surprising that none of the 108 control women had detectable antibody.

2. Cell-mediated immunity

The lack of an in vitro infected target cell makes it difficult to investigate cell-mediated responses, and so most of the information comes from studies of mitogen responses of circulating lymphocytes, lymphocyte migration-inhibition tests against wart virus antigens, or delayed hypersensitivity responses using purified wart virus antigens (Lee & Eisinger, 1976; Morison, 1975; Viac et al, 1977). All this work, has been carried out with patients who have developed cutaneous wart lesions. Evidence from some of these studies might suggest that a lower reactivity of lymphocytes to wart virus antigens is seen in patients with the prolonged presence of wart lesions, and a higher lymphocyte reactivity in individuals who have regressing warts or who had warts for short periods in the past. One difficulty of these studies is that they are measuring systemic responses when local ones may be more important. A study using monoclonal antibodies against T lymphocytes, B lymphocytes, and various macrophage cells (including Langerhan cells) has investigated the type of immune cells in tissue sections from CIN lesions (Syrjanen et al, 1984). In these studies there was not a significant increase or decrease in any particular cell type no matter how severe the CIN lesion, or even during regression, although the numbers tested were small.

The lack of detectable local tissue response may be due to the fact that (i) the virus producing cells are on the wrong side of the base membrane as far as the immune response is concerned, (ii) only small amounts of viral antigens are produced — this is supported by the small amounts of mature particles seen in genital warts either by immunoperoxidase staining or electron microscopy and (iii) the infected cells may exhibit a reduced content of the histocompatibility antigens on their surface as seen with other virus induced tumours. Hence research to characterise specific genital wart virus antigens may help in elucidating the immune response to these infections.

CONCLUSIONS

Great interest has been generated in papillomaviruses owing to the recently detected association of the genital papillomaviruses with various dysplasias and malignant carcinomas of the lower genital tract. Research has been hampered by the fact that the viruses cannot be grown in tissue culture and so genetic manipulative techniques are used, and there is to date no animal model for these genital lesions. The evidence for a causal association of genital papillomas with lesions in the lower genital tract is at present more convincing than it is for herpesviruses, but it remains possible that these viruses are only coincidentally associated with the dysplasias and carcinomas, as both exist in or are transmitted by sexually promiscuous individuals.

REFERENCES

Baird P J 1983 Serological evidence for the association of papillomavirus and cervical neoplasia. Lancet ii: 17–18

Chen E Y, Howley P M, Levinson A D, Seeburg P H 1982 The primary structure and genetic organization of the bovine papillomavirus type 1 genome. Nature 299: 529–534

Chesters P M, McCance D J 1985 Human papillomavirus type 16 recombinant DNA is maintained as an autonomously replicating episome in monkey kidney cells. Journal of General Virology 66: 615–620

Danos O, Katinka M, Yaniv M 1982 Human papillomavirus 1a complete DNA sequence: a novel type of genome organization among papovaviridae. EMBO Journal 1: 231–236

Gissmann L, de Villier E-M, zur Hausen H 1982 Analysis of human genital warts (condylomata acuminata) and other genital tumours for human papillomavirus type 6 DNA. International Journal Cancer 29: 143–146

Gissmann L, Wolnik L, Ikenberg H, Koldovsky U, Schnurch H G, zur Hausen H 1983 Human papillomavirus type 6 and 11 DNA sequences in genital and laryngeal papillomas and in some cervical cancers. Proceedings of the National Academy of Sciences 80: 560–563

Jablonska S, Orth G, Lutzner M A 1982 Immunopathology of papillomavrius-induced tumours in different tissues. Springer Seminars in Immunopathology 5: 33–62

Jacobson E R, Maldinich C R, Clubb S, Sundberg J P, Lancaster W D 1983 Papilloma-like virus infection in an African Gray parrot. Journal of the American Veterinary and Medical Association 183: 1307–1308

Jarrett W F H, McNeil P E, Laird H M, O'Neil B W, Murphy J, Campo M S, Moar M H 1981 Papilloma viruses in benign and malignant tumours of cattle. In: Essex M, Todaro G, zur Hausen H (ed) Cold Spring Harbor Laboratory, Cold Spring Harbor, New York, p 215–222

Kremsdorf D, Jablonska S, Favre M, Orth G 1983 Human papillomaviruses associated with Epidermodysplasia Verruciformis. II Molecular cloning and biochemical characterization of human papillomavirus 3a, 8, 10 and 12 genomes. Journal of Virology 48: 340–351

Kremsdorf D, Favre M, Jablonska S, Obalek S, Rueda L A, Lutzner M A, Blanchet-Bardon C, Van Voorst Vader P C, Orth G 1984 Human papilloma viruses (HPVs) associated with Epidermodysplasia Verruciformis. III Molecular cloning and characterization of the genome of nine newly recognized HPV types (HPV14, 15, 17, 19, 20, 21, 22, 23 and 24). Journal of Virology 52(3): 1013–1018

Kurman R J, Sanz L E, Jenson A B, Perry S, Lancaster W D 1982 Papillomavirus infection of the cervix. I Correlation of histology with viral structural antigens and DNA sequences. International Society of Gynaecological Pathology 1: 17–28

La Porta R F, Taichman L B 1982 Human papilloma viral DNA replicates as a stable episome in cultured epidermal keratinocyes. Proceedings of the National Academy of Sciences 79: 3393–3397

Law M-F, Lowy D R, Dvoretzky I, Howley P M 1981 Mouse cells transformed by bovine papillomavirus contain only extrachromosomal viral DNA sequences. Proceedings of the National Academy of Sciences 78: 2727–2731

Leavy J J, Brigati D J, Ward D C 1983 Rapid and sensitive colorimetric method for visualising biotin-labelled DNA probes hybridized to DNA or RNA immobilized on nitrocellulose: bio-blots. Proceedings of the National Academy of Sciences 80: 4045–4049

Lee A K Y, Eisinger M 1976 Cell-mediated immunity (CMI) to human wart virus and wart-associated tissue antigens. Clinical and Experimental Immunology 26: 419–424

Lutzner M A, Croissant O, Ducasse M-F, Kreis H, Grosnier I, Orth G 1980 A potentially oncogenic human papillomavirus (HPV5) foci in two renal allograft recipients. Journal of Investigative Dermatology 75: 353–356

Lutzner M A, Orth G, Dutronquay V 1983 Detection of GPV type 5 DNA in skin cancers of an immunosuppressed renal allograft recipient. Lancet ii: 422–424

Matthews R S, Shirodaria P V 1973 Study of regressing warts by immunofluorescence. Lancet i: 689–691

McCance D J, Walker P G, Dyson J L, Coleman D V, Singer A 1983 Presence of human papillomavirus DNA sequences in cervical intraepthelial neoplasia. British Medical Journal 287: 784–788

McCance D J, Clarkson P K, Dyson J L, Walker P G, Singer A 1985 Human papillomavirus types 6 and 16 in multifocal intraepithelial neoplasias of the female lower genital tract. British Journal of Obstetrics and Gynaecology 92(11): 1101–1105

Medical News 1984 Papillomavirus invades oesophages, incidence seems to be increasing. Journal of the American Medical Association 251: 2185–2187

Meisels A, Fortin R 1976 Condylomatous lesions of the cervix and vagina. I Cytologic patterns. Acta Cytologica 20: 505–509

Morison W L 1975 Cell-mediated immune responses in patients with warts. British Journal of Dermatology 93: 553–556

Nakabayashi Y, Chattopadhyay S K, Lowy D R 1983 The transforming function of bovine papillomavirus DNA. Proceedings of the National Academy of Sciences 80: 5832–5836

Orth G, Jablonska S, Breitburd F, Favre M, Croissant O 1978 The human papillomaviruses. Bulletin of Cancer 65: 151–164

Osterhaus A D M E, Elleus D J, Horzinek M C 1977 Identification and characterization of a papillomavirus from birds (Frigillidae). Intervirology 8: 351–359

Pfister H, zur Hausen H 1978 Sero-epidemiological studies of human papillomavirus (HPV1) infections. International Journal of Cancer 21: 161–165

Purola E, Savia E 1977 Cytology of gynaecologic condyloma acuminatum. Acta Cytologica 21: 26–31

Rigby P W S, Dieckman M, Rhodes C, Berg P 1977 Labelling deoxyribonucleic acids to high specific activity in vitro by nick translation with DNA polyomas I. Journal of Molecular Biology 113: 237–251

Rous P, Beard J W 1935 The progression to carcinoma of virus induced rabbit papilloma (Shope). Journal Experimental Medicine 62: 523–548

Schneider V, Kay S, Lee H M 1983 Immunosuppression as a high-risk factor in the development of condyloma acuminatum and squamous neoplasia of the cervix. Acta Cytologica 27: 220–224

Schwarz E, Durst M, Demankowski C, Latterman O, Zech R, Wolfsperger E, Suhai S, zur Hausen H 1983 DNA sequence and genome organization of genital human papillomavirus type 6b. EMBO Journal 2: 2341–2348

Shelley W B, Wood M G 1981 Transformation of the common wart into squamous cell carcinoma in a patient with primary lymphedema. Cancer 48: 820–824

Shirodaria P V, Matthews R S 1975 An immunofluorescence study of warts. Clinical and Experimental Immunology 21: 329–338

Shokri-Tabibzadeh S, Koss L G, Molinar J, Romney M D 1981 Association of human papillomavirus with neoplastic processes in the genital tract of four women with impaired immunity. Gynaecological Oncology 12: 5129–5140

Singer A, Walker P G, McCance D J 1984 Genital wart virus infections: nuisance or potentially lethal? British Medical Journal 288: 735–737

Southern E M 1975 Detection of speciific sequences among DNA fragments separated by gel electrophoresis. Journal of Molecular Biology 98: 503–517

Spencer E S, Andersen H K 1970 Clinically evident, non terminal infections with herpesvirus and the wart virus in immunosuppressed renal allograft recipients. British Medical Journal 3: 251–254

Spencer E S, Andersen H K 1979 Viral infections in renal allograft recipients treated with long term immunosuppression. British Medical Journal 2: 829

Spradbrow P B, Beardmore G L, Francis J 1983 Virions resembling papillomaviruses in hyperkeratotic lesions from un-damaged skin. Lancet i: 189

Syrjanen K, Vayrynen M, Castren O, Mantyjarvi R, Yliskoski 1984 The relation between the type of immunoreactive cells found in human papillomavirus (HPV) lesions of the uterine cervix and the subsequent behaviour of these lesions. Archives of Gynaecology 234: 189–196

Syverton J T 1952 The pathogenesis of the rabbit papilloma-to-carcinoma sequence. Annals of the New York Academy of Sciences 54: 1126–1140

Vanselow B A, Spradbrow P B 1982 Papillomaviruses, papillomas and squamous cell carcinomas in sheep. Veterinary Record 110: 561–562

Vanselow B A, Spradbrow P B 1983 Squamous cell carcinoma of the vulva, hyperkeratosis and papillomaviruses in a ewe. Australian Veterinary Journal 60: 194

Viac J, Thivolet J, Hegazy M R, Chardonnet Y, Dambuyant C 1977 Comparative study of delayed hypersensitivity skin reactions and antibodies to human papillomavirus (HPV). Clinical and Experimental Immunology 29: 240–246

zur Hausen H, Gissmann L, Schlehofer J R 1984 Viruses in the aetiology of human genital cancer. Progress in Medical Virology 30: 170–186

7. Genital papillomavirus infections: clinical manifestations

J. D. Oriel

EPIDEMIOLOGY OF GENITAL WARTS

Incidence in adults

In 1981, 29 704 patients with 'condylomata acuminata', 18 807 men and 10 897 women, attended clinics for sexually transmitted diseases (STD) in England (Chief Medical Officer, 1984): it should be noted that although the term 'condyloma acuminatum' describes a type of tumour with a characteristic histology, many authors use 'condylomata acuminata' as synonymous with 'genital warts'. The incidence per 100 000 population was 82.63 (men), 45.36 (women and 63.49 (total). This is a large increase over 1971, when the incidence per 100 000 population was 39.81 (men), 20.32 (women) and 29.79 (total) (Chief Medical Officer, 1973). The total national incidence of genital warts in England is unknown, but it is likely to be much higher than these returns from STD clinics indicate, as they do not include cases seen by urologists, gynaecologists, dermatologists or general practitioners, or patients who have been treated in the armed services. Moreover, cervical wart virus infections which can be detected only by colposcopy or cytology are not usually reported.

Under-reporting of genital warts also occurs in the USA (Katz et al, 1984) but, as in England, the available data suggest a substantial increase in the number of new cases. An analysis by the Centers for Disease Control (Editorial note, 1983) shows that the number of consultations with office based physicians for condylomata acuminata increased five-fold between 1966 and 1981. More consultations were requested by women than by men, and 65% were by people aged 15–29 years, the highest risk group being aged 20–24 years. In public health clinics in the USA 3.4 cases of genital warts were diagnosed in men for every 100 visits, compared with 3.4 cases of genital herpes and 24.0 of gonorrhoea; the incidence was higher in whites than in blacks (Editorial note, 1983).

An epidemiological study was undertaken among residents of Rochester, Minnesota between 1950 and 1978 to discover trends in the incidence of condylomata acuminata: virtually all the medical care in this city is provided by the Mayo Clinic and one group practice, and a centralised diagnosis retrieval system is in operation (Chuang et al, 1984a). During the 24 year period the number of cases diagnosed each year rose until 1975, after which it declined somewhat. The mean annual incidence rate increased from 13.0 per 100 000 population in 1950–1954 to 106.5 in 1975–1978. This rate was highest in the 20–24 year old group, and female patients presented more often, and at a younger age, than men. The authors point out that the incidence rate reported in this study must be considered minimal, because many of those affected may not seek medical advice because they are unaware that the disease is present. A different approach to estimating the prevalence of genital warts was adopted by

127

Daling et al (1984). They asked a group of 771 married women who had had children in King County, Washington between 1971 and 1981 whether they had ever had genital warts; 6% said that they had, and this figure was fairly consistent among the 5 year age groups from ages 20–34 years.

Human papilloma virus (HPV) infection of the cervix is much commoner than was formerly thought. Meisels et al (1977) reported typical cellular changes in about 1% of cervical smears from all patients screened in Quebec, with peak prevalence in younger age groups. Reid et al (1980) found that over a 6 month period 1.3% of smears taken at George V Hospital in Sydney showed the features of HPV infection. Syrjänen et al (1984) compared the sexual behaviour of 146 women with HPV infections of the cervix with an age-matched group who were free from this infection. The HPV-infected women differed from the control group in an earlier onset of sex activity. more numerous partners, higher frequency of casual relationships and a history of more attacks of STD.

Infectivity in adults
Since genital warts are contagious, the presence of subclinical lesions in male partners of women with condylomatous and non-condylomatous cervical HPV infection is of particular interest. Levine et al (1984) examined sex partners of 34 women with warts of the lower genital tract or cervical intraepithelial neoplasia (CIN). External lesions were detected in 18 (53%) of the men, mostly on the shaft of the penis and arranged in small slightly raised clusters; one man had a lesion in the urethral meatus. The authors emphasise the importance of examination of partners of patients with genital warts.

Associated infections in adults
The association between condylomata acuminata and other STD is familiar. Kinghorn (1978) detected gonorrhoea in 10%, and 'non-specific genital infection' in 17% of a group of men attending an STD clinic with genital warts. N. gonorrhoeae was reco-vered from 12%, and T. vaginalis from 12% of female patients with warts. In a population-based study performed in the USA by Chuang et al (1984b), concurrent STD was less often found. Of the male patients with warts 1% had gonorrhoea and 2% non-gonococcal urethritis; of the female patients 1% had gonorrhoea and 8% trichomoniasis. Associated infections may be symptomatic or symptomless. Harahap (1979) noted in Indonesia that 23 (34%) of 67 male patients with genital warts but no urethral symptoms or signs yielded isolates of N. gonorrhoeae.

Condylomata acuminata in children
Anogenital warts were formerly rare in prepubertal children, but now appear to be commoner (Stumpf, 1980). The majority of lesions affect the vulva or perianal area rather than the penis, and the reported age of onset varies from one day to 13 years. Girls are more often affected than boys (de Jong et al, 1982).

The mode of infection is uncertain. Infants can acquire HPV from maternal genital condylomas at the time of delivery (Eftaiha et al, 1978; Zamora et al, 1983), with resulting genital or laryngeal disease (see below). However, there have been several recent reports which suggest that condylomata acuminata in young children may also be a result of sexual molestation (Storrs, 1977; Seidel et al, 1979; McCoy et al, 1982; de Jong et al, 1982). Stumpf (1980) believes that infection may also come about through close non-sexual contact within a family.

EPIDEMIOLOGY OF ANAL WARTS

Anorectal warts have received remarkably little attention recently (Schlappner & Shaffer, 1978), yet the disease is common, particularly among homosexual men. Carr & Williams (1977) reported that homosexual or bisexual men with anal warts were more likely to give a history of anoreceptive intercourse than those without anal warts. The average age of onset of anal lesions in the patients in this study was 23 years, and the authors confirmed previous reports that in homosexual men anal warts are several times commoner than penile warts. Perianal condylomata acuminata in a one-year-old child were described by Baruah et al (1984). Although the infant's mother had no history or clinical evidence of genital or non-genital warts, the father had had penile condylomata acuminata for 6 months, and an accidental infection from him seemed likely.

MANIFESTATIONS OF INFECTION OF THE GENITAL TRACT BY HPV

Manifestations in men
Genital warts are pleomorphic. It has been suggested that the lesions in men may sometimes be so inconspicuous as to escape recognition unless magnification is used. Warts of this kind, resembling 'flat condylomas' of the cervix, have been described by Meisels et al (1977) and Levine et al (1984), but their prevalence is unknown.

Between 0.5% and 5% of men with penile warts have urethral condylomas (Wein & Benson, 1977). Nearly 80% of these are in the distal 3 cm of the urethra, but growths can affect any part (de Benedictis et al, 1977). Dean et al (1983) examined 25 squamous papillomas of the penile meatus both histologically and for the presence of HPV antigen with an immunochemical technique. All the tumours had the characteristics of HPV-associated squamous metaplasia, particularly koilocytosis, and 11 (44%) of the 25 were positive for viral antigen. The authors suggest that male urethral papillomas may play an important role in the sexual transmission of HPV. Pollack et al (1978) described the radiological appearance of urethral condylomas. They can be seen well by either retrograde or voiding urethrography. The latter, following intravenously injected contrast medium, is recommended. Not only are the condylomas well displayed, but the need for urethral instrumentation, with the attendant risk of retrograde spread of infection, is avoided. A case of condyloma acuminatum of the bladder in an elderly man was described by Massé et al (1981). The tumour was excised, but recurred 11 months later. Cytology of urine samples showed moderate numbers of atypical cells, chiefly of transitional type.

Manifestations in women
Vulva and vagina
Roy et al (1981) performed colposcopic studies, and stated that the vagina is more often affected by HPV-induced lesions that the vulva, although less often than the cervix. On the vulva, only florid condylomas could be identified. Schmauz & Owor (1980), in a histological study, also noticed the predominance of proliferative exophytic

condylomas on the vulva, although they were able to identify a few 'flat condylomas' on the vulva and vagina. Roy et al (1981) described several varieties of vaginal wart. Florid condylomas are dense white lesions with finger-like projections; hyperkeratosis is usually present. These tumours are usually multiple and readily identified with the naked eye, but sometimes they are hard to see without a colposcope. Flat vaginal condylomas are white, with a granular surface and no visible blood vessels; these lesions are usually multiple, and may accompany florid condylomas. The 'spiked condyloma' is intermediate between the florid and flat varieties and is white, with asperities containing visible capillary tips. Histologically, vaginal condylomas show koilocytotic cells in the superficial layers, and transmission electron microscopy often shows papillomavirus particles in their nuclei.

Papillomavirus antigens have been identified in vulval and vaginal warts by Kurman et al (1981). They screened 40 cases of vulval condyloma with a genus-specific peroxidase-antiperoxidase method, and found that 20 (50%) gave positive reactions. Similar results were obtained by Woodruff et al (1980), who with a similar technique identified viral antigen in 10 of 20 vulval and in two of six vaginal condylomas.

The differential diagnosis of vulval and vaginal warts is not usually difficult. However, Altmeyer et al (1982) described lesions of the vulva in two sexually active women which at first appeared to be fine condylomata acuminata; more detailed examination showed that the structures were actually harmless malformations which closely resembled hirsutes papillaris penis.

Cervix

COLPOSCOPY

The colposcopic changes indicating HPV infection of the cervix were described by Meisels et al (1977); subsequently the diagnostic criteria were refined (Meisels et al, 1982). The florid, or exophtic condyloma shows a thick white epithelium with finger-like projections in which capillary loops are visible. Florid condylomas are usually multiple and visible with the naked eye, but a colposcope may be needed to identify small lesions. The 'spiked condyloma' has a thin white epithelium with sharp borders and an irregular uneven surface: vessels are sometimes visible in the 'spikes'. The flat condyloma appears as a flat white epithelium with or without a granular surface, and fine punctation may be seen. Meisels et al (1977) believed that these lesions had formerly been wrongly categorised as mild dysplasia.

Reid et al (1980) introduced the term 'non-condylomatous wart virus infection' (NCWVI) to described macroscopically flat cervical lesions produced through HPV infection. Although the colposcopic features of NCWVI, consisting mostly of epithelial opacity and vascular atypia, often lead to confusion with CIN, differences in surface contour, colour, vascular patterns and topography generally allow colposcopic differentiation. They pointed out, however, that NCWVI and CIN often coexist. A different view was taken by Kirkup et al (1982), who did not believe that colposcopy could reliably distinguish between NCWVI and CIN. Walker et al (1983c) examined 200 women who were referred for colposcopy because of abnormal cervical smears. Comparison between the results of colposcopy and histology suggested that it was possible to identify epithelial changes which were likely to be due to an HPV infection, including an epithelium which appeared shiny white after the application of acetic acid, often with a raised and roughened surface. In a subsequent paper Walker et al (1983b) noted that about 50% of women with vulval warts showed evidence of cervical HPV infection. Like Kirkup et al, they concluded that it is not possible by colposcopy to make a complete distinction between the lesions of HPV infection and those of CIN.

HISTOPATHOLOGY

Meisels et al (1977, 1982) differentiated four histological types of cervical condyloma, of which the first three correspond to the colposcopic classification described above. The exophytic condyloma is histologically identical to classical condyloma acuminatum of the penis, vulva and anus. The diagnostic features are acanthosis, papillomatosis, elongation and thickening of the rete pegs, and parakeratosis. Koilocytosis is present in the upper epithelial layers. In the 'spiked condyloma' blood vessels push upwards through the epithelium, producing the characteristic 'spikes' which are covered by only a few layers of dyskeratotic cells. The epithelium often lacks differentiation, and contains clear cells with irregular nuclei. The flat condyloma shows a squamous epithelium which may appear normal but is often of increased thickness. There is evidence of acanthosis and accentuated rete pegs. There is a marked contrast between the deeper cells, which have a dense and abundant cytoplasm, and the superficial layers, which contain many koilocytes. An 'inverted condyloma' is also described, in which the papillary growth moves into the glandular necks, obliterating the columnar epithelium; koilocytosis may be present in the depths of the glands. Meisels et al (1981) later described a special subgroup of condylomatous lesions, the 'atypical condyloma', which may be particularly difficult to differentiate from CIN (see below).

Reid et al (1980) did not delineate particular subgroups of cervical condyloma, but referred in general terms to a varied histological picture which usually included acanthosis, hyperkeratosis, parakeratosis, and sometimes basal cell hyperplasia. The most striking feature is the presence of koilocytotic cells which on occasion may show intranuclear inclusions resembling those seen in non-genital warts. One of the most important findings is the frequent presence in these condylomatous lesions of nuclear atypia which, although usually mild, may sometimes be difficult to differentiate from all grades of CIN.

Routine Papanicolaou smears have proved to be very valuable for the detection of warty lesions of the cervix (Meisels & Fortin, 1976; Purola & Savia, 1977; Reid et al, 1980). The pathognomonic cell is the koilocyte, whose nucleus is surrounded by an irregular clear area of variable size. Outside this perinuclear clearing the cytoplasm is dense and shows amphophilic staining. In addition to koilocytosis, individual cells or groups of cells may show dyskeratosis; their nuclei are enlarged, dense or pyknotic, and their cytoplasm contains keratin or its precursors, staining brilliant orange by the Papanicolaou technique. This dyskeratosis is not specific to HPV infection of the cervix. There may be difficulty in diagnosing cervical condylomatous disease when there is marked atypia and hyperchromatism, and when koilocytosis is inconspicuous. Walker et al (1983b) have pointed out that the results of colposcopy and cytology may not be in close agreement. Perhaps a colposcopic diagnosis of HPV infection which is unsupported by cytology is due to inadequate sampling of the whole transformation zone. On the other hand, an unsupported cytological diagnosis could be explained by the presence of an early HPV infection producing changes only at cellular level. The clinicopathological correlation and the dynamics of cervical wart virus infection require further study and Fletcher (1983) has critically reviewed the nature, nomenclature and taxonomy of these conditions.

VIROLOGY

Della Torre et al (1978) took colposcopically directed biopsies from eight women with histologically confirmed cervical condylomas and demonstrated intranuclear virus particles, morphologically identical with papillomavirus, in ultrathin sections in four cases. Hills & Laverty (1979) obtained a cervical smear which showed appearances suggestive of HPV infection. The smear was reprocessed for electron microscopy, and some cells were seen to contain intranuclear papillomavirus particles. Morin & Meisels (1980) reprocessed seven smears of flat condyloma lesions, and saw virus particles in three. Reid et al (1980) found typical virus particles in 24 (45%) of 53 colposcopically directed cervical biopsies in which a firm diagnosis of NCWVI had been made. Smith & Coleman (1983) have given technical details of a method which can be used to study by electron microscopy cells in which light microscopy shows suggestive cytological changes.

Immunological identification of HPV antigen in cervical condyloma tissue has been reported by several workers. Woodruff et al (1980) stained paraffin sections by a peroxidase-antiperoxidase technique and identified HPV antigen in 11 of 24 lesions. Morin et al (1981) used a similar technique to examine 35 flat cervical condylomas, and demonstrated viral antigen in 21 (60%). Antigen-positive nuclei were found in the upper layers of the epithelium. Electron microscopy of five reprocessed antigen-positive sections showed in every case papillomavirus particles in the nuclei of cells in the superficial layers of the epithelium. Syrjänen & Pyrhönen (1982) used an indirect immunoperoxidase technique to demonstrate HPV antigen in eight of 10 cervical condylomas, the antigen being mostly within the nuclei of koilocytes and dyskeratotic cells. Gupta et al (1983) reported a study in which they used the avidinbiotin complex method and a cross-reactive anti-HPV antiserum on paired Papanicolaou-stained smears and tissue sections from 45 cases of histologically confirmed cervical condylomas. Both preparations gave positive reactions in 53% of the cases, but only a small proportion of condylomatous cells showed viral antigen. Mariuzzi et al (1983) used an immunoperoxidase technique and demonstrated HPV antigen in 10 (37%) of 27 cervical condylomas. Dyson et al (1984) examined biopsy specimens from 139 women who had been referred to a colposcopy clinic because of abnormal smears. They used a broadly cross-reactive antiserum raised by the immunisation of rabbits with purified plantar wart virions and an indirect immunoalkaline phosphatase technique. Histochemical staining was seen in 28 (20%) of the specimens. Histological examination of adjoining sections from the same blocks showed a wide range of abnormality Koilocytes were present in all the cells which gave positive reactions. Individual cell keratinisation was present in 10 (36%) of the 28 cases. The accompanying epithelial findings ranged from normal to CIN3.

The distribution of nuclear DNA in vulval and cervical condylomas has been the subject of much recent research, and has been described in the preceding chapter. HPV6 and HPV11 are found in exophytic condylomas of the penis, vulva, vagina and cervix, and are also found in flat condylomas of the cervix. HPV16 and HPV18 are more often detected in the higher grades of CIN, but are occasionally present in condylomata acuminata.

All these results indicate that there is a wide range of cervical pathology associated with HPV infection. However, about half of typical vulval, vaginal and cervical condylomas do not show papillomavirus particles on electron microscopy or HPV antigen by immunochemistry, although unintegrated DNA can be found in the majority of these lesions. The reasons for this phenomenon are not well understood. Failure to detect virions or viral antigen may be due simply to their sparseness in condyloma tissue (Reid et al, 1980) Alternatively, genital wart tissue may at times, for unknown reasons, be non-permissive; it would not then allow complete HPV maturation, although unintegrated DNA was present (Meisels et al, 1982). Reid (1984) has pointed out that late viral expression is tied to squamous differentiation and keratinisation of cells: because genital epithelia have a limited capacity to keratinise, viral replication may not proceed to the point of capsid protein production or virion assembly. This is not to suggest that particle- or antigen-negative koilocytes need necessarily have a non-viral aetiology. Indeed, Bender & Pass (1981) have considered the possibility that intact virus particles may not be necessary for the sexual transmission of genital warts.

The natural history of cervical condylomas is uncertain. Meisels et al (1982) state that in their experience 68% regress either spontaneously or following treatment. Another 27% remain unchanged after a mean follow-up period of 14.5 months. Progression to more advanced lesions (CIN 2–3 and invasive cancer) was seen in 10% of patients with 'atypical' condylomas and in 5% of those with other histological types of condyloma. Laverty (1980) states that in his experience NCWVI usually remains flat for many months or even years. Walker et al (1983a) undertook a prospective study of 50 women with vulval warts, of whom 28 had colposcopic evidence of a cervical epithelial abnormality. It was possible to re-examine 19 of these patients after 6 months, when it was found that the epithelial abnormality had persisted in 14. These authors believe that lesions of the cervix associated with HPV infection show little sign of short-term regression.

HPV infections in pregnancy
Lecatsas (1983) performed electron microscopy on centrifuged urine specimens from 2500 pregnant women, and found that 8 (0.32%) contained particles of the size and morphology of papillomavirus. None of the women had visible condylomas, and these results are so far unexplained.

Chuang et al (1984b) undertook a retrospective review of 500 women with condylomata acuminata, and evaluated the outcome of 51 pregnancies which occurred in the group. There were four elective abortions, four miscarriages, three premature births and one stillbirth. The authors state that although this study was uncontrolled the figures for unfavourable outcome of pregnancy are not unduly high. Of 42 live infants, 28 were evaluated for a year or more, and 11 developed an atopic disease; the authors suggest that HPV infections may be commoner among atopic individuals, and that this trait may be inherited. The relationship between juvenile laryngeal papillomatosis and maternal genital warts is discussed in detail below.

HPV AND GENITAL NEOPLASIA

The most serious complication of infection of the genital tract by HPV is malignancy, and this has been the subject of much recent research. The carcinogenic potential of papillomaviruses had been proved in tumours such as the Shope papilloma of and bovine papillomas of the oesophagus and intestine: a co-factor is often involved (Rous et al, 1953; Jarrett, 1980). In man, epidermodysplasia verruciformis (EV) is a disease in which progression of benign warty lesions to squamous-cell carcinoma occurs (Lutzner, 1978). Several HPV types have been identified in EV, but HPV5 is specifically associated with malignant progression, and HPV5 has been identified in skin cancers in patients with EV (Ostrow et al, 1982; Jablonska & Orth, 1983). In EV the development of malignancy seems to depend on genetic susceptibility to HPV infection, infection with a specific viral type, and probably exposure to ultraviolet light which acts as a co-factor (Jablonska & Orth, 1983). Juvenile laryngeal papillomatosis is often associated with the 'genital' HPV11 type; carcinoma of the larynx can follow spontaneously, but radiation therapy appears to act as a co-factor.

In the genital tract the development of giant condyloma, carcinoma in situ or squamous-cell carcinoma in association with genital warts has often been described (Oriel, 1977). In a follow-up evaluation of 500 women with condylomata acuminata Chuang et al (1984b) noted the development of one invasive squamous-cell carcinoma, 13 carcinomas in situ, six severe dysplasias and 21 moderate to mild dysplasias of the cervix and, less often, of the vagina; these occurred in 8% of the subjects studied. Only one of 246 men with genital warts had genital anaplasia, in the form of carcinoma in situ of the glans and prepuce. Of these 42 anaplasias, six were concurrent with active condylomas, the remaining 36 developing subsequently.

Giant condyloma

Over 100 cases of giant condyloma (Buschke-Loewenstein tumour) have been reported; usually the penis is affected, but sometimes the vulva and anus (Baird et al, 1979). The disease runs a prolonged course, the tumour is locally invasive but non-metastasising, and histologically consists of only condyloma acuminatum tissue. Ananthakrishnan et al (1981) described 24 cases, and discussed their differentiation from squamous-cell carcinoma. Tessler & Applebaum (1982), however, believe that giant condyloma is probably a well-differentiated carcinoma from the beginning; areas of anaplasia which develop subsequently probably represent a loss of differentiation in a previously well-differentiated carcinoma rather than malignant degeneration of a benign lesion. Partridge et al (1980) discussed the distinction between giant condyloma and verrucous carcinoma, and stressed the need for large biopsy specimens in order to identify unequivocally malignant areas. The same point was made by Tropé et al (1982). One of their patients, a 49-year-old woman, had huge vulval and perianal masses; after radical surgery it was found that while most of the tumour was typical condyloma acuminatum there were two areas of squamous-cell carcinoma.

The apparent histological identity between giant condyloma and condyloma acuminatum suggests the possibility of a common viral aetiology. Papillomavirus particles have not been seen by electron microscopy, but recently Gissmann et al (1982) identified HPV6 DNA in each of three tumours. Whether other factors are also involved is unknown.

Vulval, vaginal and penile neoplasia

Vulval intra-epithelial neoplasia (VIN) shows lesions which are single or multiple, erosive or papular, and pigmented or non-pigmented. In the past these lesions have received various names, including Bowen's disease, bowenoid papulosis, carcinoma in situ, and erythroplasia of Queyrat. These familiar eponyms are still used by clinicians, but histologically VIN lesions are now graded VIN 1–3, according to the amount of pleomorphism within the epithelium (Ridley, 1983). They are generally aneuploid (Fu et al, 1981). These categories may not directly correspond to increasing risk of invasive carcinoma; other factors, including the age and immune status of the patient and the area of the lesion must also be considered.

Intraepithelial neoplasia of the lower genital tract is often associated, perhaps causally, with HPV. Carcinoma in situ may accompany or follow condylomata acuminata of the vulva or penis (Grussendorf & Bär, 1977; Laohadtanaphorn et al, 1979; Kimura, 1980). Wade et al (1979) reported 34 cases of bowenoid papulosis, 28 in men and six in women; there was a history of antecedent condylomata acuminata in 12 patients. Invasive carcinoma has also been described in association with condylomata acuminata (Shafeek et al, 1979). Daling et al (1984) observed a strong association between condylomata acuminata and squamous carcinoma of the vulva.

In virological studies Katz et al (1978) and Kimura et al (1978) noted that some bowenoid papulosis lesions contained spherical particles which resembled papillomaviruses on electron microscopy. Braun et al (1983) detected HPV antigen by an immunoperoxidase technique in two of 21 bowenoid lesions, and Guillet et al (1984) in one of two lesions. Crum et al (1982a) attempted immunoperoxidase location of HPV antigen in 68 vulval intraepithelial lesions, of which 39 were also analysed for nuclear DNA content. Overall, four (6%) of the 68 specimens gave positive staining for HPV. Of the 39 specimens tested for DNA, 35 (90%) were aneuploid, and of these 35 one (3%) stained for HPV. In contrast, two (50%) of four polyploid lesions gave positive staining reactions. The authors concluded that HPV is detected infrequently in aneuploid lesions, probably because epithelial maturation is needed for viral assembly.

In a further paper Crum et al (1982b) pointed out that abnormal mitoses and cytologically atypical nuclear enlargement were specific predictors of aneuploidy, and were therefore reliable for distinguishing VIN from condyloma acuminatum.

In 1982 Zachow et al used the Southern blot technique to search for HPV DNA in three types of genital tumour: Bowen's disease, bowenoid papulosis and squamous-cell carcinoma. They detected HPV-related sequences in four of eight cases of Bowen's disease, in each of two cases of bowenoid papulosis (one penile and one vulval) and in each of two cases of verrucous carcinoma (one penile and one vulval). Ikenberg et al (1983) used P-labelled DNA of HPV16 to screen cellular DNA from 20 biopsies of Bowen's disease or bowenoid papulosis. HPV16 DNA or related sequences were identified in six of 10 cases of Bowen's disease and in eight of 10 cases of bowenoid papulosis. These workers also analysed a large number of normal genital tissue samples, and failed to find HPV DNA in any of them. Okagaki et al (1984) identified HPV genomes in two cases of verrucous carcinoma of the vagina.

Multiple primary squamous, mainly intraepithelial neoplasms of the lower genital tract are common (Choo & Morley, 1980). The majority of VIN in premenopausal women is also multifocal, and often accompanied by overtly condylomatous lesions of the vulval skin (Stanbridge & Butler, 1983). These facts must influence clinicians who are treating patients for either viral condylomas or intraepithelial neoplasia of the anogenital region. The importance of examining sex partners of patients with these disorders is emphasised in a case report by Stein (1980). A woman had been treated for vulval condylomata acuminata for 6 years when biopsy revealed several non-contigous areas of carcinoma in situ, and vulvectomy was performed. Two years before this her husband had developed two subpreputial warty lesions; he was circumcised, and histology showed extensive carcinoma in situ of the prepuce.

Carcinoma of the cervix

During the last few years the relationship between HPV and cervical neoplasia has been intensively studied. The precursors of carcinoma of the cervix are regarded as a continuum, cervical intraepithelial neoplasia (CIN). CIN has a variable course: regression is commoner in early (Grade 1) lesions, and progression is commoner in Grades 2 and 3 (Crum et al, 1984). Many cervical lesions which were formerly classified as CIN are really subclinical papillomavirus infections, and these often regress (Meisels et al, 1977). Subclinical papillomavirus infection of the cervix can be associated with dysplasia of all grades of severity up to invasive squamous-cell carcinoma (Syrjänen, 1980; Pilotti et al, 1981; Schmauz et al, 1983), and areas of transition between the two types of lesion have been seen (Reid et al, 1982). A geographic correlation between the incidence of condylomata acuminata and of cervical carcinoma was reported from Uganda by Schmauz et al (1983).

Cervical smears from women with histologically verified severe dysplasia, carcinoma in situ or invasive carcinoma have shown the presence of cytological features of wart virus infection in between 20% and 30% of cases, the association being more noticeable in younger age groups (Syrjänen et al, 1981; Pilotti et al, 1982). Reid et al (1982) studied a series of women who had been treated surgically for invasive or preinvasive cervical neoplasia and showed that 91% of these patients, but only 12.5% of age-matched controls, showed histological evidence of HPV infection. Reid et al (1984) analysed a series of colposcopically directed biopsies by 24 validated mutually exclusive histological parameters and found that the histological expression of papillomavirus infection decreased with increasing degrees of premalignant change.

The possibility of designating a subset of cervical papillomaviral lesions in which there is a particular risk of malignant transformation was discussed by Meisels et al (1981). The distinction between these 'atypical condylomas' and conventional flat condylomas can be made by analysis of their nuclear DNA content and histology. Lesions which are euploid or polyploid rarely progress, whereas lesions which are aneuploid often proceed to higher grades of CIN. The presence of abnormal mitoses is the most reliable histological criterion for aneuploidy (Fu et al, 1981). Crum et al (1984) examined koilocytotic cervical lesions thought to be induced by HPV for abnormal mitoses and viral antigen. They reported that although the biology of these lesions is not well defined the presence of abnormal mitotic figures may identify a subgroup of HPV-induced cervical changes which represent a transition between flat condylomas and CIN. The nature of the deep epithelial cellular disturbances associated with HPV infection and CIN has been discussed by Fletcher & Norval (1983) and Morris et al (1983).

Further evidence of a possible connection between HPV infection and CIN has come from the identification of viral antigen in biopsy specimens. Both Kurman et al (1981) and Syrjänen (1983) used the immunoperoxidase technique and identified antigen in approximately 50% of biopsy specimens associated with all degrees of epithelial atypia. Fu et al (1983) studied cervical lesions by the Feulgen technique for nuclear DNA quantitation and by an immunoperoxidase test for viral antigen. All banal HPV cervical lesions, without atypia, had a diploid or polyploid nuclear DNA distribution, and 61% had detectable HPV antigen. Among 31 lesions with atypia, 14 (45%) were aneuploid, two (14%) of which contained cells with viral antigen; on the other hand, 17 (55%) had diploid or polyploid nuclei, and of these 10 (59%) showed antigen. Syrjänen et al (1983) examined a series of cervical biopsies histologically and with an immunoperoxidase technique; they found an association between dysplasia and morphological and histochemical evidence of HPV involvement, and noted that it became less easy to detect HPV antigen as the degree of epithelial atypia became worse. Guillet et al (1983) reported similar results, and commented that evidence that viral production diminishes as the cervical lesion worsens does not exclude the possibility that HPV is involved in the aetiology of CIN, as cells transformed by the virus could easily stop producing mature virus yet still harbour the viral genome. Walker et al (1983d), using an immunoalkaline phosphatase technique, showed viral antigen in two (14%) of 14 cases of CIN, five (25%) of 20 of CIN 2, 11 (17%) of 64 of CIN 3 and in neither of two cases of invasive cancer.

It has recently become possible to identify HPV DNA in the lesions of CIN. Gissmann et al (1982) found HPV6 in two of six atypical condylomas of the cervix. Okagaki et al (1983) found that 15 (79%) of 19 samples of CIN and VIN contained HPV6, and 10 (53%) of 19 contained HPV3. McCance et al (1983) examined biopsy specimens from 22 patients referred to a colposcopy clinic, 17 because of abnormal cytology and five because of a suspicious cervical lesion, and found HPV6 in 13 (59%) of them. An important development was reported by Dürst et al (1983). They isolated a new viral DNA, HPV16, from a biopsy specimen of carcinoma of the cervix, then found it in 11 (61%) of 18 cervical cancer specimens from German women and in 8 (35%) of 23 specimens from women in Kenya and Brazil. Another new virus type, HPV18, has also been recovered from some malignant cervical tumours (zur Hausen, quoted by Singer et al, 1984). Crum et al (1984) analysed 23 flat condylomas for the presence of HPV16 and other HPV types, and correlated the results with the histology. Of 10 lesions with abnormal mitotic figures, seven contained HPV16 and one another type of HPV. Of 13 lesions without abnormal mitotic figures, only one contained HPV16, and seven other types of HPV. The authors conclude that the presence of HPV16 correlated with abnormal mitotic figures in flat warts of the cervix, and that this kind of lesion is a precursor of invasive cancer.

This evidence linking HPV with cervical neoplasia is supported by data from Baird (1983), who screened sera from patients with genital warts, CIN and invasive cancer of the cervix with an enzyme-linked immunosorbent assay for IgG antibody to a group-specific HPV antigen. All these groups had higher antibody titres than the control groups, and patients with invasive cancer has a higher geometric mean titre than those with CIN or genital warts. Studies in this rapidly expanding field suggest that some HPV types, notably HPV16 and HPV18, may be involved in the pathogenesis of cervical neoplasia; whether other factors are also involved is not yet known. These problems have been discussed by Reid et al (1982, 1983, 1984), zur Hausen (1982) and Singer et al (1984).

The question has been asked: is the differentiation of 'warty' from 'non-warty' dysplasia of practical clinical value? Grunebaum et al (1983) performed a matched pairs analysis of a group of patients attending a colposcopy clinic and found that in 69 pairs the distribution of CIN was the same whether or not there was evidence of HPV infection. Cheetham et al (1984) studied a group of 30 women with cervical lesions associated with HPV, and 25 controls, prospectively for up to 2 years and found that resolution or persistence of the viral infection appeared to make no difference to the development of the CIN lesion. Kaufman et al (1983) concluded that until more information on the natural history of these lesions is available dysplasia associated with clinical or cytological evidence of wart virus infection should be treated no differently from dysplasia without evidence of such infection.

It has been observed that condyloma acuminatum, VIN and CIN are all commoner in immunosuppressed patients than in others (Leckie & Cotton, 1977; Schneider et al, 1983). This immunosuppression may be iatrogenic, as in renal transplant recipients, or a part of a disease process, as in lymphoma (Shokri-Tabibzadeh et al, 1981).

Comment

It has been known for many years that carcinoma of the cervix and female sexual behaviour are related. The key epidemiological factors appear to be the debut of intercourse at an early age and multiple sex partners (Harris et al, 1980). The possibility that a sexually transmissible agent acts as a factor or co-factor in cervical carcinogenesis is generally admitted, and the evidence described above suggests that this agent may be a papillomavirus, particularly HPV16 and HPV18 (zur Hausen et al, 1984). Briefly, this evidence comes from the epidemiological, histological and cytological association of wart virus infection with CIN, the identification of viral antigen in dysplastic cervical biopsies, and the presence of viral DNA, particularly relating to HPV16 and HPV18, in cervical carcinoma and its precursor lesions. As this evidence accumulates, it becomes increasingly unlikely that the association between HPV and cervical neoplasia is simply a marker of promiscuity; it is probably causal.

The natural history of cervical neoplasia is still uncertain. It has been suggested that HPVs do not act alone in pathogenesis and that other factors such as infection by Herpes simplex virus, or cigarette smoking, may be involved (zur Hausen, 1982). The role of the male sex partner has also been discussed. There is evidence that the husbands of women with cervical dysplasia or carcinoma show an early debut of intercourse, and have had multiple sex partners (Buckley et al, 1981), and women whose husbands have previously been married to partners with cervical neoplasia have an increased risk of developing the disease themselves (Kessler, 1976). The concept of a 'high risk male' in the aetiology of cervical cancer has been proposed by Singer et al (1976).

Campion et al (1985) reported an increased risk of cervical neoplasia in the consorts of men with penile condylomata acuminata. Hauser et al (1985) point out that condylomata acuminata are particularly associated with HPV6 and HPV11, viruses which are found in only 20% of invasive cervical cancers, and favour the hypothesis that bowenoid papulosis, strongly associated with HPV16 and HPV18, and often clinically inconspicuous, is a high risk lesion in the aetiology of cervical cancer. The detection and clinical characterisation of penile lesions containing HPV16 and HPV18 is clearly of great importance, and studies in this field are now in progress.

HPV INFECTION OF THE ANUS AND ANAL CANAL

The distribution of anal warts was studied by Schlappner & Shaffer (1978). They reported that of 26 homosexual men with perianal condylomata acuminata 19 (73%) had internal condylomas, 19 in the anal canal and five in the rectum, above the pectinate line. In five cases persistence of internal condylomas was noted after the perianal lesions had been eradicated. Ten heterosexual men with perianal warts had no internal lesions.

Medley (1984) undertook a cytological study to determine the incidence of non-condylomatous wart virus infection of the anal canal. Anal smears processed by the Papanicolaou technique. Of 102 homosexual men 45 (44%) showed cytological features of HPV infection. Many of the patients had previously had treatment for anal warts, but only five still had them. Medley noted the existence of a transformation zone with the capacity for metaplastic change.

Complications

South et al (1977) reported a case of giant condyloma of the anus in a 38-year-old man; despite major resections the tumour spread into the pelvis, with a fatal outcome. Histologically, it was uniformly benign. Ejeckam et al (1983) described the malignant transformation of anal condylomata acuminata to squamous-cell carcinoma in a 61-year-old man, and stressed the importance of histological examination of anal warts to exclude malignant change.

HPV INFECTION OF THE RESPIRATORY TRACT

Lesions of the oral cavity

Condylomata acuminata of the mouth have been regarded as rare, but recently several case reports have appeared in which condylomas have been described affecting the lip, tongue and palate (McClatchley et al, 1979; Shaffer et al, 1980; Judson, 1981; Swan et al, 1981; Choukas & Toto, 1982; Lutzner et al, 1982; Anneroth et al, 1982). Some patients had concurrent genital or anal warts, and some gave a history of oral sex with partners with condylomata acuminata. These oral condylomas appear to be viral. Intranuclear virus particles have been seen by electron microscopy, and immunoperoxidase techniques have given positive reactions in many cases (Jenson et al, 1982; Lutzner et al, 1982). Transmission of HPV by orogenital contact is clearly possible, but non-sexual transmission may also occur (Ashiru, 1984).

An analogous disease is focal oral epithelial hyperplasia (Heck's disease). This occurs mostly in American Indians, South Africans and Eskimos (Jablonska & Orth, 1983). Histologically the lesions resemble flat cervical condylomas, but a distinct viral type, HPV 13, is present, and Heck's disease is not thought to be sexually transmissible.

Lesions of the larynx

Squamous papillomas of the larynx are a serious clinical problem, particularly in the first years of life. Papillomatosis runs a prolonged course, recurrence after treatment is common, and malignancy can develop (Bewtra et al, 1982; von Krogh, 1984). There is recent evidence linking laryngeal papillomas in infants with genital warts in their mothers. Quick et al (1980) reported that 21 (68%) of the mothers of children with laryngeal papillomas had had genital warts during pregnancy or parturition.

The infectivity of genital warts to infants may be low (Cohn et al, 1981), but in view of the serious nature of the laryngeal disease there has been discussion about the desirability of screening for genital warts in pregnancy, and even prophylactic caesarian section (Leading Article, 1980).

Papillomavirus particles have only rarely been seen in juvenile laryngeal papillomas, but genus-specific antigen has been demonstrated in approximately 50% of lesions (Lack et al, 1980; Quick et al, 1980; Costa et al, 1981; Lancaster & Jenson, 1981). HPV6 and HPV11, both commonly associated with vulval and cervical condylomas, have been recovered from laryngeal papillomas (Gissmann et al, 1983). Mounts & Kashima (1984) identified HPV6 in respiratory papillomas from both adults and infants. They distinguished four viral subtypes, and noted variations in the behaviour of the lesions according to the subtype involved.

Steinberg et al (1983) analysed biopsy specimens from 20 patients with a history of laryngeal papillomas. All the tumours examined contained HPV DNA sequences, but in addition four samples from uninvolved sites in two patients with active disease and eight samples from patients in remission also contained viral DNA. The authors comment that these results explain the clinical pattern of frequent recurrences in laryngeal papillomatosis, even after long periods of remission, and raise the possibility that many infants exposed to HPV from maternal condylomas may develop 'silent' infections which are not expressed as condylomas. Papillomavirus sequences have also been detected in normal skin adjacent to anogenital condylomata (Ferenczy et al 1985).

REFERENCES

Altmeyer P, Chilf G-N, Holzmann H 1982 Hiruties papillaris vulvae (pseudo-condylomata of the vulva). Hautarzt 33: 281–283

Ananthakrishnan N, Ravindran R, Veliath A J, Parkash S 1981 Loewenstein-Buschke tumour of penis — a carcinomimic. Report of 24 cases with review of the literature. British Journal of Urology 53: 460–465

Anneroth G, Anniko M, Romander H 1982 Oral condyloma acuminatum. A light and electron microscopic study. International Journal of Oral Surgery 11: 260–264

Ashiru J O, Ogunbawjo B O, Rotowa N A, Adeyemi-Doro F A B, Osoba A O 1983 Intraoral condylomata acuminata. British Journal of Venereal Diseases 59: 325–326

Baird P J 1983 Serological evidence for the association of papillomavirus and cervical neoplasia. Lancet ii:17–18

Baird P J, Elliott P, Stening M, Korda A 1979 Giant condyloma acuminatum of the vulva and anal canal. Australian and New Zealand Journal of Obstetrics and Gynaecology 19: 119–122

Baruah M C, Sardari L, Selvaraju M, Veliath A J 1984 Perianal condylomata acuminata in a male child. British Journal of Venereal Diseases 60: 60–61

Bender M E, Pass F 1981 Papillomavirus and cutaneous malignancy. International Journal of Dermatology 20: 468–474

Bewtra C, Krishnan R, Lee S S 1982 Malignant changes in non-irradiated juvenile laryngotracheal papillomatosis. Archives of Otolaryngology 108: 114–116

Braun L, Farmer E R, Shah K V 1983 Immunoperoxidase localisation of papillomavirus antigen in cutaneous warts and Bowenoid papulosis. Journal of Medical Virology 12: 187–193

Buckley J D, Harris R W, Doll R 1981 Case control study of the husbands of women with dysplasia and carcinoma of the cervix uteri. Lancet 11: 1010–1012

Campion M J, Singer A, Clarkson P K, McCance D J 1985 Increased risk of cervical neoplasia in the consorts of men with penile condylomata acuminata. Lancet i 943–945

Carr G, William D C 1977 Anal warts in a population of gay men in New York City. Sexually Transmitted Diseases 4: 56–57

Cheetham D, Smith J, Wilson C, Munday P E, Coleman D V 1984 Clinical significance of human papillomavirus infection of the uterine cervix in the development of cervical intraepithelial neoplasia. British Journal of Venereal Diseases 60: 182–185

Chief Medical Officer 1973 Sexually transmitted diseases. Extract from annual report of the Chief Medical

Officer to the Department of Health and Social Security for the year 1971. British Journal of Venereal Diseases 49: 89–95

Chief Medical Officer 1984 Sexually transmitted diseases. Extract from annual report of the Chief Medical Officer to the Department of Health and Social Security for the year 1981. British Journal of Venereal Diseases 60: 199–203

Choo Y C, Morley G W 1980 Multiple primary neoplasms of the anogenital region. Obstetrics and Gynecology 56: 365–369

Choukas N C, Toto P D 1982 Condylomata acuminata of the oral cavity. Oral Surgery 54: 480–485

Chuang T-Y, Perry H O, Kurland L T, Ilstrup D M 1984a Condyloma acuminatum in Rochester Minnesota 1950–78 1. Epidemiology and clinical features. Archives of Dermatology 120: 469–475

Chuang T-Y, Perry H O, Kurland L T, Ilstrup D M 1984b Condyloma acuminatum in Rochester Minnesota 1950–78 2. Anaplasia and unfavourable outcomes. Archives of Dermatology 120: 476–483

Cohn A M, Kos J T, Taber L H, Adam E 1981 Recurring laryngeal papilloma. American Journal of Otolaryngology 2: 129–132

Costa J, Howley P M, Bowling M C, Howard R, Bauer W C 1981 Presence of human papilloma virus antigens in juvenile multiple laryngeal papilloma. American Journal of Clinical Pathology 75: 194–197

Crum C P, Ikenberg H, Richart R M, Gissmann L 1984 Human papillomavirus type 16 and early cervical neoplasia. New England Journal of Medicine 310: 880–883

Crum C P, Braun L A, Shah K V, Fu Y S, Levine R U, Fenoglio C M, Richart RM, Townsend DE 1982a Vulval intraepithelial neoplasia: correlation of nuclear DNA content and the presence of a human papilloma virus (HPV) antigen. Cancer 49: 468–471

Crum C P, Fu Y S, Levine R U, Richart R M, Townsend D E, Fenoglio C M 1982b Intraepithelial squamous lesions of the vulva: biologic and histologic criteria for the distinction of condylomas from vulval intraepithelial neoplasia. American Journal of Obstetrics and Gynecology 144: 77–83

Daling J R, Chu J, Weiss N S, Emel L, Tamini H K 1984 The association of condylomata acuminata and squamous carcinoma of the vulva. British Journal of Cancer 50: 533–535

Daling J R, Weiss N S, Sherman K J 1984 History of genital warts in a selected population. Lancet i 157–158

Dean P, Lancaster W D, Chun B, Jenson A B 1983 Human papillomavirus structural antigens in squamous papilloma of the male urethra. Journal of Urology 129: 873–875

de Benedictis T J, Marmar J L, Praiss D E 1977 Intraurethral condyloma acuminata: management and a review of the literature. Journal of Urology 118: 767–769

de Jong A R, Weiss J C, Brent R L 1982 Condylomata acuminata in children. American Journal of Diseases of Children 136: 704–706

Della Torre G, Pilotti S, de Palo G, Rilke F 1978 Viral particles in cervical condylomatous lesions. Tumori 64: 549–553

Dürst M, Gissmann L, Ikenberg H, zur Hausen H 1983 A papillomavirus DNA from a cervical carcinoma and its prevalence in cancer biopsy samples from different geographic regions. Proceedings of the National Academy of Science 80: 3812–3815

Dyson J L, Walker P G, Singer A 1984 Human papillomavirus infection of the uterine cervix: histological appearances in 28 cases identified by immunohistological techniques. Journal of Clinical Pathology 37: 126–130

Editorial Note 1983 Condyloma acuminatum — United States 1966–1981. Journal of the American Medical Association 250: 336

Eftaiha M S, Amshel A L, Shonberg I L 1978 Condylomata acuminata in an infant and a mother: report of a case. Diseases of the Colon and Rectum 21: 369–371

Ejeckam G C, Idikio H A, Nayak V, Gardiner J P 1983 Malignant transformation in an anal condyloma acuminatum. Canadian Journal of Surgery 26: 170–173

Ferenczy A, Mitao M, Nagai N et al 1985 Latent papillomavirus and recurring genital warts. New England Journal of Medicine 313: 784–788

Fletcher S 1983 Histology of papillomavirus infection of the cervix uteri: the history, taxonomy, nomenclature and reporting of koilocytotic dysplasia. Journal of Clinical Pathology 36: 616–624

Fletcher S, Norval M 1983 On the nature of the deep cellular disturbances in human papillomavirus infection of the squamous cervical epithelium. Lancet ii 546–549

Fu Y S, Reagan J W, Richart R M 1981 Definition of precursors. Gynecologic Oncology 12: S220–231

Fu Y S, Braun L, Shah K V, Lawrence W D, Robboy S J 1983 Histologic, nuclear DNA and human papillomavirus studies of cervical condylomas. Cancer 52: 1705–1711

Fu Y S, Reagan J W, Townsend D E, Kaufman R H, Richart R M, Wentz W B 1981 Nuclear DNA study of vulval intraepithelial and invasive squamous neoplasia. Obstetrics and Gynecology 57: 643–652

Gissmann L, de Villiers E M, zur Hausen H 1982 Analysis of human genital warts (condylomata acuminata) and other genital tumours for human papillomavirus DNA. International Journal of Cancer 29: 143–146

Gissmann L, Wolnik L, Ikenberg H, Koldovsky U, Schnürch H G, zur Hausen H 1983 Human papillomavirus types 6 and 11 DNA sequences in genital and laryngeal papillomas and in some cervical cancers. Proceedings of the National Academy of Science USA 80: 560–563

Grunebaum A N, Sedliz A, Sillman F, Fruchter R, Stanek A, Boyce J 1983 Association of human papillomavirus infection and cervical intraepithelial neoplasia. Obstetrics and Gynecology 62: 448–455

Grussendorf E T, Bar T 1977 Condylomata acuminata associated with morbus Bowen (carcinoma in situ). A light and electron microscopic study. Dermatologica 155: 50–58

Guillet G Y, Braun L, Shah K, Ferenczy A 1983 Papillomavirus in cervical condylomas with and without associated cervical intraepithelial neoplasia. Journal of Investigative Dermatology 81: 513–516

Guillet G Y, Braun L, Massé R, Aftimos J, Geniaux M, Texier L 1984 Bowenoid papulosis. Demonstration of human papilloma virus (HPV) with anti-HPV serum. Archives of Dermatology 120: 514–516

Gupta J W, Gupta P K, Shah K V, Kelly D P 1983 Distribution of human papilloma virus antigen in cervicovaginal smears and cervical tissues. International Journal of Gynecological Pathology 2: 160–170

Harahap M 1979 Asymptomatic gonorrhoea among patients with condylomata acuminata. British Journal of Venereal Diseases 55: 450

Harris R W C, Brinton L A, Cowdell R H, Skegg D C, Smith P G, Vessey M P, Doll R 1980 Characteristics of women with dysplasia or carcinoma in situ of the cervix uteri. British Journal of Cancer 42: 359–369

Hauser B, Gross G, Schneider A, de Villiers E-M, Gissmann L, Wagner D 1985 HPV-related bowenoid papulosis. Lancet 1, 106.

Hills E, Laverty C R 1979 Electron microscopic detection of papilloma virus particles in selected koilocytotic cells in a routine cervical smear. Acta Cytologica 23: 53–56

Ikenberg H, Gissmann L, Gross G, Grussendorf-Conen, zur Hausen H 1983 Human papilloma virus type 16-related DNA in genital Bowen's disease and in bowenoid papulosis. International Journal of Cancer 32: 563–565

Jablonska S, Orth G 1983 Human papillomaviruses. In: Rook A J, Maibach H I (eds) Recent advances in dermatology. Churchill Livingstone, Edinburgh, ch 1, 1–36

Jarrett W F H 1980 Papillomaviruses in benign and malignant tumours in cattle. In: Essex M, Todero G, zur Hausen H (eds) Viruses in naturally occurring cancers, vol A, Cold Spring Harbor Laboratory, 215–222

Jenson A B, Lancaster W D, Hartmann D-P, Shaffer E L 1982 Frequency and distribution of papillomavirus structural antigens in verrucae, multiple papillomas and condylomata of the oral cavity. American Journal of Pathology 107: 212–218

Judson F N 1981 Condyloma acuminatum of the oral cavity: a case report. Sexually Transmitted Diseases 8: 218–219

Katz R L, Anderson M D, Weiss K M 1984 Diagnosis and epidemiology of condyloma acuminatum. Journal of the American Medical Association 251: 1028–1029

Katz H I, Posalaky Z, McGinley D 1978 Pigmented penile papules with carcinoma in situ changes. British Journal of Dermatology 99: 155–162

Kaufman R, Koss L G, Kurman R J, Meisels A, Okagaki T, Patten S F, Reid R, Richart R M, Wied G L 1983 Statement of caution in the interpretation of papillomavirus-associated lesions of the epithelium of the uterine cervix. American Journal of Obstetrics and Gynecology 146: 125

Kessler II 1976 Human cervix cancer as a venereal disease. Cancer Research 36: 783–791

Kimura S 1980 Condylomata acuminata with pigmented papular lesions. Dermatologica 160: 390–397

Kimura S, Hirai A, Harada R, Nagashima M 1978 So-called multicentric pigmented Bowen's disease. Dermatologica 157: 229–237

Kinghorn G 1978 Genital warts: incidence of associated genital infections. British Journal of Dermatology 99: 405–409

Kirkup W, Evans A S, Brough A K, Davis J A, O'Loughlin T, Wilkinson G, Monaghan J M 1982 Cervical intraepithelial neoplasia and 'warty' atypia: a study of colposcopic, histological and cytological characteristics. British Journal of Obstetrics and Gynaecology 89: 571–577

Kurman R J, Shah K H, Lancaster W D, Jenson A B 1981 Immunoperoxidase localisation of papillomavirus antigens in cervical dysplasias and vulvar condylomas. American Journal of Obstetrics and Gynecology 140: 931–935

Lack E E, Jenson A B, Smith H G, Healy G B, Pass F, Vawter G F 1980 Immunoperoxidase localisation of human papillomaviruses in laryngeal papilloma. Intervirology 14: 148–154

Lancaster W D, Jenson A B 1981 Evidence for papillomavirus genus-specific antigens and DNA in laryngeal papilloma. Intervirology 15: 204–212

Laohadtanaphorn S, Hunter J C, Ansell I D 1979 Multicentric pigmented carcinoma in situ in the vulva in association with vulval condylomata acuminata. Australian and New Zealand Journal of Obstetrics and Gynaecology 19: 249–252

Laverty C 1980 Noncondylomatous wart infection of the cervix: cytologic, histologic and electron microscopic features. Obstetric and Gynecologic Survey 34: 820–822

Leading Article 1980 Multiple papillomas of the larynx in children. Lancet i: 367

Lecatsas G 1983 Papillomavirus in urine in pregnancy and following renal transplantation. Progress in Clinical and Biological Research 105: 143–148

Leckie G B, Cotton R E 1977 Simultaneous in situ carcinoma of the cervix, vulva and perineum after immunosuppressive therapy for renal transplantation. British Journal of Obstetrics and Gynaecology 84: 143–148

Levine R U, Crum C P, Herman E, Silvers D, Ferenczy A, Richart R M 1984 Cervical papillomavirus infection and intraepithelial neoplasia: a study of male sexual partners. Obstetrics and Gynecology 64: 16–20

Lutzner M A 1978 Epidermodysplasia verruciformis: an autosomal recessive disease characterised by viral warts and skin cancer. A model for viral oncogenesis. Bulletin of Cancer (Paris) 65: 169–182

Lutzner M A, Kuffer R, Blanchet-Bardon C, Croissant O 1982 Different papillomaviruses as the causes of oral warts. Archives of Dermatology 118: 393–399

McCance D J, Walker P G, Dyson J L, Coleman D V, Singer A 1983 Presence of human papillomavirus DNA sequences in cervical intraepithelial neoplasia. British Medical Journal 287: 784–788

McCoy C R, Applebaum H, Besser A S 1982 Condylomata acuminata: an unusual presentation of child abuse. Journal of Pediatric Surgery 17: 505–507

McClatchley K D, Colquitt W N, Robert R C 1979 Condyloma acuminatum of the lip: report of a case. Journal of Oral Surgery 37: 751–752

Mariuzzi G M, Beltrami C A, di Loreto C, de Nictolis M, Stramazotti D, Portolani M, Borgatti A M, Morresi A 1983 Human papillomavirus in cervical condylomata: an immunohistochemical study. Ricordo Clinici Laboratorio 13: 255–260

Massé S, Tosi-Kruse A, Carmel M, Elhilali M 1981 Condyloma acuminatum of the bladder. Urology 17: 381–382

Medley G 1984 Anal smear test to diagnose occult anorectal infection with human papillomavirus in men. British Journal of Venereal Diseases 60: 205

Meisels A, Fortin R 1976 Condylomatous lesions of the cervix and vagina I Cytologic patterns. Acta Cytologica 20: 505–509

Meisels A, Fortin R, Roy M 1977 Condylomatous lesions of the cervix and vagina II Cytologic, colposcopic and histopathologic study. Acta Cytologica 21: 379–390

Meisels A, Morin C, Casas-Cordero M 1982 Human papillomavirus infection of the cervix. International Journal of Gynecological Pathology 1: 75–94

Meisels A, Roy M, Fortier M, Morin C, Casas-Cordero M, Shah K V, Turgeon H 1981 Human papillomavirus infection of the cervix. The atypical condyloma. Acta Cytologica 25: 7–14

Morin C, Meisels A 1980 Human papillomavirus infection of the uterine cervix. Acta Cytologica 24: 82–84

Morin C, Braun L, Casas-Cordero M, Shah K V, Roy M, Fortier M, Meisels A 1981 Confirmation of the papillomavirus etiology of condylomatous cervical lesions by the peroxidase-antiperoxidase technique. Journal of the National Cancer Institute 66: 831–835

Morris H H, Gatter K C, Sykes G, Cazemore V, Mason D Y 1983 Langerhans' cells in human cervical epithelium: effects of wart virus infection and intraepithelial neoplasia. British Journal of Obstetrics and Gynaecology 90: 412–420

Mounts P, Kashima H 1984 Association of human papilloma virus subtype and clinical course in respiratory papillomatosis. Laryngoscope 94: 28–33

Okagaki T, Twiggs L B, Zachow K R, Clark B A, Ostrow R S, Faras A J 1983 Identification of human papillomavirus DNA in cervical and vaginal intra-epithelial neoplasia with molecularly cloned virus specific DNA clones. International Journal of Gynecologic Pathology 2: 153–159

Okagaki T, Clark B A, Zachow K R, Twiggs L B, Ostrow R S, Pass F, Faras A J 1984 Presence of human papillomavirus in verrucous carcinoma (Ackerman) of the vagina. Archives of Pathology and Laboratory Medicine 108: 567–570

Oriel J D 1977 Genital warts. Sexually Transmitted Diseases 4: 153–159

Ostrow R S, Bender M, Niimura M, Seki T, Kawashima M, Pass F, Faras A J 1982 Human papillomavirus DNA in cutaneous primary and metastasised squamous-cell carcinoma from patients with epidermodysplasia verruciformis. Proceedings of the National Academy of Science USA 79: 1634–1638

Partridge E E, Murad T, Shingleton H M, Austin J M, Hatch K D 1980 Verrucous lesions of the female genitalia 1. Giant condyloma. American Journal of Obstetrics and Gynecology 137: 412–418

Pilotti S, Rilke F, Alasio L, Fontanelli R 1982 Histologic evidence for an association of cervical intraepithelial neoplasia and human papillomavirus infection. Diagnostic Gynecology and Obstetrics 4: 357–362

Pilotti S, Rilke F, de Palo G, Della Torre G, Alasio L 1981 Condyloma of the uterine cervix and koilocytosis of intraepithelial neoplasia. Journal of Clinical Pathology 34: 52–54

Pollack H M, de Benedicits T J, Marmar J L, Praiss D E 1978 Urethrographic manifestations of venereal warts (condylomata acuminata). Radiology 126: 643–646

Purola E, Savia E 1977 Cytology of gynecologic condyloma acuminatum. Acta Cytologica 21: 26–31

Quick C A, Watts S L, Krzyzek R A, Faras A J 1980 Relationship between condylomata and laryngeal papillomata. Clinical and molecular virological evidence. Annals of Otology, Rhinology and Laryngology 89: 467–471

Reid R 1984 Papillomavirus and cervical neoplasia. Modern implications and future prospects. Colposcopy and Gynecologic Laser Surgery 1: 3–34

Reid R 1983 Genital warts and cervical cancer. II Is human papillomavirus infection the trigger to cervical carcinogenesis? Gynecologic Oncology 15: 239–252

Reid R, Laverty C R, Coppleson M, Isarangkul W, Hills E 1980 Non-condylomatous cervical wart virus infection. Obstetrics and Gynecology 55: 476–483

Reid R, Stanhope C R, Herschmann B R, Booth E, Phibbs G D, Smith J P 1982 Genital warts and cervical cancer. I Evidence of an association between subclinical papillomavirus infection and cervical malignancy. Cancer 50: 377–387

Reid R, Crum C P, Herschmann B R, Fu Y S, Braun L, Shah K V, Agronow S J, Stanhope C R 1984 Genital warts and cervical cancer. III Subclinical papillomavirus infection and cervical neoplasia are linked by a spectrum of continuous morphologic and biologic change. Cancer 53: 943–953

Ridley C M 1983 Vulval dysplasia. Journal of Hospital Medicine 30: 223

Rous P, Kidd J G, Smith W E 1953 Experiments on the cause of the rabbit carcinomas derived from virus-induced papillomas. Journal of Experimental Medicine 96: 159–174

Roy M, Meisels A, Fortier M, Morin C, Casas-Cordero M 1981 Vaginal condylomata — a human papillomavirus infection. Clinical Obstetrics and Gynecology 24: 461–483

Schlappner O L A, Shaffer E A 1978 Anorectal condylomata acuminata: a missed part of the condyloma spectrum. Canadian Medical Association Journal 118: 172–173

Schmauz R, Owor R 1980 Condylomatous tumours of the vulva, vagina and penis. Relationship between histological appearance and age. Journal of Clinical Pathology 33: 1039–1046

Schneider V, Kay S, Lee H M 1983 Immunosuppression as a high-risk factor in the development of condyloma acuminatum and squamous neoplasia of the cervix. Acta Cytologica 27: 220–224

Seidel J, Zonana J, Totten E 1979 Condylomata acuminata as a sign of sexual abuse in children. Journal of Pediatrics 95: 553–554

Shafeek M A, Osman M I, Hussein M A 1979 Carcinoma of the vulva arising in condylomata acuminata. Obstetrics and Gynecology 54: 120–123

Shaffer E L, Reimann B E F, Gysland W B 1980 Oral condyloma acuminatum. A case report with light microscopic and ultrastructural features. Journal of Oral Pathology 9: 163–173

Shokri-Tabibzadeh S, Koss L G, Molnar J, Romney S 1981 Association of human papillomavirus with neoplastic processes in the genital tract of four women with impaired immunity. Gynecologic Oncology 12: 129–140

Singer A, Reid B L, Coppleson M 1976 The role of the high risk male in the aetiology of cervical cancer — a correlation of epidemiology and molecular biology. American Journal of Obstetrics and Gynecology 126: 110–116

Singer A, Walker P G, McCance D J 1984 Genital wart virus infections: nuisance or potentially lethal? British Medical Journal 288: 735–736

Smith J, Coleman D V 1983 Electron microscopy of cells showing viral cytopathic effects in Papanicolaou smears. Acta Cytologica 27: 605–613

South L M, O'Sullivan J P, Gazet J C 1977 Giant condyloma of Buschke and Loewenstein. Clinical Oncology 3: 107–115

Stanbridge C M, Butler E B 1983 Human papillomavirus infection of the lower female genital tract: association with multicentric neoplasia. International Journal of Gynecologic Pathology 2: 264–274

Stein D S 1980 Transmissible venereal neoplasia: a case report. American Journal of Obstetrics and Gynecology 137: 864–865

Steinberg B M, Topp W C, Schneider P S, Abramson A L 1983 Laryngeal papillomavirus infection during clinical remission. New England Journal of Medicine 308: 1261–1264

Storrs F J 1977 Spread of condylomata acuminata to infants and children. Archives of Dermatology 113: 1294

Stumpf P G 1980 Increasing occurrence of condylomata acuminata in premenarchal children. Obstetrics and Gynecology 56: 262–264

Swan R H, McDaniel R K, Dreiman B B, Rome W C 1981 Condyloma acuminatum involving the oral mucosa. Oral Surgery 51: 503–508

Syrjänen K J 1980 Current views on the condylomatous lesions in the uterine cervix and their possible relationship to cervical squamous cell carcinoma. Obstetric and Gynecologic Survey 35: 685–694

Syrjänen K J 1983 Human papillomavirus lesions in association with cervical dysplasias and neoplasias. Obstetrics and Gynecology 62: 617–624

Syrjänen K J, Pyrhönen S 1982 Demonstration of human papilloma virus antigen in the condylomatous lesions of the uterine cervix by immunoperoxidase technique. Gynecologic and Obstetric Investigation 14: 90–96

Syrjänen K J, Heinonen U-M, Kauraniemi T 1981 Cytologic evidence of the association of condylomatous lesions with dysplastic and neoplastic changes in the uterine cervix. Acta Cytologica 25: 17–22

Syrjänen K J, Väyrnen M, Castrén O, Mäntyjärvi R, Pyrhönen S, Yliskoski M 1983 Morphological and immunohistochemical evidence of human papillomavirus involvement in the dysplastic lesions of the uterine cervix. International Journal of Gynecology and Obstetrics 21: 261–269

Syrjänen K J, Väyrnen M, Castrén O, Yliskoski M, Mäntyjärvi R, Pyrhonen S, Saarikoski S 1984 Sexual behaviour of women with human papillomavirus lesions of the uterine cervix. British Journal of Venereal Diseases 60: 243–248

Tessler A N, Applebaum S M 1982 The Buschke-Loewenstein tumour. Urology 20: 36–39

Tropé C, Grundsell H, Henrikson H, Johnsson J-E, Lindahl B, Simonsson E 1982 Giant condyloma acuminatum with focal malignant degeneration. Acta Obstetrica Gynecologica Scandinavia 61: 93–95

Von Krogh G 1984 The association between condyloma acuminatum, airway papillomata and squamous-cell carcinomata: a preventive-therapeutic challenge. European Journal of Sexually Transmitted Diseases 1: 119–123

Wade T R, Kopf A W, Ackerman A B 1979 Bowenoid papulosis of the genitalia. Archives of Dermatology 115: 306–308

Walker P G, Singer A, Dyson J L, Oriel J D 1983a Natural history of cervical epithelial abnormalities in patients with vulval warts. A colposcopic study. British Journal of Venereal Diseases 59: 327–329

Walker P G, Colley N V, Grubb C, Tejerina A, Oriel J D 1983b Abnormalities of the uterine cervix in women with vulval warts. British Journal of Venereal Diseases 59: 120–123

Walker P G, Singer A, Dyson J L, Shah K V, Wilters J, Coleman D V 1983c Colposcopy in the diagnosis of papillomavirus infection of the uterine cervix. British Journal of Obstetrics and Gynaecology 90: 1082–1086

Walker P G, Singer A, Dyson J L, Shah K V, To A, Coleman D V 1983d The prevalence of human papillomavirus infection in patients with cervical epithelial neoplasia. British Journal of Cancer 48: 99–101

Wein A J, Benson G S 1977 Treatment of urethral condyloma acuminatum with 5-fluorouracil cream. Urology 9: 413–415

Woodruff J D, Braun L, Calavieri R, Gupta P, Pass F, Shah K V 1980 Immunologic identification of papillomavirus antigen in condyloma tissues from the female genital tract. Obstetrics and Gynecology 56: 727–732

Zachow K R, Ostrow R S, Bender M, Watts S, Okagaki T, Pass F, Faras A J 1982 Detection of human papillomavirus DNA in anogenital neoplasia. Nature 300: 771–773

Zamora S, Baumgartner G, Shaw M 1983 Condyloma acuminatum in a 2½-year-old girl. Journal of Urology 129: 145–146

zur Hausen H 1982 Human genital cancer: synergism between two virus infections or synergism between a virus infection and initiating events? Lancet ii: 1370–1372

zur Hausen H, Gissmann L, Schlehofer J R 1984 Viruses in the aetiology of human genital cancer. Progress in Medical Virology 30: 170–186

8. Genital papillomavirus infections: treatment

G. R. Kinghorn

The management of condylomata acuminata presents a problem of increasing magnitude to genito-urinary medicine, dermatology, gynaecology and urology clinics and continues to be a formidable therapeutic challenge. The well-known cliché that it is easier to treat skin cancer than venereal warts still holds true. Evidence of this difficulty is provided by the innumerable types of medical, surgical, immunological and psychotherapeutic approaches to treatment. The medical literature abounds with uncontrolled studies of various treatments, each with enthusiastic advocates, in which significant cure rates are claimed yet the spontaneous, unpredictable and ill understood resolution of condylomata acuminata provides an uncertain base upon which to judge the efficacy of any individual treatment. Some recent controlled studies have questioned the value of several long established therapies.

GENERAL MANAGEMENT

Condylomata accuminata display a marked variability in their responsiveness to any treatment and particular problems may occur with intraurethral, anorectal, cervico-vaginal and oral warts. In pregnancy, where physiological changes favour wart proliferation, chemotherapeutic treatments are contraindicated.

The proliferation of warts remains poorly understood but appears to be favoured by local conditions which promote warmth and humidity (Oriel, 1971) and general conditions which impair cell mediated immunity (Powell, 1978). All patients with genital warts should be screened for other sexually transmitted diseases. The recognition and treatment of these local or systemic conditions is clearly important in facilitating optimal therapeutic response. It is also beneficial to give advice routinely about the maintenance of genital hygiene and means of preventing reinfection. Sexual consorts should be encouraged to attend for examination and the use of the condom advocated until both partners are wart-free.

The role of emotional factors in accelerating or inhibiting spontaneous wart remissions remains controversial and has received scant scientific study. They are believed by some to be responsible for the many lay treatments of warts, for which there are impressive claims of success. It has been argued, based on the variable success rates of wart treatments, that the method of treatment is less important than the person who applies it (Allington, 1952). Advocates of the treatment of warts by psychotherapy and hypnosis believe that, under the influence of suggestion, affective responses induced in the patient produce skin physicochemical and blood flow changes which result in wart regression (Ullman, 1959). The cure of condylomata acuminata in four patients by hypnosis alone was claimed by Ewin (1974) and Straatmeyer & Rhodes (1983) were able to use hypnotic suggestion to eradicate resistant genital

147

warts in a woman. Whilst the efficacy of psychotherapy alone remains unproven, it is clearly desirable that the use of suggestion as an adjunct to other treatments in the general management of HPV infections be further investigated.

CHEMOTHERAPY

Podophyllin, obtained as a resin from the rhizomes of the mayapple and mandrake plants, has been the most widely used cytotoxic treatment of genital warts since the initial enthusiastic reports of its use by Culp & Kaplan (1944). This caustic agent has a colchicine-like action, initiating mitotic activity in prickle cell skin layers and then arresting cell division in the metaphase. Cellular swelling and pyknosis ensue which can make difficult the histological distinction between podophyllin treated condylomatous lesions and intraepithelial neoplasia (Fitzgerald et al, 1974). Concern has been expressed that podophyllin may be carcinogenic, following the report of vulval dysplasia developing in a podophyllin treated wart (Gueson et al, 1971). Certainly lesion biopsy, where indicated, and cervical cytology smears should be performed prior to podophyllin application. The growing evidence of the oncogenic potential of HPV in the genital tract (Ludwig et al, 1981; Fenoglio & Ferenczy, 1982; Reid et al, 1982, 1984) strongly suggests that podophyllin treatment of cervical and vaginal warts is best avoided.

The topical application of podophyllin in a 10 to 40% solution in spirit or tincture of benzoin may produce painful ulceration at treatment sites, especially with anal warts. Local side effects can be minimised by careful application by clinic personnel, beginning treatment with weaker solutions and shorter intervals before the paint is washed off, and gradually increasing these according to patient response. The purified active ingredient of the resin, podophyllotoxin, has fewer local side effects (Von Krogh, 1978, 1981). Von Krogh found that 49% of 214 men with penile warts treated with podophyllotoxin for up to 7 days were wart free at 3 months. The cure rate for preputial warts was higher than for meatal warts and penile skin warts. Flat hyperkeratotic lesions also respond poorly (Oriel, 1977). Simmonds (1981) investigated the effect of differing concentrations of podophyllin on the eradication of penile warts. He found that of 109 patients treated at weekly intervals, with either 10% of 25% podophyllin in benzoin, only 22% were wart free at 3 months, the results being unaffected by the concentration of the application.

The limitations of topical podophyllin in terms of variable and often slow response, the frequency of recurrences and local side effects, are compounded by the occurrence of systemic toxicity. Podophyllin is potentially teratogenic (Cullis, 1962; Karol et al, 1980) and has resulted in fetal death after cutaneous application in late pregnancy (Chamberlain et al, 1972). Its use should be avoided in all stages of pregnancy. Systemic toxicity is more common after oral ingestion, or topical administration of large amounts to vascular or traumatised lesions (Montaldi et al, 1974; Stoehr et al, 1978). Neurotoxicity is most commonly reported. Slater et al (1978) described a 16-year-old girl who developed a reversible encephalopathy, manifest as progressive stupor leading to coma, and a residual peripheral neuropathy, following application of 5 ml of 25% podophyllin in spirit to vaginal warts. Myocardial, hepatic and renal toxicity (Ward et al, 1954) may also occur.

These shortcomings of podophyllin treatment of condylomata acuminata require medical supervision and regular reassessment of patients undergoing treatment, and transfer to other therapy if genital warts show little response after weekly treatment for one month.

Of the other topical cytotoxic preparations, both Powell (1972) and Kovar (1979) recommend trichloracetic acid which when applied to warts has an instant coagulant and dessicant action leading to necrosis of superficial skin layers. Although systemic absorption is not a problem, pain on application is common, and careless use can result in deep ulcers which heal with considerable scarring. Gabriel & Thin (1983) reported a double blind study in which they compared topical treatment by a combination of 25% podophyllin and 50% trichloracetic acid with 25% podophyllin alone in the management of anogenital warts in men. Although combination treatment required significantly fewer applications to achieve wart eradication, local side effects were more common and at 3 months the mean clearance rate of 32% was not significantly different in either treatment group.

Caustic agents are relatively ineffective for meatal and urethral warts, and can cause chemical urethritis and meatal stenosis. Many topical chemotherapeutic agents have been employed, including chloropactin, colchicine, methotrexate, thiotepa and bleomycin for warts in this site. Most reports favour the use of 5-fluouracil (5FU) (Brenner et al, 1983). This fluorinated pyrimidine has an antimetabolic action by inducing thymine deficiency in rapidly metabolising cells which interferes with DNA synthesis. Hursthouse (1975) showed in a double-blind study that 5% 5FU was superior to a placebo in the treatment of common warts. Uncontrolled trials of 5FU use in penile (Haye, 1974) meatal (Nel & Fourie, 1973) and vulval warts (Handojo & Pardjono, 1973) have been reported. The effect of 1% 5FU, applied twice daily for 3 weeks, on penile warts was studied by Von Krogh (1978). The cure rates after 3 months were 25% for meatal, 36% for preputial, and 71% for penile skin warts. Mild local side effects, consisting of itching or superficial erosions at the site of application, were reported by 58% of patients. Dretler & Klein (1975) successfully treated 19 of 20 patients with intraurethral warts with 5% 5FU cream instilled per urethram after each voiding and at bedtime for 3–8 days. The single failure occurred with warts sited proximal to the external sphincter. Weimar et al (1978) used 5FU urethral suppositories, inserted twice daily for 7–10 days, to treat sucessfully 12 patients and avoid the irritative effects of urethral spillage of 5FU cream on adjacent genital skin. Pereira & Arruda (1982) were able to achieve intraurethral wart eradication in 15 patients with three daily instillations of 5FU cream in courses lasting 5–15 days. In none of these studies was systemic toxicity reported, although transient dysuria and meatitis were not uncommon. A patient in whom an intense urethritis, leading to urinary retention, followed topical 5FU was reported by Cetti et al (1984). The relatively long duration of treatment and frequent recurrences after treatment are also limitations of 5FU (Debenedictus et al, 1977).

The use of topical antiviral agents in treating papillomavirus induced lesions has been of limited success. Idoxuridine in 10%, 20% and 40% solutions has been investigated by Morrison (1975); Kinghorn (unpublished data) did not find 5% acyclovir cream of value in treating penile condylomata. There have been more encouraging reports of the use of systemic interferon in the treatment of HPV associated lesions. Interferons inhibit a broad spectrum of both DNA and RNA viruses as well as stimulating natural killer cell activity and other components of the immune system. In vitro studies have shown that they are capable of ridding cultures of bovine papilloma virus-transformed cells of extrachromosomal virus (Turek et al, 1982). Systemic lymphoblastoid interferon (IFN-α), administered by intramuscular injection, is effective in inducing regression of HPV-associated laryngeal papillomata (Haglund et al, 1981; McCabe & Clarke, 1983).

Topical treatment with IFN-α in an ointment base eradicated vulval warts significantly more frequently and rapidly than a placebo in a double-blind trial (Ikic et al, 1983). Preliminary uncontrolled studies of systemic IFN-α have indicated efficacy against condylomata acuminata (Einhorn et al, 1983); Alewattagama & Kinghorn (1984) reported a dramatic response of vaginal warts to intramuscular IFN-α administered three times weekly for up to 6 weeks.

Fibroblast interferon was found too painful for intralesional treatment of anogenital warts (Scott & Csonka, 1978). In a preliminary open study, Schonfield and his colleagues (1984) found limited efficacy and acceptability of both intralesional and topical IFN-β and found IM preferable to subcutaneous administration. In a subsequent double-blind controlled investigation, 22 women with previously untreated anogenital warts were given 10 consecutive daily IM injections of 2 mega units IFN-β or placebo. The lesions in nine of 11 women on active treatment resolved completely in 5–8 weeks compared to only two of 11 women given placebo. Moreover, eight of the nonresponders including the two without complete response with their first IFN-β treatment were subsequently successfully treated with an open 10 day course of IFN-β. After 12 months follow-up none of the responders has had a recurrence. Side effects of systemic interferon in the low dosages used for treating condylomata acuminata are usually mild. Transient pyrexia and influenzal symptoms are not uncommon and may be accompanied by a moderate reversible leucopenia and thrombocytopenia which requires dosage reduction or temporary cessation of therapy. Caution is advised in elderly patients and those with pre-existing cardiovascular disease, especially where high dosage therapy is given.

The potential advantages of interferon in eradicating HPV justify further studies to determine its efficacy and place in the treatment of condylomata acuminata. As well as being considered for extensive and resistant anogenital warts, further investigation of an effect on cervical intraepithelial neoplasia associated with HPV is desirable. Both Schonfield et al (1984) and Alewattegama & Kinghorn (1984) found individual patients where systemic interferon treatment of anogenital warts was associated with coloposcopic and histological regression of CIN associated with noncondylomatous wart virus infection of the cervix.

SURGERY

The consensus concerning surgical techniques is that they also have a variable success rate, and that they should be reserved for oral lesions, and for anogenital lesions unresponsive to other treatments (Margolis, 1982). Curettage, under local anaesthetic, rapidly removes isolated hyperkeratotic warts which resist chemotherapy. Circumcision produces a less humid environment in which persistent subpreputial warts are less likely to recur. Electrocauterisation and excision have most often been used as the final treatment of extensive or resistant warts but may require a general anaesthetic with its small attendant risks. Secondary infection, haemorrhage and scarring are additional recognised complications of surgical techniques. Electrocautery of anal warts may result in rectal stenosis (Grace, 1974). A scissor-dissection technique which spares normal tissue, prevents scarring, and has a good cosmetic result was described by Thompson & Grace (1978). In this method, a saline and adrenaline solution is infiltrated to separate the warts and allow their accurate removal. Gollock et al (1982) reported a primary cure rate of 71% in 34 patients with peri- and intra-anal warts treated by scissor excision. The recurrence rate was 9%.

Cryotherapy, which requires no prior anaesthetic and causes little or no scarring, was advocated by Ghosh (1977) and Balsdon (1978) and has become a widely available outpatient procedure for treating anogenital warts. It is particularly useful where there are few lesions and small heavily keratinised warts (Oriel, 1981), meatal warts which can be fully exposed, and for the treatment of warts in pregnancy. Outpatient treatment of anogenital warts by cryotherapy was as effective, but more acceptable, than electrocautery to patients treated by Simmons et al (1981). Anorectal warts were successfully eradicated in 21 patients treated by Dodi et al (1982) in one to three cryotherapy sessions, with a subsequent recurrence rate of 10%.

In gynaecological surgery, the carbon dioxide laser has many advantages over electrocautery (Powell, 1982; Ferenczy, 1983). Use of the instrument with colposcopic guidance gives greater precision over the site and depth of treatment, and leaves a sterile wound in which healing is more rapid and scarring less likely; post-operative bleeding and pain is less. The carbon dioxide laser emits a beam of radiant energy in a narrow spectrum of wavelengths, between 9.6–10.6 M, which induces vibrational shifts in water molecules, creating heat. The energy transformation results in immediate boiling of intracellular water with disruption and vaporisation of cytoplasmic and nuclear material. Whether it also kills intracellular HPV is still debated. Hoye et al (1967) found viable cells in the laser emission plume which has raised questions about the possible inhalational hazards to operators and the risk of dissemination of virus infected cells. However, Bellina et al (1983) were unable to detect any biologic activity on extensive investigation of the emission plume from condylomata acuminata treated with a continuous waveform carbon dioxide laser. High success rates, of 91–95%, have been reported in the laser treatment of anogenital warts (Baggish, 1980; Hahn, 1981; Calkins, 1982; Grundsell et al, 1984). Treatment failure and recurrence rates in these studies were low. Bellina (1982) obtained an overall cure rate of 97% in 243 patients treated by CO_2 laser over an 8 year period with a recurrence rate of only 3% during a prolonged follow-up period. The safe use of the laser in pregnancy was reported by Hahn (1981), Malfetano et al (1983). The best results are obtained when laser treatment is administered in the final trimester (Ferency, 1984). These investigators have emphasized the need for routine examination of male consorts in order to reduce recurrence rates following apparently successful laser treatment, and Malfetano et al (1983) recommended the routine colposcopic examination of the consort's penis to detect small warts which were often hard to visualise without magnification. The CO_2 laser also has advantages over other surgical techniques in the treatment of urethral condylomata by requiring only a single application and causing a minimum of discomfort and stricture formation (Fuselier et al, 1980; Rosemberg et al, 1981). However, in the treatment of anorectal warts, Billingham & Lewis (1982) found that recurrences were more common after CO_2 laser therapy than after electrocautery.

A characteristic of Buschke-Loewenstein tumours is their poor response to conventional wart treatments (Powell, 1978). In 1983, Harvey et al reported a case which recurred after treatment with 5FU and electrocautery, and subsequently required subtotal penile amputation. Apfelberg and his colleagues (1983) successfully treated three patients with either giant perineal condylomata or verrucous carcinoma with the CO_2 laser with excellent functional and cosmetic results.

Undoubtedly the CO_2 laser will become more widely used in the treatment of genital warts and intraepithelial neoplasia. In future research it will be important to establish whether the procedure kills rather than disseminates HPV in condylomata, and to compare the cost benefits of this expensive but effective treatment with those of the longer established therapies.

IMMUNOTHERAPY

Deficiencies in cell mediated immunity in patients with persistent condylomata acuminata have been demonstrated (Lee & Eisenger, 1976; Seski et al, 1982). Attempts to enhance the immune response, by the use of an autogenous vaccine, in patients with common warts were made by Bilberstein (1944) and the technique was revived by Powell (1970) for use in patients with anogenital warts. In uncontrolled studies, success rates varying between 80–95% have been claimed (Nel & Fourie, 1973; Ablin & Curtis, 1975; Abcarian, Smith & Sharon, 1976).

The vaccine is prepared as the sterile lysate from a homogenised suspension of the patient's warts and is administered subcutaneously at weekly intervals for up to 6 weeks. In 1982, Abcarian & Smith reported upon the long term efficacy of immunotherapy in treating anorectal warts. During an 8 year period, they treated 200 patients with autogenous vaccine and achieved cure rates of 95%. Follow-up of 186 patients for an average of 4 years showed that there were no significant side effects and all remained wart-free. Eftaiha et al (1982) reported that the recurrence rate of 16% after use of autogenous vaccine following surgical removal of giant or recurrent anal warts was lower than the 28–65% recurrence rates for similar lesions conventionally treated in one or more episodes by surgical excision with or without concomitant podophyllin. In other studies, non-specific vaccines prepared from milk, saline or bovine warts have given equally impressive results (Rowson & Mahy, 1967) but have not been subjected to controlled studies. The sole controlled study of immunotherapy (Malison et al, 1982) failed to demonstate a significant benefit from autogenous wart vaccine as compared with a placebo vaccine prepared from normal skin. In this crossover study 12 of 30 patients treated with wart vaccine were eventually cured. Duration of disease was an important determinant for curability. Whereas cure rates of 86% were obtained with either wart or placebo vaccines for condylomata present for less than 12 months, the cure rate was zero for warts present for longer than this. The clinical response did not appear to be influenced by the protein concentrations of the wart vaccine.

Thus the value of autogenous vaccine remains unproven, despite the impressive results described by some authors. If the active constitutent of these vaccines can be shown to be HPV antigen, then the future development of in vitro antigen production via tissue culture or DNA replication might allow the production of standardised vaccines of sufficient potency to justify further investigations of the role of immunotherapy in the treatment of anogenital warts.

Treatment of genital warts by non-specific stimulation of cell-mediated immunity has also been subject to open studies. Van Krogh (1981) found that sensitisation of 66 patients with 2,4 dinitrochlorobenzene applied to the forearm had no significant effect on wart remission, and repeated BCG immunisation was unsuccessful in eradicating longstanding warts in six patients (Malison & Salkin, 1981). The immune modulatory properties of cimetidine, 400 mg for times daily for 4 weeks, used as an adjunct to podophyllin treatment did not appear to hasten wart remission nor justify further randomised prospective study (Rampen & Van Everdingen, 1982).

As yet no universally effective, safe and acceptable treatment for genital HPV infection exists. It is vital that more effective therapies are found, especially in view of the growing knowledge associating HPV infection with anogenital malignancy and juvenile laryngeal papillomata. It is to be hoped that the widening interest in genital warts as a model for virus induced tumours will stimulate additional investigations of the biochemical and immunological mechanisms associated with their proliferation and remission and that this knowledge might be translated into more precise chemotherapy, surgical techniques and immunotherapy. New treatment will require carefully controlled studies of efficacy and safety before they become more widely used. An effective treatment for genital warts is a major priority in the field of sexually transmitted diseases; the rewards of success, both in the more cost-effective use of clinic facilities and personnel and the long-term gain to the health of patients, are potentially enormous.

REFERENCES

Abcarian H, Sharon N 1982 Long-term effectiveness of the immunotherapy of anal condyloma acuminatum. Dis. Colon Rectum 25: 648–651

Abcarian H, Smith D, Sharon N 1976 The immunotherapy of anal condyloma acuminatum. Dis. Colon Rectum 19: 237–244

Ablin R J, Curtis W W 1975 Condyloma accuminatum: treatment by autogenous vaccine. Ill. Medical Journal 147: 343–346

Alewattegama A, Kinghorn G R 1984 Systemic interferon in the treatment of reistant genital warts. Lancet i: 1468

Allington H V 1951 Review of the psychotherapy of warts. Arch. Dermatol. Syphilol. 62: 316–326

Appelberg D B, Maser M R, Lash H, Drunker D 1983 CO_2 laser resection for giant perineal condyloma and verrcuous carcinoma. Annals Plastic Surgery 11: 417–423

Baggish M S 1980 Carbon dioxide laser treatment for condylomata accuminata veneral infections. Obstet. Gynecology 55: 711–715

Balsdon M J 1978 Cryosurgery of genital warts. British Journal of Venereal Diseases 54: 352–355

Bellina J H 1983 The use of carbon dioxide laser in the management of condyloma acuminatum with eight year follow-up. American Journal Obstetrics and Gynecology 147: 375–378

Bellina J H, Stjernholm R L, Kurpel J E 1982 Analysis of plume emissions after papovavirus eradication with the carbon dioxide laser. Journal of Reproductive Medicine 27: 268–270

Biberstein H 1944 Immunization therapy of warts. Arch. Dermatol. Syphilol. 48: 12–22

Billingham R P, Lewis F G 1982 Laser versus electrical cautery in the treatment of condolyomata acuminata of the anus. Surg. Gynecology Obstetrics 155: 865–867

Brenner M, Johnson C M, Nulf T H, Rheinfranr R E 1983 Intraurethral condyloma acuminatum. Current management. Journal of American Osteopath Assoc. 82: 611–615

Calkins J W, Masterton B J, Magrina J F, Capen C V 1982 Management of condylomata acuminata with the carbon dioxide laser. Obstetrics and Gynecology 59: 105–108

Cetti N E 1984 Condyloma acuminatum of the urethra; problems in eradication. British Journal of Surgery 71: 57

Chamberlain M J, Reynolds A L, Teoman W B 1972 Toxic effects of podophyllum application in pregnancy. British Medical Journal 3: 391–392

Cullis J E 1962 Congenital deformities and herbal slimming tablets. Lancet ii: 511–512

Culp O S, Kaplan I W 1944 Condylomata acuminata. Two hundred cases treated with podophyllin. Annal of Surgery 120: 251–256

Debenedictus T J, Marmar J L, Praiss D E 1977 Intraurethral condylomas acuminata: management and review of the literature. Journal of Urology 118: 767–769

Dodi G, Indanrino A, Moretti R, Scalco G, Lise M 1982 Crytotherapy of anorectal warts and condylomata. Cryobiol. 19: 287–288

Dretler S P, Kelin L A 1975 The eradication of intraurethral condyloma acuminata with 5 percent fluouracil cream. Journal of Urology 113: 195–198

Eftaiha M S, Amshel A C, Sonberg L, Batshon B 1982 Giant and recurrent condyloma acuminatum; appraisal of immunotherapy. Dis. Colon Rectum 25: 136–138

Einhorn N, Ling P, Strander H 1983 Case Report. Systemic interferon Alpha treatment of human condylomata acuminata. Acta Obstet. Gynecol. Scand. 62: 285–287

Ewin D M 1974 Condyloma acuminatum. Successful treatment of four cases by hypnosis. American Journal of Clinical Hypnosis 17: 73–83

Fenoglio C M, Ferenczy A 1982 Etiologic factors in cervical neoplasia. Seminars in Oncology 9: 349–372

Ferenczy A 1983 Using the laser to treat vulvar condylomata acuminata and intraepidermal neoplasia. Canadian Medical Assoc. J 128: 135–137

Ferenczy A 1984 Treating genital condylomas during pregnancy with the carbon dioxide laser. American Journal of Obstetrics and Gynecology 148: 9–12

Fitzgerald D M, Hamit H F 1974 The variable significance of condylomata acuminata. Ann. Surg. 179: 328–331

Fuselier H A, McBurney E I, Brannan W, Randruf E R 1980 Treatment of condylomata acuminata with carbon dioxide laser. Urology 15: 265–266

Gabriel G, Thin R N T 1983 Treatment of anogenital warts. Comparison of trichloracetic acid and podophyllin versus podophyllin alone. British Journal of Venereal Diseases 59: 124–126

Ghosh A K 1977 Cryosurgery of genital warts in cases in which podophyllin treatment failed or was contraindicated. British Journal of Venereal Diseases 53: 49–53

Gollock J M, Slatford K, Hunter J M Scissor excision of anogenital warts. British Journal of Venereal Diseases 58: 400–401

Grundsell H, Larsson G, Bekassy Z 1984 Treatment of condylomata acuminata with the carbon dioxide laser. British Journal of Obstetrics and Gynecology 91: 193–196

Gueson E J, Liu C T, Emrich J P 1971 Dysplasia following podophyllin treatment of vulvar condylomata acuminata. Journal of Reproductive Medicine 6: 159–163

Haan G A 1981 Carbon dioxide laser surgery in treatment of condylomata. American Journal of Obstetrics and Gynecology 141: 1000–1008

Haglund S, Ludquist P G, Cantell K, Strander H 1981 Interferon therapy in juvenile laryngeal papillomatosis. Arch Otolaryngol 107: 327–332

Handojo I, Pardjono A 1973 Treatment of condylomata acuminata with 5 percent 5-fluorouracil ointment. Asian Journal of Medicine 9: 162–166

Haye K R 1974 Treatment of condyloma acuminata with 5 percent 5-fluouracil (5FU) cream. British Journal of Venereal Diseases 50: 466–467

Hoye R C, Ketcham A S, Riggle G C 1967 The airborne dissemination of viable tumour by high energy neodymium laser. Life Science 6: 119–124

Harvey J M, Glen E, Watson G S 1983 Buschke Loewenstein tumour of the penis. A case report. British Journal of Venereal Diseases 59: 273–276

Hursthouse M W 1975 A controlled trial on the use of topical 5-Fluoracil on viral warts. British Journal of Dermatology 92: 93–96

Ikic D, Trajer D, Cupak K et al 1981 The clinical use of human leukocyte interferon in viral infections. Int. J. Clin. Pharmacol. Therapy Toxicology 19: 495–505

Karol M D, Conner C S, Watanabe A S, Murphrey K J 1980 Podophyllum: suspected teratogenicity from topical application. Clinical Toxicology 16: 283–286

Kovar W R 1979 Condyloma Acuminatum. Diagnosis, precautions, treatment. Nebraska Medical Journal 60: 306–308

Lee Axy, Eisenger M 1976 Cell-mediated immunity (CMI) to human wart virus and wart-associated tissue antigens. Clin. Exp. Immunol. 26: 419–424

Ludwig M E, Lowell D M, Livolsi V A 1981 Cervical condylomatous atypia and its relationship to cervical neoplasia. American Journal of Clinical Pathology 76: 255–262

Malfetano J H, Marin A C, Malfetano J H 1983 Carbon dioxide laser treatment of condyloma acuminata. Arizona Medical 40: 467–469

Malison M D, Salkin D 1981 Attempted BCG immunotherapy for condylomata acuminata. British Journal of Venereal Diseases 57: 148

Malison M D, Morris R, Jones L W 1982 Autogenous vaccine for condylomata acuminatum. A double-blind controlled study. British Journal of Venereal Diseases 58: 62–65

Margolis S 1982 Therapy for condyloma acuminatum: a review. Review of Infectious Diseases 4: Suppl: S829–S836

McCabe B F, Clark K F 1983 Interferon and laryngeal papilloma. The Iowa experience. Ann. Otolaryngol. 92: 2–7

Montaldi D H, Giambionne J P, Cowey N G 1974 Podophyllin poisoning associated with treatment of condylomata acuminata. A case report. American Journal of Obstetrics and Gynecology 119: 1130–1131

Nel W S, Fourie E D 1973 Immunotherapy and 5 percent topical 5-fluouracil ointment in the treatment of condyloma acuminata. South African Medical Journal 47: 45–49

Oriel J D 1977 Genital warts. Sexually Transmitted Diseases 4: 153–159

Oriel J D 1981 Genital warts. Sexually Transmitted Diseases 8: 326–329

Powell J L 1982 Carbon dioxide laser surgery for condylomata acuminata. Journal of the Medical Association of Georgia 71: 697–699

Powell L C, Pollard M, Jinkins J L 1970 Treatment of condyloma acuminata by autogenous vaccine. South African Medical Journal 63: 202–205

Powell L C 1978 Condyloma acuminatum: recent advances in development, carcinogenesis and treatment. Clinical Obstetrics and Gynecology 21: 1061–1079

Pereira B R, Arruda A 1982 5-Fluouracil cream 5 percent in the treatment of intraurethral condylomata acuminata. British Journal of Venereal Diseases 54: 295

Reid R, Crum C P, Herschman B R et al 1984 Genital warts and cervical cancer. Cancer 53: 943–953

Rampen F H J, Van Everdingen J J E 1987 Inefficacy of cimetidine in condylomata acuminata. British Journal of Venereal Diseases 58: 275

Reid R, Stanhope R, Herschman B R et al 1982 Genital warts and cervical cancer. Cancer 50: 377–387

Rosemberg S K, Jacobs H, Fuller T 1982 Some guidelines in the treatment of urethral condylomata with carbon dioxide laser. Journal of Urology 127: 907–908

Rowson K E K, Mahy B W J 1967 Human papova (wart) virus. Bacteriology Review 31: 110–115

Schonfield A, Schattner A, Crespi M, Levavi H, Shoham J et al 1984 Intramuscular human interferon B injections in the treatment of condylomata acuminata. Lancet i: 1038–1041

Scott M B, Csonka G W 1979 Effect of injections of small doses of human fibroblast interferon into genital warts. A pilot study. British Journal of Venereal Diseases 55: 442–445

Seski J C, Reinhalter E R, Silva J 1978 Abnormalities of lymphocyte transformations in women with condylomata acuminata. Obstetrics and Gynecology 51: 188–192

Simmonds P D 1981 Podophyllin 10 percent and 25 percent in the treatment of anogenital warts. British Journal of Venereal Diseases 57: 208–209

Simmonds P D, Langlet F, Thin R N T 1981 Cryotherapy versus electrocautery in the treatment of genital warts. British Journal of Venereal Diseases 57: 273–274

Slater G E, Rumack B H, Peterson R G 1978 Podophyllin poisoning: systemic toxicity following cutaneous application. Obstetrics and Gynecology 52: 94–96

Stoehr G P, Peterson A L, Taylor W J 1978 Systemic complications of local podophyllin therapy. Ann. Intern. Med. 89: 362–363

Straatmeyer A J, Rhodes N R 1983 Condylomata acuminata: results of treatment using hypnosis. J. Am. Acad. Dermatol. 9: 434–436

Turek L P, Bryne J C, Lowry D R, Dvoretsky I, Friedman R M, Howley P M 1982 Interferon induces morphological reversion with elimination of extrachromosomal viral genomes in bovine papilloma virus-transformed cells. Proceedings of the National Academy of Scientists of the USA 79: 7914–7918

Ullman M 1959 On the psyche and warts. Psychosomatic Medicine 21: 473–488

Von Krogh G 1978 The beneficial effect of one percent 5-fluouracil in 7 percent ethanol on therapeutically refractory condylomas in the preputial cavity. Sexually Transmitted Diseases 5: 137–140

Von Krogh G 1978 Topical treatment of penile condylomata acuminata with podophyllin, podophyllotoxin and colchicine. A comparative study. Acta Derm. Venerol. (Stockh.) 58: 163–168

Von Krogh G 1981 Penile condylomata acuminata: an experimental model for evaluation of topical self-treatment with 0.5 percent — 1 percent ethanolic preparations of podophyllotoxin for 3 days. Sexually Transmitted Diseases 8: 179–186

Ward J W, Clifford M S, Monaco A R 1954 Fatal systemic poisoning following podophyllin treatment of condyloma acuminata. South African Medical Journal 47: 1204–1206

Weimar G W, Milleman L A, Reiland T L, Culp D A 1978 5-Fluouracil urethral suppositories for the eradication of condyloma acuminata. Journal of Urology 120: 174–175

9. Chronic hepatitis B virus infection: treatment and prevention

Howard C. Thomas   David M. Novick

1. INTRODUCTION

Chronic infection with the hepatitis B virus (HBV) may result in a variety of hepatic lesions, ranging from chronic active and lobular hepatitis leading to cirrhosis, chronic persistent hepatitis, to a carrier state with virtually normal histology (Fig. 9.1). There

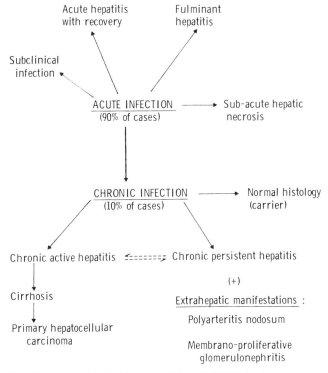

Fig. 9.1 Clinical syndromes associated with acute and chronic HBV infection.

are two phases of the chronic infection. In the first, which lasts several years and during which the patient's serum contains hepatitis B e antigen (HBeAg), the virus replicates and the serum and other body fluids are infectious. Serum transaminases tend to be elevated, and hepatic histology reveals an active inflammatory lesion. During the second stage, viral replication ceases, the patient develops hepatitis B e antibody (anti-HBe) and clones of hepatocytes containing integrated hepatitis B viral DNA continue to secrete hepatitis B surface antigen (HBsAg) (Fig. 9.2). Serum transaminases tend to normalise and the inflammatory activity in the liver decreases.

Mechanisms of liver damage

Several histological lesions are seen in these patients at different times during infection (Thomas et al, 1982b). Focal liver cell necrosis, which is seen throughout the lobule, occurs when active viral replication is subsiding. At this stage, the histological features are similar to those seen in acute viral hepatitis. It seems probable that 'focal necrosis' represents immune lysis of hepatocytes which are actively replicating the virus. Current evidence suggests that this is mediated by cytotoxic T cells (Eddleston et al, 1982; Montano et al, 1983). If this phase of destruction of hepatocytes containing replicating

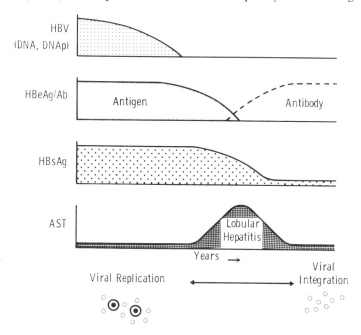

Fig. 9.2   Natural history of chronic HBV infection. During the period of active viral replication, HBe antigen and HBs antigen are found in serum. Several years after the onset of infection, hepatitis B virus replication ceases, HBe antigen is cleared from the serum and HBe antibody is produced. The continued production of HBs antigen at this stage occurs because of integration of HBs gene sequences into the patient's liver cell. Note that there is an exacerbation of the hepatitis during clerance of hepatitis B virus from the serum.

virus is protracted then hepatic fibrosis will ensue. In other individuals, elimination of hepatocytes containing replicating virus is rapidly achieved and these patients then develop either chronic persistent hepatitis or become carriers with normal liver histology.

In some patients viral replication initiates an autoimmune process similar to that seen in lupoid chronic active hepatitis (Eddleston & Williams, 1974). These patients, probably because of a relative deficiency of suppressor cell function (Thomas et al, 1982a), develop liver membrane reactive antibodies (Thomas et al, 1982b; Wiedmann et al, 1984) which result in piecemeal necrosis of periportal hepatocytes. If this process continues for a prolonged period of time cirrhosis will develop. In general, the degree of piecemeal necrosis seen in these patients is minor compared to that seen in lupoid chronic active hepatitis. This may account for the relatively slower progression of the HBV-induced form of the disease.

After several years of infection the patient will develop clones of cells containing integrated hepatitis B viral DNA (Brechot et al, 1981; Fowler et al, 1983). These cells will continue to produce HBsAg after elimination of cells which are actively replicating virus. It is probable that some of these cells which contain the integrated viral genome will undergo malignant transformation leading to the development of primary liver cell cancer.

Liver injury in patients with chronic HBV infection may be accelerated by co-existent infection with the hepatitis D virus (HDV; formerly called the delta agent). HDV is an incomplete RNA virus which requires the presence of the hepatitis B virus in order to replicate and express its viral proteins. HDV was first described in the South of Italy (Rizzetto, Shih & Gerin, 1980), but has now been shown to be prevalent amongst Northern European haemophiliacs and drug addicts with chronic HBV infection (Weller et al, 1983b). Patients with persistent infection with HDV and HBV have chronic liver disease which is rapidly progressive and more severe than would be expected on the basis of chronic HBV infection alone (Rizzetto, 1983).

2. TREATMENT

The aim of therapy in patients with chronic HBV infection is to eradicate the virus in both its replicating and non-replicating forms, thereby preventing the development of progressive liver disease and liver cell cancer. The approach to therapy will depend on the phase of the infection (HBeAg or anti-HBe), the predominant lesion (focal lobular or periportal piecemeal necrosis) and the presence or absence of clones of cells containing integrated HBV-DNA.

During the HBeAg positive phase of infection, when there is active viral replication and focal liver cell necrosis, attempts at therapy are directed towards inhibition of viral replication. The specific aims of therapy are seroconversion from HBeAg to anti-HBe and disappearance of HBV-DNA and DNA polymerase from the serum. These changes are associated with an initial rise and subsequent normalisation of serum transaminase and reduction of inflammatory activity in the liver. In evaluating drugs with antiviral activity, it must be recognised that these events do occur spontaneously (Realdi et al, 1980; Hoofnagle et al, 1981; Viola et al, 1981; Liaw et al, 1983). Although all of the factors which influence the spontaneous HBeAg to anti-HBe seroconversion rate are not known, in males sexual preference appears to be of major importance. In a study from Taiwan (Liaw et al, 1983) in which there were no homosexual men, the annual seroconversion rate was 17%. In contrast, among 100 British HBsAg carriers, 77% of whom were homosexual men and 62% of whom were HBeAg-positive, fewer than 5% per year spontaneously seroconverted from HBeAg to anti-HBe (Viola et al, 1981).

An additional factor which complicates evaluation of antiviral therapy for the HBeAg-positive phase is reactivation of chronic HBV infection. Two groups of investigators from the USA have reported patients who have spontaneously lost HBeAg, DNA polymerase and/or HBV-DNA but several months later developed an exacerbation of their chronic liver disease and reappearance of these viral markers (Davis et al, 1984; Perrillo et al, 1984). Signs and symptoms of hepatic failure developed in some such patients. One group has noted an association of reactivation of HBV infection with male homosexuality (Perrillo et al, 1984). In addition, two patients have been described who lost HBeAg after treatment with adenine arabinoside mono-phosphate (ARA-AMP) but several months later reverted to an HBeAg-positive state (Hoofnagle et al, 1984). These observations necessitate that patients who are considered to have responded to antiviral therapy be followed for at least one year after their response to ensure that reactivation has not occurred.

Once the patient has ceased to replicate the virus (anti-HBe positive phase), the level of inflammatory necrosis of hepatocytes usually subsides and no therapy is necessary. If the patient has already developed cirrhosis by the time viral replication has ceased, there is a significant risk of development of primary liver cell cancer (Beasley, Hwan & Lin, 1981), presumably because of the presence of clones of cells containing integrated HBV-DNA (Thomas, 1983). Attempts to eliminate these cells usually involve either stimulation of the host's immune system (Thomas, 1979) or passive immunisation with antiviral globulins (Thomas et al, 1982b).

If inflammatory necrosis continues in an anti-HBe positive patient, coexistent infection with HDV should be strongly suspected. Rarely, a patient with anti-HBe and chronic active liver disease who does not have concomitant HDV infection will be seen. Such patients may have continuing HBV replication manifested by the presence of hepatitis B core antigen (HBcAg) in liver cell nucleii (Lok et al, 1984a) and antiviral therapy may be indicated. A suitable period of observation, probably one year, is necessary in this circumstance to be sure that such patients have not recently serocon-verted from HBeAg to anti-HBe, in which case the hepatic histology may yet improve. Another small group of anti-HBe positive patients without HDV infection will have continuing inflammatory necrosis without detectable HBcAg display in the liver. These are likely to have an autoimmune diathesis allowing the development of liver membrane reactive antibodies (Thomas et al, 1982b). After a period of careful monitoring this group of patients may respond to moderate doses of prednisolone (Weller et al, 1982b).

Certain pretreatment factors may have a major impact on the outcome of antiviral therapy, since all studies have shown that only some patients respond. We recently reviewed the first 38 male HBeAg-positive patients who had received antiviral therapy (with ARA-MP) at the Royal Free Hospital and who had been followed for one year or longer (Novick et al, 1984c). We found that only two of 19 (11%) homosexual men had had a favourable response, defined as loss of HBeAg and HBV-DNA, as compared with ten of 19 (53%) heterosexual men. This difference between responsive-ness in homosexual and heterosexual men is highly significant and may be related to more severe immunologic abnormalities in the homosexual group (Regenstein et al, 1983; Novick et al, 1984a). Serum transaminse levels were also higher in responders, a finding also noted by investigators from the USA (Scullard et al, 1981b), but homosex-uality was associated with a poor response independent of transaminase levels (Novick et al, 1984c). These observations are particularly relevant to studies of antiviral therapy in Northern Europe and the USA, where a large proportion of patients with chronic HBV infection will be homosexual men.

Inhibition of hepatitis B viral replication

Interferon

Interferons are polypeptides which are produced in response to virus infection and induce an antiviral state in non-infected cells. There are three main types, designated

α, β and γ. Initially the interferons were produced by stimulation of cell lines with either viruses or synthetic polynucleotides. Genetic engineering has now allowed the insertion of the α- and γ- interferon genes into various bacteria or yeasts which then produce large amounts of the protein. Although much of the current research is being conducted with interferons which are a mixture of polypeptides produced from either normal leucocytes or lymphoblastoid cell lines, future work will be undertaken with the genetically engineered interferons which are homogenous single proteins (Smith et al, 1983).

Human leucocyte interferon either alone or in combination with adenine arabinoside (ARA-A) has been used to treat chronic HBV infection (Scullard, Andres & Greenberg, 1981a). In these uncontrolled studies, 37% of patients lost HBeAg and DNA polymerase activity and seroconverted to anti-HBe. A few treated patients also cleared HBsAg. These changes in viral markers were accompanied by improvement in symptoms, biochemistry and histology. Since two drugs were used, it is not clear whether human leucocyte interferon or ARA-A, or both, are responsible for the response. A controlled study using human leucocyte interferon alone at a much lower total dose failed to show any long-term inhibition of viral replication (Weimar et al, 1980). Controlled studies are still required with more protracted and higher-dose regimens of this type of interferon.

Lymphoblastoid interferon is a mixture of at least eight polypeptides. It has recently been used to treat a small number of patients at the Royal Free Hospital and has been shown to have similar effects to human leucocyte interferon (Weller et al, 1982d). Further studies indicate that thrice weekly injections are as effective as the daily regimen in suppressing HBV replication and are better tolerated (Lok et al, 1984b). Two large-scale studies of lymphoblastoid interferon are currently in progress, and it is clear that some patients have developed permanent inhibition of HBV replication (Lok et al, unpublished observations; Novick et al, 1984b) (Fig. 9.3).

Fibroblast interferon (IFN-) has been shown to have no significant antiviral activity in chronic HBV infection (Weimer et al, 1979). This lack of effect may be related to the greater instability of this compound and further studies are necessary. The -interferons (IFN-γ) have not yet been produced in sufficient quantities to be examined for therapeutic effect, but there is great interest in them because they may possess more potent immunomodulatory effects than other interferons (Dolei et al, 1983).

Side effects with interferon therapy include febrile reactions, headache and myalgia (Scott et al, 1981). These symptoms usually subside within the first week of therapy. Other effects related to interferon include leucopenia and thrombocytopenia and are dose-related.

Synthetic antiviral agents

ADENINE ARABINOSIDE
Adenine arabinoside (ARA-A) is a synthetic purine nucleoside with a broad spectrum of antiviral activity against DNA viruses (Shannon, 1975). Early uncontrolled studies indicated that ARA-A had activity against HBV (Chadwick et al, 1978; Pollard et al, 1978). In a randomised controlled study of ARA-A (Bassendine et al, 1981), four of seven treated HBeAg positive patients lost DNA polymerase activity, and three lost HBeAg associated with a significant decrease in HBsAg concentration and aspartate

transaminase. No such changes occurred in the control group. Although ARA-A has a low toxicity relative to other antiviral agents (Keeney, 1975), its usefulness is limited by insolubility and the need for continuous intravenous administration. Adenine arabinoside monophosphate (ARA-AMP), the synthetic easter of ARA-A, is at least 400 times more water-soluble. In eight HBeAg positive patients with chronic liver disease, ARA-AMP given intravenously or intramuscularly at 6- or 12-hourly intervals produced inhibition of viral replication (Weller et al, 1982a). In five patients

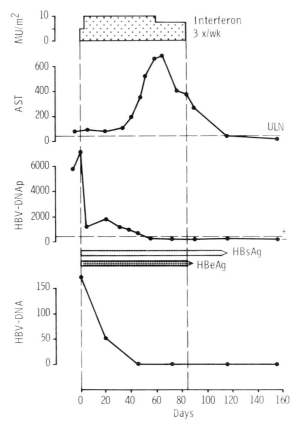

Fig. 9.3 Lymphoblastoid interferon given thrice weekly for a period of three months produces long term inhibition of viral replication. Note that clerance of the virus is associated with an exacerbation of the hepatitis, but is then followed by a remission. In this patient, HBe and HBs antigen were cleared from the serum.

given a short course of therapy with 10 or 15 mg/kg per day, this effect was transient, and in two thrombocytopenia occurred. In a further four consecutive cases given a longer course of 5 mg/kg per day as a twice daily intramuscular injection, thrombocytopenia was not seen and inhibition of viral replication was permanent (Craxi et al, 1983; Weller et al, 1982a). These patients lost DNA polymerase activity, viral DNA and HBeAg from the serum, developed anti-HBe, and HBsAg concentration decreased (Fig. 9.4). There was a transient four- to fivefold increase in transaminase associated with this decrease in viral replication, but then transaminases returned to within the normal range. This rise in transaminases has also been observed by other workers

(Bassendine et al, 1981; Scullard, Andres & Greenberg, 1981) and may predict permanent response to therapy. ARA-AMP has now been assessed in a randomised controlled clinical trial (Weller et al unpublished observations), in which four of 15 treated, but none of 14 untreated, patients showed permanent inhibition of replication.

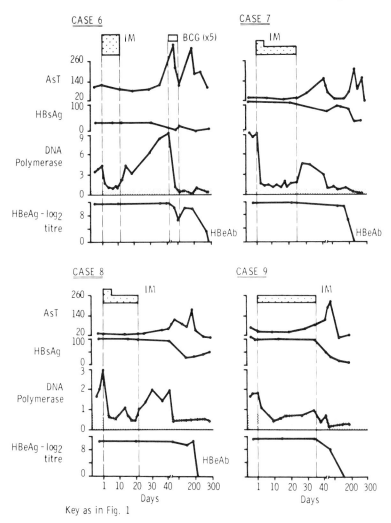

Fig. 9.4 Adenine arabinoside monophosphate given twice daily for 28 days produces long term inhibition of HBV replication in approximately a quarter of patients. There is an exacerbation of the hepatitis during clerance of the virus followed by remission.

In an attempt to produce higher response rates, more protracted therapeutic regimens are being examined. The limiting factor now appears to be the development of severe but reversible sensory polyneuropathy.

ACYCLOGUANOSINE (ACYCLOVIR)

Acycloguanosine (acyclovir) inhibits Herpes simplex virus replication in vitro and in vivo, its action being dependent on phosphorylation of the drug by a virus-coded thymidine kinase (Elion et al, 1977; Fyfe et al, 1978). In vitro studies have also shown activity against cytomegalo- and Epstein-Barr viruses, but at much higher drug concentrations (Colby et al, 1980; Tymes, Scamons & Nairm, 1981). These DNA viruses, like HBV, lack the virus-coded thymidine kinase enzyme. Recently, acycloguanosine has also been shown to inhibit HBV replication in vivo (Weller et al, 1982c, 1983a). Extreme care should be taken in patients with pre-existing renal impairment or dehydration, as nephrotoxicity may occur (Brigden, Roseling & Woods, 1983). Further studies in chronic HBV infection are needed to establish a suitable regimen.

INTERCALATING AGENTS

Intercalating agents such as choloroquine, primacrine, and chlorpromazine can inhibit the HBV-DNA polymerase reaction in vitro, probably by acting as DNA template blockers (Hirschman & Garfunkel, 1978). They do not seem to be active in vivo (Thomas, Bassendine & Weller, 1980).

TRISODIUM PHOSPHONOFORMATE

Trisodium phosphonoformate is a pyrophosphate analogue which inhibits the HBV-DNA polymerase reaction in vitro (Helgstrand et al, 1980), but as yet there has been no report of its use in vivo.

Manipulation of the immune response

The hepatitis B virus is not directly cytopathic: patients with chronic viral replication (HBeAg HBV-DNA and DNA polymerase positive) may have normal transaminases and liver histology. In acute heptatitis B the immune response to either viral antigens or virus-modified host antigens results in elimination of the infected hepatocytes (Fig. 9.5). In patients with chronic infection and inflammatory liver disease, there is a balance between the continued replication of the virus and the attempts of the patient's immune response to lyse infected cells. It seems probable that different components of the immune response are involved in lysis of hepatocytes containing replicating and non-replicating integrated HBV-DNA (Thomas, 1983, Fig. 9.6).

In chronically infected patients attempts have been made to manipulate the immune response by active and passive processes, including immunostimulation and immuno-suppression. Our knowledge of the immunopathogenesis of this disease is still incomplete, so these approaches to therapy have been largely empirical.

Enhancement of cell-mediated immunity with levamisole has been tried in HBV-induced chronic liver disease (Chadwick et al, 1981). There was an increase in T-cell concentrations and a transient rise in transaminases but no effect on viral replication. Transfer factor has also been used in these patients. In one controlled study (Jain et al, 1977), a transient increase in transaminases, similar to that seen with levamisole, was observed and interpreted as an increase in cell-mediated immunity with destruction of infected liver cells. An uncontrolled study showed no effect (Tong et al, 1976).

Enhancement of humoral immunity by infusion of conventional (Reed, Eddleston & Cullens, 1973) or monoclonal anti-HBs (Thomas et al, unpublished observations) produced only a transient decrease in HBsAg titre.

Enhancement of both cell-mediated and humoral immunity has been produced with complete Freund's adjuvant (Kassur, Babiuch & Brzosko, 1977) and BCG

(Brzosko, Deboski & Derecka 1978, Bassendine et al, 1980). Complete Freund's adjuvant was used to immunise a group of 16 patients who had HBsAg positive chronic liver disease. In three cases HBsAg disappeared from the serum and in a

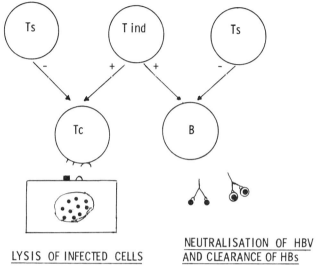

Fig. 9.5 Resolution of hepatitis B virus infection is dependent on lysis of HBV infected cells by cytotoxic T cells (TC) and production of virus-neutralising antibody by primed B cells. These effector cells of the immune system are controlled by regulatory T cells of the inducer and suppressor type (Tn and Ts respectively).

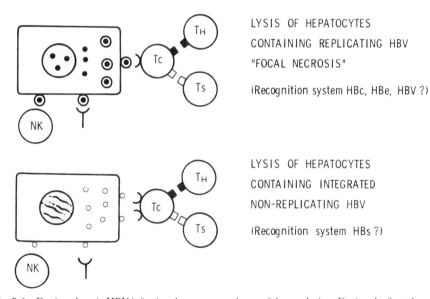

Fig. 9.6 During chronic HBV infection there are two phases of the resolution. During the first phase, hepatocytes supporting HBV replication are lysed by cytotoxic T cells sensitised to the HB core/HBe antigen system. During the second phase, hepatocytes containing integrated non-replicating HBV are lysed by cytotoxic T cells sensitised to HBs. In many patients, the first phase is successfully achieved but the second elimination process does not occur. These patients become HBe antibody positive carriers who are at risk of developing primary liver cell cancer.

further five there was a significant reduction. However, the side effects of treatment with this agent make its use undesirable. Similar results were obtained in children given BCG (Brzosko, Deboski & Derecka, 1978).

Intradermal BCG has also been used in a pilot study at the Royal Free Hospital (Bassendine et al, 1980). In two of five HBeAg positive males given intradermal BCG over a period of 10–20 weeks, there was inhibition of viral replication. These changes were associated with a rise in aspartate transaminase similar to that seen with antiviral therapy. A further patient developed anti-HBe 1 year after therapy, without a rise in liver enzymes. Of four anti-HBe positive patients treated with BCG, one lost HBsAg and developed anti-HBs. BCG seems to be the most promising immunostimulant therapy tried so far, but clearly controlled trials are now required. This form of treatment is of theoretical interest because it is potentially effective in eliminating hepatocytes containing both replicating and integrated virus (Thomas et al, 1980).

Immunosuppression with prenisolone allows increased HBV replication (Scullard et al, 1981c, Weller et al, 1982b) in patients who are actively replicating the virus. These groups also noted that, in patients already on prednisolone, stopping treatment resulted in cessation of viral replication. This has led investigators to consider using a short course of steroid administration as antiviral therapy for HBeAg positive patients. The danger of precipitating severe liver cell necrosis exists and these investigations should proceed cautiously.

Elimination of hepatocytes containing integrated HBV-DNA

The clearance of these cells can only be achieved by stimulation of the endogenous immune lytic systems or by administration of specific lytic agents. Their clearance is necessary in patients who have already developed cirrhosis but not in carriers with normal histology, since the former, unlike the latter, run the risk of malignant transformation of these cells.

Immunostimulation with BCG (see earlier) has produced encouraging results in uncontrolled studies (Brzosko et al, 1978; Bassendine et al, 1980) and further efforts are needed.

More recently, following the observation that native or toxin-conjugated monoclonal anti-HBs will inhibit the growth of malignantly transformed hepatocytes containing integrated HBV-DNA (Thomas et al, 1982b; Shouval et al, 1982; Oladapo et al, 1984, Fig. 9.7), it has become apparent that monoclonal anti-HBs may have some role in the elimination of hepatocytes containing integrated HBV, and further studies are now in progress.

Treatment of autoimmune component in anti-HBe positive HBsAg carriers with chronic active hepatitis

In a minority of patients, inflammatory activity continues after cessation of HBV replication. This may be caused by superinfection with HDV or by an autoimmune reaction initiated by the virus (Eddleston & Williams, 1974; Montano et al, 1983). Once HDV infection has been excluded by serological tests, a trial of 10–15 mg of prednisolone daily should be considered after a period of careful observation. In previous studies at the Royal Free Hospital, 14 anti-HBe positive patients treated with prednisolone/azathioprine had a significant decrease in serum aspartate transaminase (Weller et al, 1982b).

Immunosuppressant drugs such as prednisolone and azathoprine have been widely used in the treatment of chronic active hepatitis and are of proven benefit in the primary autoimmune (lupoid) type (Cook, Mulligan & Sherlock, 1971; Kirk et al, 1980). In a single-blind randomised controlled trial (Lam et al, 1981), prednisolone treatment of HBsAg positive patients produced a decrease in serum bilirubin and

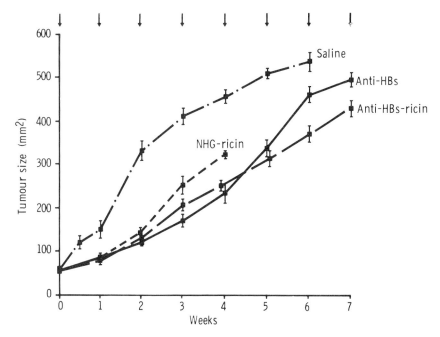

Fig. 9.7   Therapeutic attempts to destroy hepatocytes containing integrated HBV sequences with monoclonal native and ricin conjugated anti-HBs. Alexander tumours (hepatocellular carcinoma cells containing integrated hepatitis B virus sequences and screting HBs antigen) implanted into athymic mice were used in these studies. Monoclonal antibodies were then injected to try to influence tumour growth. Anti-HBs and anti-HBs ricin caused significant inhibition of tumour growth as indicated.

globulin but no change in transaminase levels. Furthermore, the complication and death rates were increased, and there was unfortunately no attempt to differentiate between HBeAg and anti-HBe positive patients. In a study at the Royal Free Hospital, potentiation of HBV replication was observed in HBeAg positive patients given predni-solone (Weller et al, 1982b). Results obtained by other groups (Sagnelli et al, 1980; Muller, Vido & Schmidt, 1981; Scullard et al, 1981c) also support the view that immunosuppression serves only to potentiate viral replication in HBeAg positive patients and is therefore contraindicated in this group.

3. PREVENTION OF HBV INFECTION

There are probably more than 175 million HBsAg carriers in the world today. Not only are these individuals at risk of developing chronic liver disease and primary liver cell carcinoma, but also they comprise a large reservoir from which HBV infection may be transmitted to others. An approach based on prevention of HBV infection is essential if the prevalence of this condition is to be significantly decreased. Prevention of HBV infection has two components: pre-exposure and post-exposure prophylaxis. The former is carried out by active immunisation with hepatitis B vaccine, and the latter by passive immunoprophylaxis using hepatitis B immune globulin. Although safe and effective products are currently available for both pre- and post- exposure prophylaxis, further improvements are expected as a result of recombinant DNA technology or improved chemical synthetic processes (Zuckerman, 1982; Seeff & Koff, 1984).

In China and Japan infection occurs in the perinatal period (Beasley et al, 1983), in Africa in the first two years of life (Greenfield et al, 1984) and in Northern Europe and North America in adult life as a result of sexual activity or drug abuse. Infection may also occur at any age by exposure to blood or blood products used therapeutically. In the hospital, exposure is related to contact with blood during professional activities. The risk of infection is dependent on the amount of virus in the inoculum. The availability of HBV-DNA probes (Weller et al, 1982) allows direct quantitation of virus in body fluids and gives a measure of potential infectivity (Karayiannis et al, 1984). Body fluids from HBe antigen positive patients contain several fold more virus than those from anti-HBe positive carriers. An example of this variable risk is that children of HBe antigen positive mothers are virtually always infected whereas 5% of children of anti-HBe positive mothers are infected.

The policies followed in the prevention of HBV infection are varied because of variation in availability of resources, globulins and vaccines. Clearly, exposure to HBe antigen positive blood always requires prophyactic measures.

Hepatitis B vaccine

A vaccine for prevention of HBV infection must be immunogenic, effective and safe. The currently available hepatitis B vaccine, which consists of HBsAg particles derived from the plasma of healthy carriers using plasmaphoresis, meets these criteria (CDC 1982a; Gerety & Tabor 1983; Schwartz 1984). It is indicated for persons at high risk of contracting HBV infection (Table 9.1). Although expensive ($100; cost in £ varies with exchange rates), its administration to high-risk groups is cost-effective to society (Adler et al, 1983). The vaccine is given as three injections, the second and third succeeding the first by one and six months, respectively. Immunosuppressed and haemodialysis patients should receive double doses.

The immunogenicity and efficacy of the hepatitis B vaccine have been established in randomised controlled trials (Szmuness et al, 1981b; Crosnier et al, 1981; Francis et al, 1982). Antibody to hepatitis B surface antigen (anti-HBs) developed in 85–95% of subjects and has remained detectable for at least 3 years. It is not known whether booster doses will be needed to ensure long-term immunity. The efficacy of the vaccine in preventing HBV infection was 80–95%, and in patients who received all three doses and developed anti-HBs, it was virtually 100%. The immunogenicity and efficacy may be reduced in immunosuppressed patients.

Numerous steps are taken to ensure the safety of the hepatitis B vaccine (CDC, 1982a). Vaccine plasma donors must be asymptomatic, must have normal haemoglobin, haematocrit and serum protein levels, and must undergo a physical examination. In addition, their transaminase levels must be stable, although they may be elevated. The production of the vaccine includes biophysical and biochemical processes to purify the immunogen (the 22 nm HBsAg particle) and to remove or inactivate the infectious HBV particles. The HBsAg is isolated using a double ultracentrifugation procedure, isopyknic and rate zonal. Then, it is subjected to pepsin digestion at pH 2.0 for 18 hours, followed by 8 M urea for 4 hours and finally formalin treatment. These biochemical procedures will inactivate all known groups of animal viruses. In addition, each lot of hepatitis B vaccine is safety tested in chimpanzees.

Table 9.1   Groups at high risk for HBV infection, in whom hepatitis B vaccine may be indicated

1. Health Care Personnel★
    Dentists
    Physicians and Surgeons
    Nurses
    Paramedical personnel
    Dental nurses and hygienists
    Laboratory and blood bank workers
    Students

2. Patients and Patient Contacts
    Haemodialysis patients
    Recipients of blood products†
    Patients in mental institutions
    Household and sexual contacts of HBsAg carriers
    Immigrants to areas of high HBV prevalence
    Morticians and embalmers

3. Persons whose lifestyle predisposes to HBV infection
    Homosexual men
    Female prostitutes
    Prisoners
    Parenteral drug abusers

4. Children born to HBsAg positive mothers

★ Indicated only for those who have frequent direct contact with blood or blood products

† Frequent or large-volume

Additional concern about the safety of the hepatitis B vaccine has arisen following description of the acquired immune deficiency syndrome (AIDS). AIDS is manifested by opportunistic infections, malignancies, and profound abnormalities of T helper cell number and function (Pinching, 1984). AIDS is epidemiologically restricted to certain groups — homosexual men, parenteral drug abusers, and recipients of blood products — which also have high HBsAg carrier rates. Since at least some vaccine plasma donors are from high-risk groups for AIDS, it has been suggested that these individuals might have pre-clinical or asymptomatic AIDS at the time of plasmapheresis. The plasma used in the vaccine could thus contain the causative agent of AIDS. As noted above, however, the inactivation steps in manufacturing the vaccine destroy all known classes of viruses (CDC, 1982a). Retroviruses, which have recently been associated with AIDS (Gallo et al, 1984; Barre-Sinoussi et al, 1983), are inactivated by formalin (CDC, 1982a). In addition, retrospective analysis of homosexual men in the controlled trials of hepatitis B vaccine disclosed no increased incidence of AIDS in vaccine recipients (Stevens, 1983). There is no evidence to date that the hepatitis B vaccine can transmit AIDS, and there is clear evidence that it is effective in preventing HBV infection. Therefore, susceptible persons at high risk for HBV infection (Table 9.1) should be vaccinated. Both authors of this chapter have received the vaccine.

Side effects of the hepatitis B vaccine have been minimal. Pain at the injection site is the most common side effect. Low-grade fever may occur transiently.

Because the hepatitis B vaccine is expensive, pre-vaccination serologic screening has been proposed to prevent needless administration of the vaccine to HBsAg carriers or persons already immune to HBV infection (CDC, 1982b). Serologic screening is cost-effective in high-risk groups with a high prevalence of HBV infection, e.g. homosexual men or parenteral drug abusers (Mulley et al, 1982). From an economic point of view, groups with a low prevalence of HBV infection but a high risk for this disease, e.g. new surgical or dental trainees, may be immunised without prior serologic screening. There is no risk in administering the vaccine to HBsAg carriers (Dienstag et al, 1982) or to persons immune to HBV. Only one test, either anti-HBs or antibody to the hepatitis B core antigen (anti-HBc), should be used for screening. Anti-HBc may be preferable, particularly in groups with high HBsAg carrier rates, because it is positive both in carriers and in persons immune to HBV. Anti-HBc testing will not distinguish between these two groups, however. Anti-HBs detects immune subjects but not HBsAg carriers. Rarely, it may be present in low titre as a non-specific and non-protective antibody, usually in the absence of anti-Hbc (Sherertz et al, 1983; Linnemann & Askey, 1984; Seeff & Koff, 1984). It may therefore be advisable to perform anti-HBc in subjects with low titre anti-HBs and to consider them immune only if both antibodies are present (Seeff & Koff, 1984).

Hepatitis B immune globulin (HBIG)

HBIG is derived from plasma of anti-HBs positive donors and consequently contains high titres of anti-HBs (CDC, 1982c; Seeff & Koff, 1984). HBIG is recommended for prophylaxis following perinatal, percutaneous (needlestick) or mucous membrane exposure to known HBsAg-positive material. It should be administered to susceptible (anti-HBs negative) individuals as soon as possible after exposure. For perinatal exposure, doses of 0.5 ml of HBIG are given intramuscularly at birth and at age 3 and 6 months. The frequency of administration of HBIG needed to prevent perinatal HBV infection is still under evaluation. The child born to the HBe antigen positive mother is at much greater risk than the child born to the anti-HBe positive carrier. Some recommend HBIG only for the former. Active immunisation should be started at the same time as passive immunisation. For percutaneous or transmucosal exposure, 0.06 ml/kg is given immediately and again in one month. HBIG may also be considered for use following sexual contact with HBsAg-positive persons, but further studies are needed.

Exposures frequently occur to blood for which the HBsAg status is not known. If the source of the blood is an individual at high risk of being HBsAg-positive, 0.06 ml/kg HBIG or standard immune globulin (IG) should be given immediately (Seeff & Koff, 1984). If HBsAg is found to be positive on subsequent testing, HBIG should be given again in one month and also immediately to those treated initially with IG. If the source is of low risk of being HBsAg-positive (e.g. an average hospital patient), either no prophylaxis or a single dose of 0.06 ml/kg IG may be given.

Many susceptible persons who require HBIG for post-exposure prophylaxis will also be candidates for the hepatitis B vaccine. Studies have shown that passive immunisation with HBIG does not interfere with the immunogenicity (Szmuness et al, 1981a) or efficacy (Besley et al, 1983) of the vaccine. It is therefore reasonable to administer the first dose of the vaccine concurrently with the first dose of HBIG.

4. SUMMARY

In HBeAg positive patients with a high level of viral replication, antiviral therapy is the treatment of choice. The most promising agents at the moment are ARA-AMP and interferon, and both are being assessed in controlled clinical trials. In the anti-HBe positive patients, in whom continued HBs antigenaemia is due to the presence of clones of cells containing integrated virus, some form of immune manipulation may be necessary. In some cases stimulation of the endogenous immune response may be adequate, but in others passive immunisation may be needed. In rare cases in whom continuing inflammatory activity is related to an autoimmune reaction, low-dose prednisolone may be beneficial.

Although these forms of therapy are currently experimental, some are now entering phase 3 clinical trials. It seems probable that the ultimate regimen will include antiviral drugs and immune manipulation for the adequate elimination of hepatocytes containing replicating and integrated virus. The latter is essential if we are to deal with the problem of neoplasia as well as infectivity and inflammatory liver disease.

A safe and effective vaccine for prevention of HBV infection is now available, but its high cost prohibits its use on a large scale worldwide. It is likely that recent advances in biochemistry and molecular biology will lead to the development of a vaccine with similar efficacy but which can be produced in large quantities at low cost. Then, eradication of HBV infection will become a realistic possibility.

REFERENCES

Adler M W, Belsey E M, McCutchan J A, Mindel A 1983 Should homosexuals be vaccinated against hepatitis B virus? Cost and benefit assessment. British Medical Journal 286: 1621–1624

Barre-Sinoussi F, Chermann J C, Rey F et al 1983 Isolation of a T-lymphocyte retrovirus from a patient at risk for acquired immune deficiency syndrome (AIDS). Science 220: 868–871

Bassendine M F, Weller I V D, Murray A, Summers J, Thomas H C, Sherlock S 1980 Treatment of HBsAg positive chronic liver disease with Bacillus Calmette Guerin (BCG). Gut 21: A915

Bassendine M F, Chadwick R G, Salmeron J, Shipton U, Thomas H C, Sherlock S 1981 Adenine arabinoside therapy in HBsAg-positive chronic liver disease: a controlled study. Gastroenterology 80: 1016–1021

Beasley et al 1983 Prevention of perinatally transmitted hepatitis B virus infections with hepatitis B immune globulin and hepatitis B vaccine. Lancet ii: 1099–1102

Beasley R P, Hwang L Y, Lin C C 1981 Hepatocellular carcinoma and hepatitis B virus: a prospective study of 22,707 men in Taiwan. Lancet 2: 1129–1133

Brechot C, Scotto J, Charnay P, Hadchouel M, Degos F, Trepo C, Tiollais P 1981 Detection of hepatitis B virus DNA in liver and serum. A direct appraisal of the chronic carrier state. Lancet 2: 765–767

Brigden D, Whiteman P 1983 The mechanism of action, pharmacokinetics and toxicity of acyclovir — a review. Journal of Infection 6 (suppl 1): 3–9

Brzosko W J, Deboski R, Derecka K 1978 Immunostimulation for chronic active hepatitis. Lancet 2: 311

Centers for Disease Control 1982a Hepatitis B virus vaccine safety: report of an inter-agency group. Morbidity and Mortality weekly report 31: 465–467

Centers for Disease Control 1982b Inactivated hepatitis B virus vaccine: recommendation of the immunisation practices advisory committee. Annals of Internal Medicine 97: 379–383

Centers for Disease Control 1982c Immune globulin for protection against viral hepatitis: recommendations of the immunisation practices advisory committee. Annals of Internal Medicine 96: 193–197

Chadwick R G, Bassendine M F, Crawford E, Thomas H C, Sherlock S 1978 HBs antigen positive chronic liver disease: inhibition of DNA polymerase activity by vidarabine. British Medical Journal 2: 531–537

Chadwick R G, Jain S, Cohen J, Scott G M, Thomas H C, Sherlock S 1981 Levamisole therapy for HBsAg-positive chronic liver disease. Scandinavian Journal of Gastroenterology 15: 973–978

Colby B M, Furman P A, Shaw J E, Elion G B, Pagono J S 1980 Effect of acyclovir 9-(2-hydroxyethoxymethyl) guanine on Epstein-Barr virus DNA replication. Fifth Cold Spring Harbour Meeting. Journal of Virology (abstract) 32 (2): 560–568

Cook G C, Mulligan R, Sherlock 1971 Controlled trial of corticosteroid therapy in chronic active hepatitis. Quarterly Journal of Medicine 40: 159–185

Craxi A, Weller I V D, Bassendine M F, Fowler M J F, Monjardino J, Thomas H C, Sherlock S 1983 Relationship between HBV-specific DNA polymerase and HBe antigen/antibody system in chronic HBV infection: factors determining selection of patients and outcome of antiviral therapy. Gut 24: 143–147

Crosnier J, Jungers P, Courouce A M 1981 Randomised placebo-controlled trial of hepatitis B surface antigen vaccine in French haemodialysis units: 1, medical staff. Lancet i: 455–459

Davis G L, Hoofnagle J H, Waggoner J G 1984 Spontaneous reactivation of chronic hepatitis B virus infection. Gastroenterology 86: 230–235

Dienstag J L, Stevens C E, Bhan A K, Szmuness W 1982 Hepatitis B vaccine administered to chronic carriers of hepatitis B surface antigen. Annals of Internal Medicine 96: 575–579

Dolei A, Capobianchi M R, Ameglio F 1983 Human Interferon-γ enhances the expression of Class I and Class II major histocompatibility complex products in neoplastic cells more effectively than interferon-β and interferon-α. Infection and Immunity 40: 172–176

Eddleston A L W F, Williams R 1974 Inadequate antibody response to HB antigen or suppressor T-cell defect in development of active chronic hepatitis. Lancet 2: 1543–1545

Eddleston A L W F, Modelli M, Mieli-Vergani G, Williams R 1982 Lymphocyte cytotoxicity to autologous hepatocytes in chronic HBV infection. Hepatology 2: 122S–127S

Elion G B, Furman P A, Fyfe J A, De Miranda P, Beauchamp L, Schaeffer H J 1977 Selectivity of action of an anti-hepatic agent q-(2-hydroxyethoxymethyl) guanine. Proceedings of the National Academy of Sciences, USA, 74: 5716–5720

Fowler M J F, Monjardino J, Weller I V D, Lok A S F, Thomas H C 1983 An analysis of the molecular state of HBV-DNA in the liver and serum of patients with chronic hepatitis or primary liver cell carcinoma and the effect of therapy on adenine arabinoside. Gut 25: 611–618

Francis D P, Hadler S C, Thompson S E et al 1982 The prevention of hepatitis B with vaccine: report of the Centers for Disease Control Multicenter efficacy trial among homosexual men. Annals of Internal Medicine 97: 362–366

Fyfe J A, Keller P M, Furman P A, Miller R L, Elion G B 1978 Thymidine kinase from Herpes simplex virus phosphorylates, the new antiviral compound 9-(2-hydroxyethoxymethyl) guanine. Journal of Biological Chemistry 253: 8721–8727

Gallo R C, Salahuddin S Z, Popovic M et al 1984 Frequent detection and isolation of cytopathic retroviruses (HTLV-III) from patients with AIDS and at risk for AIDS. Science 224: 500–503

Gerety R J, Tabor E 1983 Newly licensed hepatitis B vaccine: known safety and unknown risks. JAMA 249: 745–746

Greenfield C, Musoke R, Mati R, Osiendo V, Tukei P M, Galpin S, Karayiannis P, Thomas H C. In utero and perinatal HBV infection in Kenya: relationship to HBeAg/Ab and HBV-DNA status of mother (in preparation)

Helgstrand E, Flodh H, Lernestedt J O, Lundstrom J, Oberg B 1980 Trisodium phosphonoformate: antiviral activities, safety evaluation and preliminary clinical results. In: Collier, L H, Oxford J (eds) Developments in antiviral therapy. Academic Press, London, p. 63–83

Hirschman S Z, Garfunkel E 1978 Inhibition of hepatitis B DNA polymerase by intercalating agents. Nature 271: 681–683

Hoofnagle J, Dusheiko G M, Seef L B 1981 Seroconversion from hepatitis B antigen to antibody in chronic type B hepatitis. Annals of Internal Medicine 94: 744–748

Hoofnagle J H, Hanson R G, Minuk G Y, Chris Pappas S, Schafer D F, Dusheiko G M, Straus S E, Popper H, Jones E A 1984 Randomised controlled trial of adenine arabinoside monophosphate for chronic type B hepatitis. Gastroenterology 86: 150–157

Jain S, Thomas H C, Sherlock S 1977 Transfer factor in the attempted treatment of patients with HBsAg-positive chronic liver disease. Clinical and Experimental Immunology 30: 10–15

Karayiannis P, Novick D M, Lok A S F, Fowler M J F, Monjardino J, Thomas H C HBV-DNA in saliva, urine and semen of chronic HBe antigen positive carriers. Journal of Hepatology (Abstract) 1984

Kassur B, Babiuch L, Brzosko W J 1977 Treatment of patients with chronic hepatitis B with specific immunostimulation. Archives of the Hellenic Medical Society 3 (suppl): 4

Keeney R E 1975 Human tolerance of adenine arabinoside. In: Paven-Lagston D, Buchanan R A, Alford C A (eds) Adenine arabinoside: an antiviral agent. Raven Press, New York

Kirk A P, Jain S, Pocock S, Thomas H C, Sherlock S 1980 Late results of the Royal Free Hospital prospective controlled trial of prednisolone therapy in hepatitis B surface antigen negative chronic active hepatitis. Gut 21: 78–84

Lam K C, Lai C I, Ng R P, Trepo C, Wu P C 1981 Deleterious effect of prednisolone in HBsAg-positive chronic active hepatitis. New England Journal of Medicine 304: 380–386

Liaw Y-F, Chu C-M, Sui S, Huang M-J, Lin D-Y, Chang-Chien C-S 1983 Clinical and histological events preceeding hepatitis B e antigen seroconversion in chronic type B hepatitis. Gastroenterology 84: 216–219

Linnemann C C, Askey P A 1984 Susceptibility to hepatitis B despite high titre anti-HBs antibody. Lancet i: 346–347

Lok A S F, Hadziyannis S J, Weller I V D, Karvoutzis M G, Karayiannis P, Montano L, Thomas H C 1984a Contribution of low level HBV replication to continuing inflammatory activity in patients with anti-HBe positive chronic hepatitis B virus infection. Gut (in press)

Lok A S F, Weller I V D, Karayiannis P, Brown D, Fowler M J F, Monjardino J, Thomas H C, Sherlock S C 1984b Thrice weekly lymphoblastoid interferon is effective in inhibiting hepatitis B virus replication. Liver 4: 45–49

Montano L, Aranquibel F, Bofill M, Goodall A, Janossy G, Thomas H C 1983 An analysis of the composition of the inflammatory infiltrate in autoimmune and hepatitis B virus induced chronic liver disease. Hepatology 3: 292–296

Muller R, Vido I, Schmidt F W 1981 Rapid withdrawal of immunosuppressive therapy in chronic active hepatitis B infection. Lancet 1: 1323–1324

Mulley A G, Silverstein M D, Dienstag J L 1982 Indications for use of hepatitis B vaccine, based on cost-effectiveness analysis. New England Journal of Medicine 307: 644–652

Novick D M, Brown D J C, Lok A S F, Lloyd J C, Thomas H C 1984a Influence of sexual preference and chronic hepatitis B virus infection of T lymphocyte subsets, natural killer activity, and suppressor cell activity. Hepatology (abstract, in press)

Novick D M, Lok A S F, Karayiannis P, Fowler M J F, Monjardino J, Sherlock S, Thomas H C 1984b Antiviral therapy of chronic hepatitis B virus infection: treatment, outcome, and influence of pretreatent factors. Gut 24: A541

Novick D M, Lok A S F, Thomas H C 1984c Diminished responsiveness of homosexual men to antiviral therapy for HBsAg-positive chronic liver disease. Journal of Hepatology (in press)

Oladapo J M, Goodall A H, DeKoning R, Parmar J, Brown D, Thomas H C 1984 In vitro and in vivo cytotoxic activity of native and ricin-conjugated monoclonal antibodies to HBs antigen for Alexander primary liver carcinoma cells and tumours. Gut 25: 619–623

Perrillo R P, Campbell C R, Sanders G E, Regenstein F G, Bodicky C J 1984 Spontaneous clearance and reactivation of hepatitis B virus infection among chronic type B hepatitis. Annals of Internal Medicine 100: 43–46

Pinching A J 1984 The acquired immunodeficiency syndrome — a review. Clinical and Experimental Immunology 56: 1–13

Pollard R B, Smith J L, Neal A, Gregory P B, Merigan T C, Robinson W S 1978 The effect of vidarabine on chronic hepatitis B virus infection. Journal of the American Medical Association 239: 1648–1650

Realdi G, Alberti A, Rugge M, Bortolotti F, Rigoli A M, Tremolada R, Ruol A 1980 Seroconversion from hepatitis B 'e' antigen to anti-HBe in chronic hepatitis B virus infection. Gastroenterology 79: 195–199

Reed W D, Eddleston A L W F, Cullens H 1973 Infusion of hepatitis B antibody in antigen-positive active chronic hepatitis. Lancet 2: 1347–1351

Regenstein F G, Roodman S T, Perrillo R P 1983 Immunoregulatory T cell subsets in chronic hepatitis B virus infection: the influence of homosexuality. Hepatology 3: 951–954

Rizzetto M, 1983 The delta agent. Hepatology 3: 729–737

Rizzetto M, Shih J W K, Gerin J L 1980 The hepatitis B virus-associated -antigen — isolation from liver, development of solid-phase radioimmunoassays for -antigen and anti- and partial characterisation of -antigen. Journal of Immunology 125: 318–324

Sagnelli E, Maio G, Felaco F M, Izzo C M, Manzillo G, Pasquale G, Filippini P, Piccinino F 1980 Serum levels of hepatitis B surface and core antigens during immunosuppressive treatment of HBsAg positive chronic active hepatitis. Lancet 1: 395–397

Schwartz S J and the Health and Public Policy Committee, American College of Physicians 1984 Hepatitis B vaccine. Annals of Internal Medicine 100: 149–150

Scott G, Secker D, Flowers D, Bate J, Centell K, Tyrell D 1981 Toxicity of interferon. British Medical Journal 283: 562

Scullard G H, Andres L L, Greenberg H B 1981a Antiviral treatment of chronic hepatitis B virus infection: improvement in liver disease with interferon and adenine arabinoside. Hepatology 1: 228–232

Scullard G H, Pollard R B, Smith J L, Sacks S L, Gregory P B, Robinson W S, Merigan T C 1981b Antiviral treatment of chronic hepatitis B virus infection. I. Changes in viral markers with interferon combined with adenine arabinoside. Journal of Infectious Diseases 143: 772–783

Scullard G H, Smith C I, Merigan T C, Robinson W S, Gregory P B 1981c Effects of immunosuppressive therapy on viral markers in chronic active hepatitis B. Gastroenterology 81: 989–991

Seeff L B, Koff R S 1984 Passive and active immunoprophylaxis of hepatitis B. Gastroenterology 86: 958–981

Shannon W M 1975 Antiviral activity in vitro. In: Pavan-Langston D, Buchanan R A, Alford C A (eds) Adenine arabinoside: an antiviral agent. Raven Press, New York

Sherentz R J, Spindel E, Hoofnagle J H 1983 Antibody to hepatitis B surface antigen may not always indicate immunity to hepatitis B virus infection. New England Journal of Medicine 309: 1519

Shouval D, Wands J R, Qurawshi V R, Isselbacher K J, Shafritz D A 1982 Protection against experimental hepatoma formation in nude mice by monoclonal antibodies to hepatitis B virus surface antigen. Hepatology 2: 128S–133S

Smith C I, Weisberg J, Bernhardt L, Geegory P B, Robinson W S, Merigan T C 1983 Acute Dane particle suppression with recombinant leukocyte A interferon in chronic hepatitis B virus infection. Journal of Infectious Diseases 148: 907–913

Stevens C E 1983 No increased incidence of AIDS in recipients of hepatitis B vaccine. New England Journal of Medicine 308: 1163–1164

Szmuness W, Stevens C E, Oleszko W R, Goodman A 1981a Passive-active immunisation against hepatitis B: immunogenicity studies in adult Americans. Lancet i: 575–577

Szmuness W, Stevens C E, Zang E A, Harley E J, Kellner A 1981b A controlled trial of the efficacy of the hepatitis B vaccine: a final report. Hepatology 1: 377–385

Thomas H C 1979 Immunostimulants in the treatment of HBs antigen positive chronic active liver disease. In: Eddleston A L W F, Weber P, Williams R (eds) Immune reactions in liver disease. Pitman Press, London, p 281–287

Thomas H C 1983 Pathogenesis of HBV infection. In: Lossovsky M (ed) Advanced medicine 19. Pitman Press, London

Thomas H C, Bassendine M F, Weller I V D 1980 Treatment of chronic hepatitis B virus infection. In: Collier L H, Oxford J (eds) Developments in antiviral therapy. Academic Press, London, p 88–103

Thomas H C, Brown D, Routheir G, Janossy G, King P C, Goldstein G, Sherlock S 1982a Inducer and suppressor T-cells in hepatitis B virus induced liver disease. Hepatology 2: 202–204

Thomas H C, Montano L, Goodall A, de Koning R, Oladapo J, Wiedmann K 1982b Immunological mechanisms in chronic HBV infection. Hepatology 2: 1165–1215

Tong N, Nystrom J S, Redeker A G, Marshall G J 1976 Failure of transfer factor therapy in chronic active type B hepatitis. New England Journal of Medicine 295: 209–211

Tymes A S, Scamons E M, Naim H M 1981 In vitro acitivity of acyclovir and related compounds against cytomegalovirus infection. Journal of Antimicrobial Chemotherapy 8: 65–72

Viola L A, Barrison I G, Coleman J C, Paradinas F J, Fluker J L, Murray-Lyon I M 1981 Natural history of liver disease in chronic hepatitis B surface antigen carriers: survey of 100 patients from Great Britain. Lancet 2: 1156–1159

Weimar W, Heijtink R A, Schalm S W, Schellekens H 1979 Differential effects of fibroblast and leucocyte interferon in HBsAg positive chronic active hepatitis. European Journal of Clinical Investigation 9: 336–338

Weller I V D, Bassendine M F, Craxi A, Thomas H C, Sherlock S 1982a Successful treatment of HBs and HBeAg positive chronic liver disease: prolonged inhibition of viral replication by highly soluble adenine arabinoside 5′-monophosphate (ARA-AMP). Gut 23: 717–723

Weller I V D, Bassendine M F, Murray A X, Craxi A, Thomas H C, Sherlock S 1982b The effects of prednisolone/azathioprine in chronic hepatitis B viral infection. Gut 23: 650–655

Weller I V D, Carreno V, Fowler M J F, Monjardino J, Makinen D, Thomas H C, Sherlock S 1982c Acycloguanosine inhibits hepatitis B virus replication in man. Lancet 1: 273

Weller I V D, Fowler M J F, Monjardino J, Thomas H C. The detection of HBV-DNA in serum by molecular hybridisation. Journal of Medical Virology 9: 273–280

Weller I V D, Fowler M J F, Monjardino J, Carreno V, Thomas H C, Sherlock S 1982d Inhibition of hepatitis B viral replication by lymphoblastoid interferon. Philosophical Transactions of the Royal Society (Series B), 299: 128–130

Weller I V D, Carreno V, Fowler M J F, Monjardino J, Makinen D, Vanghese Z, Sweny P, Thomas H C, Sherlock S 1983a Acycloguanosine in HBeAg-positive chronic liver disease: inhibition of viral replication and transient renal impairment with i.v. bolus administration. Journal of Antimicrobial Chemotherapy 11: 223–231

Weller I V D, Karayiannis P, Lok A S F, Bamber M, Thomas H C, Sherlock S 1983b The significance of delta-agent infection in chronic hepatitis B viral infection in Great Britain. Gut 11: 223–231

Wiedmann K H, Bartholomew T C, Brown D J C, Thomas H C 1984 Liver membrane antibodies detected by immunoradiometric assay in acute and chronic virus induced and autoimmune liver disease. Hepatology 4: 199–204

Zuckerman A J 1982 Virological approach to the prevention of primary liver cancer. Hepatology 2: 67S–71S

10. Genital ulceration in the tropics

Peter Piot   André Meheus

In the past five years, several reports have been published on genital ulcerations, a previously unrecognised or underestimated problem in most developing countries. Paradoxically, they are among the more complex clinical problems in patients with sexually transmitted diseases, yet most commonly occur in the developing world, where adequate facilities for aetiologic diagnosis and proper treatment are scarce. In this chapter we will review the literature, including abstracts or proceedings of conferences, on genital ulcerations in developing countries between 1979 and 1984. However, for papers dealing exclusively with chancroid or *Haemophilus ducreyi*, the reader is referred to Chapter 4. Genital ulcerations are defined as genital lesions characterised by a defect in the epithelium of the skin.

EPIDEMIOLOGY

Since genital ulcerations are not an aetiologic entity or a reportable condition, figures on their occurrence in the population are virtually non-existent. However, an estimate of the magnitude of genital ulcer morbidity is given by the relative frequency of combined causes of genital ulceration and by prevalence surveys in selected populations. Overall, genital ulcerations are thought to be relatively more frequent in developing countries than in Europe or North America.

According to a report by the World Health Organisation (1981), genital ulcerations are found in 10 to 70% of patients seen in clinics for sexually transmitted diseases (STD) in Asia and East Africa. In Mbabane, Swaziland, as many as 51% of male patients with a sexually transmitted disease presented with a genital ulceration at a general outpatient department (Meheus et al, 1982). Among 160 pregnant women attending an STD clinic in Harare, Zimbabwe, 18 (11%) were found to have genital ulcers (Latif et al, 1983). Among children under 11 years of age seen at the same clinic, two of 17 boys, and three of 33 girls had genital ulcerations (Latif, 1983). In Ho Chi Minh City, Vietnam, genital ulcers were present in 34% of patients at STD clinics (Minh Triet, 1982).

Several reports from Nairobi have documented the relatively high frequency of genital ulcer disease in prostitutes, and the importance of this group in the transmission of genital ulcers, particularly chancroid. Thus, Haase et al (1984) identified genital ulcerations in 24(6%) of 416 prostitutes, of whom 15 (62% of cases) had chancroid. In another survey, D'Costa et al (1983) demonstrated that the prevalence of genital ulcerations in prostitutes varied with their socio-economic status, since 7–13% of prostitutes of lower and middle class strata had ulcerations, as compared to only 1% of higher class colleagues. Both a lower frequency of sexual contact, and a higher standard of hygiene may generate this difference. Of 13 cases of genital ulceration in this survey, four were due to *Haemophilus ducreyi*, and one to Herpes simplex virus.

With the exception of chancroid, reports on specific causes of genital ulcerations in the tropics are rare. Several surveys suggest that syphilis has become an important problem in many tropical areas, where the endemic treponematoses were often controlled in the 1950s (World Health Organization, 1982; Piot & Meheus, 1983). Recent serological surveys in the general population in Swaziland (Ursi et al, 1981), South African blacks (Mahomed et al, 1984), Brazil (Pereira, 1980) Zaire (Kakiese, 1983), Rwanda (De Clercq, 1982), and Central African Republic (Widy-Wirsky & D'Costa, 1980a, b), yielded seropositivity rates for *Treponema pallidum* haemagglutination (TPHA) and Venereal Disease Research Laboratory (VDRL) or Rapid Plasma Reagin (RPR) test of between 3 and 33%. The overall annual incidence of syphilis in Swaziland was estimated at 1.25–1.4%. These high rates of infection are reflected in an increasing problem of congenital syphilis in countries such as Zambia (Hira et al, 1982a, b) and Ethiopia (Bishaw et al, 1983), where 30–60 fetal and infant deaths per 1000 pregnant women are due to syphilis. Studies from Brasilia, Brazil (Pereira, 1980), and Nairobi (Nsanze et al, 1984) report on the high prevalence of syphilis in prostitutes. In the latter survey on 462 prostitutes, two had syphilitic chancres, 37% had a positive RPR and TPHA, and 36% had a positive TPHA only, and 20% of initially seronegative women seroconverted within three months. Genital herpes, the principal cause of genital ulceration in the industrialised world, is much less commonly seen in patients at STD clinics in the tropics. However, two serologic surveys in Ibadan, Nigeria, found a 12% prevalence of Herpes simplex virus type 2 neutralizing antibodies at 20 years of age, a figure comparable to those reported from Europe (Sogbetun et al, 1979; Montefiore et al, 1980). The latter authors suggest that non-venereal transmission of Herpes simplex virus type 2 may occur under humid tropical conditions, although the experimental and epidemiological data given are not strong.

Lymphogranuloma venereum is an infrequent cause of genital ulceration, although the disease has been only occasionally studied in the tropics (Perine et al, 1980; Piot et al, 1982). Surveys on genital ulcerations in migrating workers in Southern Africa, suggest that there may be distinct geographic foci of lymphogranuloma venereum in that part of the world, with most cases originating in Swaziland and adjacent subtropical areas in Mozambique and South Africa (Ballard et al, 1982; Piot et al, 1982).

Except for chancroid, risk groups for genital ulcer disease have not been defined. In most series there was an excess of males, probably because of demographic factors and because lesions in the male are easily identified.

AETIOLOGY

Table 10.1 shows the aetiology of genital ulcerations among consecutive patients in eight series from the tropics. Chancroid was the major cause of genital ulcer disease in the four African series, and in Thailand, providing 40–60% of all cases (Meheus et al, 1983b; Ballard, 1982; Duncan et al, 1981; Nsanze et al, 1981; Taylor et al, 1984). Whereas syphilis was the main diagnosis in Ho Chi Minh City (Minh-Triet, 1982), donovanosis — a rare disease elsewhere — was the most frequent diagnosis in Papua New Guinea (Vacca & MacMillan, 1980). Genital herpes, the major cause

Table 10.1 Aetiology of genital ulcerations among conceecutive patients in the tropics

Diagnosis	Centre (% of patients with diagnosis)								
	Swaziland N = 149	Carletonville N = 149	Johannesburg N = 102	Pretoria N = 100	Nairobi N = 97	Papua-New Guinea N = 174	Bangkok N = 120	Vietnam N = 9802	Singapore N = 60
Syphilis	17	18	15	33	9	14	1	49	5
Herpes	11	3	8	4	4	—	10	8	28
Chancroid	42	54	58	28	62	—	36	11	48
Lymphogranuloma venereum	12	3	1	1	—	9	—	—	—
Donovanosis	1	1	1	1	—	22	—	5	—
Mixed aetiology	4	3	3	17	2	37	2	—	5
Other causes and unknown aetiology	13	18	14	16	13	18	51	27	14

From: Meheus et al, 1983; Ballard, 1982; Duncan et al, 1981; Crewe-Brown et al, 1982; Nsanze et al, 1981; Vacca & MacMillan, 1980; Taylor et al 1984; Minh-Triet 1982; Rajan et al, 1982 of genital ulcerations in Europe and North America, was found in only 4–11% of cases. Thus, geographic variations in the aetiology of genital ulcerations do exist. The pattern of disease may be a function of parameters such as health seeking behaviour, the availability and quality of health services, sexual practices and sexual preference, the impact of prostitution on the spread of sexually transmitted diseases, and the frequency of circumcision.

Even in the best documented studies, the aetiology of 13–30% of cases of genital ulceration remains unresolved. Occasional cases are thought to be caused by microorganisms such as *Phthirus pubis*, *Entamoeba histolytica*, *Sarcoptes scabiei*, and *Trichomonas vaginalis* (World Health Organization, 1981), and a wide variety of aerobic and anaerobic bacteria can be isolated from genital ulcers. Ursi et al (1982) isolated a fastidious microaerophilic gram-negative bacillus from genital ulcers in Swaziland, but were unable to determine its pathogenicity. This bacterium should be differentiated from *Haemophilus ducreyi*, since it grows on media currently used for the isolation of the latter.

Neisseria gonorrhoeae is infrequently isolated from genital ulcers (2.5–6.4% of cases) (Nsanze et al, 1981; Rajan et al, 1982; Meheus et al, 1983b), but its role in the pathogenesis of ulcers is not clear. Rajan et al (1984) from Singapore reported on 18 males with genital ulcers from which *N. gonorrhoeae* was the sole organism grown. Most of the cases had been clinically diagnosed as chancroid. Seven (39%) out of these 18 patients had a concomitant urethral discharge. Unfortunately, only three men without urethral discharge were cultured for *N. gonorrhoeae*. Six cases healed with single dose kanamycin 2 gm IM plus ampicillin 3.5 gm combined with probenecid 1 gm. The authors conclude that while *N. gonorrhoeae* may be a contaminant in some cases, it is the causative agent of ulceration in others.

Erosive balanoposthitis and superficial ulcers, associated with non-syphilitic spirochaetes, were reported from South Africa (Duncan et al, 1981; Piot et al, 1981). Scrapings from the lesions contained numerous bacteria and spirochaetes with morphology and movement not consistent with *T. pallidum*. Such spirochaetes were not found in men without these lesions. Serologic tests for syphilis remained negative on follow up. This condition may be similar to the balanoposthitis associated with anaerobic bacteria, as described by Ewart Cree et al (1982), but anaerobic cultures were not performed on the African patients.

Mycoplasma hominis was isolated from the ulcer base in 16% of men with genital ulcerations in Kenya and southern Africa, but there was no evidence for a causative role for this organism (Piot et al, 1983).

In general, the epidemiological and clinical features of ulcers of unknown aetiology are similar to those that are positive for *H. ducreyi*, suggesting that they are caused by undetected *H. ducreyi* (Plummer et al, 1983a and 1983b). Similarly, results from treatment trials for chancroid with drugs such as trimethoprim/sulphamethoxazole (Fast et al, 1983), amoxycillin/clavulanic acid (Fast et al, 1982), trimethoprim/sulphametrole (Plummer et al, 1983d), erythromycin and rosaramicin (Plummer et al, 1983b), rifampin, and rifampin in combination with trimethoprim (Plummer et al, 1983a), spectinomycin (Ndinya-Achola et al, 1983), yielded identical results in *H. ducreyi*-negative and *H. ducreyi*-positive ulcers. This suggests at least that the causative agents of genital ulcers of unknown aetiology in those studies were susceptible to the same antibiotics as *H. ducreyi*. A third set of data implicating *H. ducreyi* as a cause of genital ulcers of as yet unknown aetiology is provided by the study of primary sexual contacts of men with culture proven chancroid (Plummer et al, 1983d). Thus, *H. ducreyi* was isolated from eight female source contacts of men with chancroid, whereas the ulcers of the remaining two prostitutes remained culture negative.

Fixed drug eruptions on the genitalia were reported in 60 patients from India (Pandhi, 1983). Tetracycline was the most common drug responsible for this reaction.

CLINICAL PRESENTATION AND DIAGNOSIS

The clinical presentation of genital ulceration is frequently atypical, particularly in the tropics where mixed infections are common and patients tend to present at health care facilities a considerable time after the onset of their disease (Meheus & Ursi, 1982). Thus, Duncan et al (1981, 1984) found little correlation between their findings and the classical description of syphilis. Only the finding of discrete, bilateral, rubbery inguinal lymph glands associated with genital ulcerations was a reasonably sensitive indicator of infection with *T. pallidum*. They also emphasised the poor performance of serologic tests for syphilis in the differential diagnosis of genital ulcers in southern Africa, because of the high prevalence of positive test results among patients with chancroid and among controls. Genital ulcers in women were even less typical than in men. Women in Johannesburg tended to have more mixed infections than men, and inguinal lymphadenopathy was less common in women with chancroid than in men (Duncan et al, 1984).

In a study in Nairobi, the overall accuracy of a clinical diagnosis was 66% for proven causes of genital ulcers (Fast et al, 1984). However, if those cases in which no laboratory diagnosis was achieved were included, the diagnostic accuracy was reduced to 42%. Conversely, extensive laboratory investigations could determine the cause of genital ulcers in only 64% of cases. Thus, neither the laboratory, nor clinical judgement, was able to provide high diagnostic accuracy in this study. The predictive values of clinical diagnoses in men with genital ulcers with a supporting laboratory diagnosis were 84% for chancroid, 60% for syphilis, and 75% for herpes. The predictive values in female patients were 57% for chancroid and 62% for syphilis (D'Costa et al, 1983). In another study in Nairobi, 14 out of 96 men with a clinical suspicion of chancroid, actually had herpes, of whom five had a mixed infection with Herpes simplex virus and *H. ducreyi* (Hazlett et al, 1983).

Ballard et al (1982) discuss the major diagnostic problems of subpreputial genital ulcerations in uncircumcised men, in whom these are often associated with phimosis or paraphimosis.

Ulcers from which only gonococci were isolated in Singapore had a mean incubation period of 4.3 days (range 1–14 days). All ulcers were soft, half were solitatry, and 61% had a purulent base (Rajan et al, 1984).

The hallmark of lymphogranuloma venereum is unilateral or bilateral lymphadenopathy. The primary lesion of lymphogranuloma venereum is usually a small painless and often transient ulcer (Schachter & Osoba 1983), and in a series of 18 cases of lymphogranuloma venereum in Ethiopia, only three patients had a genital lesion, which was a painless small papule or abrasion (Perine et al, 1980). However, 12 patients with lymphogranuloma venereum who presented with more extensive genital ulceration were reported from Swaziland and South Africa (Piot et al, 1982). *Chlamydia trachomatis* isolates from the ulcer base in all cases were typed as serovar L$_2$ (Ballard et al, unpublished). These ulcers were fairly deep and tender with elevated edges, and had an indurated base in half of the cases. A case of lymphogranuloma venereum associated with a chlamydial urethritis was reported by Ballard et al (1982). Dan et al (1980) described a case of lymphogranuloma venereum of 20 years' duration in which *C. trachomatis* was isolated from perianal lesions. In this patient, *C. trachomatis* had apparently persisted for 20 years.

Extensive and necrotic genital herpes was a common opportunistic infection among male and female patients with the acquired immune-deficiency syndrome in Kinshasa, Zaire (Piot et al, 1984).

Men with erosive balanoposthitis associated with non-syphilitic spirochaetes were all uncircumcised, and had large, serpiginous, non-indurated, tender and purulent superficial ulcers. Inguinal lymphadenopathy and phimosis were present in a minority of patients. The mean incubation period was 9 days (range: 4–17 days) (Piot et al, 1981).

Ulcers of unknown aetiology in Kenya are clinically similar to chancroid, both in men and in women (Plummer et al, 1983a; D'Costa et al, 1983).

MANAGEMENT

Over the last 5 years, the laboratory diagnosis of chancroid has been drastically improved. Well evaluated simple and relatively cheap treatment regimens are now available for both chancroid and syphilis, and episodes of genital herpes can be effectively treated. However, between traditional academic management and reality there are numerous practical problems, particularly in the developing world. Diagnostic facilities are mostly very limited, or simply not available, the presentation is often atypical, multiple infections are common, and previous treatment further obscures the clinical picture. For these reasons, standard treatment of genital ulcerations is now advocated (Meheus et al, 1981; Duncan et al, 1981; Oriel 1983; Meheus & Piot, 1983; Meheus, 1984).

Standard management should be based on the local aetiology of genital ulcerations, and on the local effectiveness of antimicrobials against different causes of genital ulcer disease (World Health Organization, 1984). In the absence of any laboratory facilities, all genital ulcerations in the tropics should be treated with benzathine penicillin 2.4 million units intramuscularly combined with single dose therapy for chancroid such as trimethoprim/sulphamethoxazole, trimethoprim/sulphametrole, ceftriaxone or spectinomycin (AUVDT, 1983; World Health Organization, 1983). As mentioned earlier, the latter part of this therapy is also effective for ulcers of unknown aetiology. An example of standard management of genital ulcerations at basic health services level is given in Figure 10.1.

Perine et al (1980) successfully treated lymphogranuloma venereum with either tetracycline hydrochloride or co-trimoxazole for 7 to 14 days in Ethiopia. The time required for healing of genital lesions was directly related to the size of lesion. About 75% of buboes became fluctuant just before or after treatment began. Gonococcal ulcers in Singapore healed with a variety of regimens including co-trimoxazole, streptomycin, and tetracycline (Rajan et al, 1984). Erosive spirochaetal balanoposthitis was cured with benzathine penicillin (Piot et al, 1981).

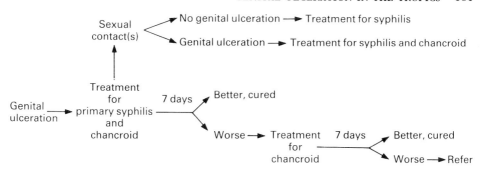

Fig. 10.1 Management of genital ulceration in the absence of diagnostic facilities (Translated from Meheus & Piot, 1983).

CONCLUSION

During the past 5 years, several studies have demonstrated that genital ulcerations are a frequent problem in various developing countries. In most surveys, chancroid was the main cause. Single dose treatment regimens were developed for chancroid, and standard management algorithms for genital ulceration were designed. More research is needed on the epidemiology of the various causes of genital ulceration, on the aetiology of ulcers of unknown origin, and on simple and cheap tests for the diagnosis of the specific causes of genital ulceration. The optimal treatment of lymphogranuloma venereum still has to be determined. Finally, it should be pointed out that our knowledge of donovanosis has hardly progressed during the last 30 years.

REFERENCES

AUVDT (African Union Against Venereal Diseases and Treponematoses) 1983 Recommendations for management and control of STD in Africa. In: Nsanze H, Widy-Wirsky R H, Ellison R H (eds) Proceedings of the Third African Regional Conference on Sexually Transmitted Diseases, Nairobi. 164–168

Ballard R C, Fehler H G, Murray L G, Msikinya B S, Meheus A, van Dyck E, Piot P 1983 Genital ulcerations in Southern Africa. Proceedings of the Third African Regional Conference on Sexually Transmitted Diseases, p 129

Ballard R C 1982 The epidemiology and immunopathology of chlamydial infections in southern Africa. PhD Thesis, University of the Witwatersrand, Johannesburg

Ballard R C, Bilgeri Y R, Fehler H G 1982 Significant inguinal lymphadenopathy associated with acute urethritis. South African Journal of Sexually Transmitted Diseases 2: 11

Ballard R C, Fehler H G, Msikinya B S 1982 Subpreputial genital ulceration — diagnostic problem. South African Journal of Sexually Transmitted Diseases 2: 34–36

Bishaw T, Tafari N, Zewdie M, Haile D, Mascola L, Brown S 1983 In: Nsanze H, Widy-Wirsky R H, Ellison R H (eds) Prevention of congenital syphilis. Proceedings of the Third African Regional Conference on Sexually Transmitted Diseases, Nairobi. 148–153

Crewe-Brown H H et al 1982 Genital ulceration in males at GA-Rankuwa hospital, Pretoria. South African Medical Journal 62: 861–867

Dan M, Rotmensch H R, Eylan E, Rubinstein A, Ginsberg R, Liron M 1980 A case of lymphogranuloma venereum of 20 years' duration. British Journal of Venereal Diseases 56: 344–346

D'Costa L, Plummer F, Bowmer I, Fransen L, Piot P, Ronald A, Nsanze H, Siongok T A 1983 Sexually transmitted diseases among Nairobi prostitutes. In: Nsanze H, Widy-Wirsky R H, Ellison R H (eds) Proceedings of the Third African Regional Conference on Sexually Transmitted Diseases, Nairobi. 19–20

D'Costa L, Plummer F, Nsanze H, Ronald A 1983 Genital ulcers in female: clinical, microbiologic and treatment studies of Kenyan women. Proceedings of the Third African Regional Conference on Sexually Transmitted Diseases, Nairobi. 96–98

De Clercq A 1982 Problemes en obstétrique et gynécologie. In: Meheus A, Butera S, Eylenbosch W, Gatera G, Kivits M, Musafili I (eds) Santé et maladies au Rwanda. Bruxelles, Administration générale de la coopération au développement. 627–656

Duncan M O, Bilgeri Y R, Fehler H G, Ballard R C 1981 The diagnosis of sexually acquired genital ulcerations in black patients in Johannesburg. South African Journal of Sexually Transmitted Diseases 1: 20–23

Duncan M O, Ballard R C, Bilger Y R, Fehler H G 1984 Sexually acquired genital ulcerations in urban black women. South African Journal of Sexually Transmitted Diseases 4: 23–27

Ewart Cree G, Willis A T, Phillips K D, Brazier J S 1982 Anaerobic balanoposthitis. British Medical Journal 284: 859–860

Fast M V, Nsanze H, Plummer F A, D'Costa L J, MacLean I W, Ronald A R 1983 Treatment of chancroid. A comparison of sulphamethoxazole and trimethoprim-sulphamethoxazole. British Journal of Venereal Diseases 59: 320–324

Fast M V, Nsanze H, D'Costa L J, Plummer F A, Karasire P, Maclean I W, Ronald A R 1982 Treatment of chancroid by clavulanic acid with amoxicillin in patients with beta-lactamase-positive *Haemophilus ducreyi* infection. Lancet 2: 509–511

Fast M V, D'Costa L J, Nsanze H, Piot P, Curran J, Karasira P, Mirza N, MacLean I W, Ronald A R 1984 The clinical diagnosis of genital ulcer disease in men in the tropics. Sexually Transmitted Diseases 11: 72–76

Hazlett D, Bowmer I, Nsanze H, Fransen L, D'Costa L 1983 In: Nsanze H, Widy-Wirsky R H, Ellison R H (ed) Herpesvirus in clinically suspected chancroid in Nairobi. Proceedings of the Third African Regional Conference on Sexually Transmitted Diseases, Nairobi. 18

Hira S K, Ratnam A V, Sehgal D, Bhat G J, Chintu C, Mulenga R C 1982a Congenital syphilis in Lusaka. 1. Incidence in a general nursery ward. East African Medical Journal 59: 241–246

Hira S K, Bhat C J, Ratnam A V, Chintu C, Mulenga R C 1982b Congenital syphilis in Lusaka. 2. Incidence at birth and potential risk among hospital deliveries. East African Medical Journal 59: 306–310

Kakiese Musumba 1983 La syphilis à Kinshasa. Thèse, Université Nationale du Zaire, Kinshasa

Latif A S 1983 Genitourinary pediatrics. In: Nsanze H, Widy-Wirsky R H, Ellison R H (eds) Proceedings of the Third African Regional Conference on Sexually Transmitted Diseases, Nairobi 14–18

Latif A S, Bvumbe S, Muongerwa J, Paraiwa E, Chikosi W 1983 Sexually transmitted diseases in pregnant women in Harare, Zimbabwe. Proceedings Third African Regional Conference on Sexually Transmitted Diseases, Nairobi 10–13

Mahomed M F, Mokaila P P, Barron C, Crewe-Brown H H 1984 The prozone phenomene in syphilis serology in antenatal patients. South African Journal of Sexually Transmitted Diseases 4: 29–31

Meheus A Z 1984 Practical approaches in developing countries. In: Holmes K K, Mardh P-A, Sparling P F, Wiesner P J (eds) Sexually Transmitted Diseases. New York, McGraw-Hill. 998–1008

Meheus A, Ursi J P, Van Dyck E, Ballard R 1981 Treatment of chancroid with single-dose doxycycline compared with a two-day course of co-trimoxazole. Annales de la Société belge de Médecine Tropicale 61: 119–124

Meheus A, Van Dyck E, Friedman F 1982 Genital infections in Swaziland. Annales de la Société belge de Médecine Tropicale 62: 361–367

Meheus A, Piot P 1983a Lutte contre les maladies sexuellement transmissibles dans les pays en développement. Annales de la Société belge de Médecine Tropicale 63: 281–311

Meheus A, Van Dyck E, Ursi J P, Ballard R C, Piot P 1983b Etiology of genital ulcerations in Swaziland. Sexually Transmitted Diseases 10: 33–35

Meheus A, Ursi J P 1982 Sexually Transmitted Diseases. Series of teaching slides. Upjohn Co, Kalamazoo, USA

Minh Triet N 1982 The problem of syphilis control in Ho Chi Minh City after liberation. M Ph thesis, Institute of Tropical Medicine, Antwerp.

Montefiore D, Sogbetun A O, Anong C N 1980 Herpesvirus hominis type 2 infection in Ibadan. Problem of non-venereal transmission. British Journal of Venereal Diseases 56: 49–53

Ndinya-Achola, D'Costa L J, Bowmer I, Fransen L, Piot P, Nsanze H, Ronald A 1983. Spectinomycin in treatment of chancroid: a comparison of 2 g versus 4 g.im In: Nsanze H, Widy-Wirsky R H, Ellison R H (eds) Proceedings of the Third African Regional Conference on Sexually Transmitted Diseases, Nairobi: 128

Nsanze H, Fast M, D'Costa L J, Tukei P, Curran J, Ronald A R 1981 Genital ulcers in Kenya: a clinical and laboratory study. British Journal Venereal Diseases 57: 378–381

Ngugi E N, Nsanze H, Haase D, Ndinya-Achola J D, D'Costa L J, Ronald A R 1984 Epidemiology of gonorrhoea and prostitution in Kenya. Abstracts of the 32nd General Assembly of the International Union against Venereal Diseases and Treponematoses, Montreal: 61

Nsanze H, Haase D, D'Costa L J, Ndinya-Achola J O, Ngugi E N, Ronald A 1984 Prevalence of syphilis among low socio-economic class prostitutes in Nairobi. Abstract of the 32nd General Assembly of the International Union against Venereal Diseases and Treponematoses, Montreal: 221

Oriel J D 1983 Management and control of genital ulcer disease. In: Nsanze H, Widy-Wirsky R H, Ellison R H (eds) Proceedings of the Third African Regional Conference on Sexually Transmitted Diseases, Nairobi. 85–92

Pandhi R K 1983 Fixed drug eruptions of genitalia in males: aetiological drugs. Program and Abstract of the International Society for STD Research, 5th International Meeting, Seattle WA: 201

Pereira M G 1980 Inquérito serologico de sifilis em adultos: Planaltina, D F, Brasil, 1977. Rev Saude Publ, S Paulo 14: 358–365

Perine P L et al 1980 Diagnosis and treatment of lymphogranuloma venereum in Ethiopia. Current Chemotherapy and Infectious Disease, American Society for Microbiology, Washington DC: 1280–1282

Piot P, Van Dyck E, Ursi J P, Lowe P, Duncan M, Ballard R C 1981 Erosive balanoposthitis associated with non-syphilitic spirochactal infection. Abstract of the 4th International Meeting for Sexually Transmitted Diseases Research, Heidelberg: 49

Piot P, Ballard R C, Fehler H G, Van Dyck E, Ursi J P, Meheus A Z 1982 Isolation of *Chlamydia trachomatis* from genital ulcerations in Southern Africa. In: Mardh P-A, Holmes K K, Oriel J D, Piot P, Schachter J (eds) Chlamydial infections, Elsevier/North Holland, Amsterdam 115–118

Piot P, Meheus A 1983 Epidémiologie des maladies sexuellement transmissibles dans les pays en développement. Annales de la société belge de Médecine Tropicale 63: 87–110

Piot P, Van Dyck E, Mårdh, P-A, Ursi J-P, Meheus A, Ballard R C, Møller B R, Fast M, Nsanze H, Ronald A 1983 Isolation of *Mycoplasma hominis* from genital ulcerations of patients in Eastern and Southern Africa. Sexually Transmitted Diseases 10: 285–288

Piot P, Quinn T C, Taelman H, Feinsod F M, Minlangu K B, Wobin O, Mbendi N, Mazebo P, Ndangi K, Stevens W 1984 Acquired Immunodeficiency syndrome in a heterosexual population in Zaire. Lancet ii: 65–69

Plummer F A, Nsanze H, D'Costa L J, Ndugga Maggara A B, Girouard Y, Karasira P, Albritton W L, Ronald A R 1983a Short course and single-dose antimicrobial therapy for chancroid in Kenya: studies with riampin alone and in combination with trimethoprim. Review of Infectious Diseases 5: S565–572

Plummer F A, D'Costa L J, Nsanze H, Maclean I W, Karasira P, Piot P, Fast M V, Ronald A R 1983b Antimicrobial therapy of chancroid: Effectiveness of erythromycin. Journal Infectious Diseases 148: 726–731

Plummer F A, D'Costa L J, Nsanze H, Dylewski J, Karasira P, Ronald A R 1983c Epidemiology of chancroid and of *Haemophilus ducreyi* in Nairobi, Kenya. Lancet ii: 1293–1295

Plummer F A, Nsanze H, D'Costa L J, Karasira P, Maclean I W, Ellison R H, Ronald A R 1983d Single-dose therapy of chancroid with trimethoprim-sulfametrole. New England Journal of Medicine 309: 67–71

Rajan V S, Doraisingham M, Sng E H, Lim A L 1982 Polymicrobial aetiology of genital ulcers. Singapore Medical Journal 23: 207–214

Rajan V S, Tham S N, Sng E H 1984 Gonococcal ulcers: A report of 18 cases. European Journal of Sexually Transmitted Diseases 1: 149–153

Schachter J, Osoba A O 1983 Lymphogranuloma inguinale British Medical Bulletin 39: 151–154

Sogbetun A O, Montefiore D, Anong C N 1979 Herpesvirus hominis antibodies among children and young adults in Ibadan. British Journal Venereal Diseases 55: 44–47

Taylor D N, Duangmani C, Suvongse C, O'Connor R, Pitarangsi C, Panikabutra K, Echeverria P 1984 The role of *Haemophilus ducreyi* in penile ulcers in Bangkok, Thailand. Sexually Transmitted Diseases 11: 148–151

Ursi J P, Van Dyck E, van Houtte C, Piot P, Colaert J, Dlamini M, Meheus A 1981 Syphilis in Swaziland. A serological survey. British Journal of Venereal Diseases 57: 95–99

Ursi J P, Van Dyck E, Ballard R C, Jacob W, Piot P, Meheus A Z 1982 The characterization of an unusual bacterium isolated from genital ulcerations. Journal of Medical Microbiology 15: 97–103

Vacca A, MacMillan L L 1980 Anogenital lesions in women in Papua New Guinea. Papua New Guinea Medical Journal 23: 70–73

Widy-Wirski R R, D'Costa J 1980a Maladies transmises par voie sexuelle dans une population rurale en Centrafique. In: Rapport final, 13ième Conférence technique, Yaounde, OCEAC, 651–654

Widy-Wirski R R, D'Costa J 1980b Prévalence des maladies transmises par voie sexuelle dans la population de femmes enceintes en milieu urbain en Centrafrique. In: Rapport final, 13ième Conférence technique, Yaounde, OCEAC. 655–660

World Health Organization 1981 Non-gonococcal urethritis and other selected sexually transmitted diseases of public health importance. Technical report series 660, Geneva, World Health Organization

World Health Organization 1982 Treponemal infections. Technical report series 671, Geneva, World Health Organization.

World Health Organization 1983 Current treatments in the control of sexually transmitted diseases. Geneva, World Health Organization: 433

World Health Organization 1984 Working group on simplified control approaches and rapid diagnostic techniques for STD. Geneva, Draft report

11. Bacterial vaginosis

C. S. F. Easmon

INTRODUCTION

The equivalent chapter in the previous volume of this series was titled '*Corynebacterium vaginale* infection'. A great deal of work has been done on this syndrome in the past seven or eight years and that title would no longer be acceptable. The bacterium has been classified as *Gardnerella vaginalis* and its precise aetiological role in bacterial vaginosis remains unclear. Various groups of anaerobic bacteria have also been implicated but their role too is uncertain. The major early work on bacterial vaginosis was done by Gardner, Dukes and their colleagues. Thirty years ago they showed the close association between the isolation of a small gram-negative bacillus and the mild vaginal condition of bacterial vaginosis (non-specific vaginitis). They called the organism *Haemophilus vaginalis* and defined the syndrome with a set of symptoms, signs and laboratory findings. Bacterial vaginosis could be produced in normal women by the inoculation of vaginal material from proven cases (Gardner & Dukes, 1955).

A similar organism had been isolated by Leopold (1953) from men with urethritis and prostatitis and from women with cervicitis. Lutz, Grootten & Wurch (1956) isolated a gram-negative bacillus from women with vaginal discharge which they called *Haemophilus vaginalis haemolyticus*.

A key part of Gardner & Dukes' work was the clear definition of the syndrome. Some of the confusion that has since arisen about many aspects of vaginosis can be linked to differences in the diagnostic criteria used by various groups. It is, therefore, an appropriate point at which to begin.

CLINICAL SYNDROME AND DIAGNOSIS

Bacterial vaginosis as originally defined by Gardner & Dukes (1955) was characterised by a homogeneous odorous vaginal discharge with a pH of 5.0 –5.5, clue cells and numerous small gram-negative bacilli, but with no inflammatory cells nor trichomonads. They stressed that symptoms should be taken as of lesser importance, there being considerable individual variation among women as to what they considered abnormal.

At an international meeting on bacterial vaginosis held in Stockholm early in 1984 (Mårdh & Taylor-Robinson, 1984) working groupos were set up to define bacterial vaginosis and to establish diagnostic criteria. The following definition of vaginosis was suggested 'A replacement of the lactobacillis of the vagina by characteristic groups of bacteria accompanied by changed properties of the vaginal fluid'.

Three of the following four criteria were proposed as the basis for diagnosis:

1. Thin/homogeneous discharge

2. pH > 4.5
3. Clue cells
4. A fishy amine odour

With the exception of the amine test described by Pheifer et al (1978), these criteria vindicated Gardner & Dukes' original observations. This definition was originally proposed by Amsel et al (1983) and supported by Ison et al (1983).

Other diagnostic criteria such as symptoms, an increased succinate lactate ratio in the vaginal washings (Spiegel et al, 1980; Piot et al, 1982) and the demonstration of amines by thin layer chromatography (Chen et al, 1979) were felt to be of value in certain situations, but not to be part of the basic clinical diagnosis.

It is hoped that the acceptance of these definitions of bacterial vaginosis will provide a standard basis for future clinical work on epidemiology, pathogenesis and therapy. They do not include the isolation of any particular organisms, merely indicating that *G. vaginalis*, *Bacteroides spp.*, anaerobic cocci, motile anaerobic curved rods and *Mycoplasma hominis* may be involved. The ability to culture some or all of these organisms is needed for those undertaking research into vaginosis but is not necessary for its routine diagnosis.

AETIOLOGY AND PATHOGENESIS

Gardner & Dukes (1955) found *G. vaginalis* in over 90% of women with vaginosis and in no women without the condition. In 1980 Gardner still felt that *G. vaginalis* was the sole aetiological agent. This view has been challenged on several grounds.

1. The isolation of *G. vaginalis* from women without vaginosis.
2. The association of a variety of anaerobic bacteria with vaginosis.
3. The failure of *G. vaginalis* to produce some of the features that characterise the condition (i.e. amines and succinate).

Several early studies refuted the view that *G. vaginalis* was exclusively associated with bacterial vaginosis (Lapage, 1961; de Louvois et al, 1975; McCormack et al, 1977). McCormack's claim that *G. vaginalis* should be considered as part of the normal vaginal flora has been supported by recent work using agreed diagnostic criteria and more sensitive cultural techniques. Spiegel et al (1980), Amsel et al (1983) and Ison et al (1983) all isolated *G. vaginalis* from a significant minority of normal women as well as from nearly all those with vaginosis. None of this excludes *G. vaginalis* from having an aetiological role in vaginosis, but it does imply that the condition has a more complex microbiological basis.

Gardner's group attempted to fulfill Koch's postulates by giving normal women either vaginal material from proven cases of bacterial vaginosis or pure cultures of *G. vaginalis*. They were significantly more successful in inducing bacterial vaginosis with the former (73% success) than with the latter (8% success). A later study by Criswell et al (1969) showed that twelve hour cultures of *G. vaginalis* produced better results than 24 hour cultures, but the very high inocula used must cast doubt on the relevance of this work to the natural disease. In the light of recent work on anaerobic bacteria and bacterial vaginosis, the difference between the efficacy of vaginal material and *G. vaginalis* in producing vaginosis may be significant.

Pheifer et al (1978) showed that vaginal discharges from women with vaginosis had high counts of non-sporing anaerobes, mainly *Bacteroides spp.* and anaerobic cocci as well as *G. vaginalis*. The common anaerobic pathogen *B. fragilis* was, however, rarely round. Successful treatment resulted in the reduction of viable counts of these anaerobic species. A number of groups have confirmed this.

Another group of anaerobic bacteria, highly motile curved rods, have also been associated with bacterial vaginosis. They are of two types, are readily seen in wet preparations and gram-stained smears of the vaginal discharge, but are more difficult to culture (Taylor & Phillips, 1982; Skarin & Mårdh, 1982; Hjelm et al 1982; Sprott et al, 1983). The presence of similar organisms in vaginal discharges was first reported over 70 years ago (Curtis, 1913). Spiegel & Roberts (1984) proposed their inclusion in a new genus, *Mobiluncus*, with two species, *Mobiluncus curtisii* and *Mobiluncus mulieris*.

The weakness of the case for an aetiological role for these anaerobic organisms is that no single species has as high an association with bacterial vaginosis as *G. vaginalis*. Against this is the possibility that there may be distinct aetiological entities within the broad definition of bacterial vaginosis. A strong point in favour of the anaerobes is that they are capable of producing two of the characteristic features of bacterial vaginosis, features that *G. vaginalis* cannot produce. Most women with vaginosis have an increased concentration of succinate in their washings (Spiegel et al, 1980). *G. vaginalis* does not appear to produce succinate while many of the anaerobes do. Similarly amines, mainly putrescine and cadaverine, that are so often daignostic of vaginosis are not produced by *G. vaginalis* but can be produced by at least some of the relevant anaerobic species. *G. vaginalis* does not have the decarboxylase enzymes necessary for the production of these amines from the parent amino acids (Chen et al, 1979).

Very little is known about the pathogenesis of vaginosis. *G. vaginalis* and nonsporing anaerobes may work together to produce a true mixed infection. It may even be that none of the organisms considered is anything more than a marker for the presence of bacterial vaginosis. Many of the diagnostic chatacteristics of bacterial vaginosis are present in both gonorrhoea and trichomonal infection (Ison et al, 1983) and an as yet unknown stimulus may precipitate vaginosis with subsequent changes in vaginal ecology.

Until recently there have been no reported attempts to reproduce bacterial vaginosis in experimental animals. Johnson et al (1984) were able to colonise Pig Tail Macacque monkeys, but neither chimpanzees nor Tamarind monkeys, with *G. vaginalis*. However, no animals developed features of vaginosis. Mårdh et al (1984) had more success with grivet monkeys. Animals given either curved anaerobic rods or these rods together with *G. vaginalis* developed a thin homogeneous discharge. It seems clear that animal models may be of value in understanding the pathogenesis of vaginosis. Work with primates is costly and requires special facilities, and is therefore only likely to be undertaken in a few centres.

The clue cell with its adherent bacteria is one of the features of vaginosis. Both *G. vaginalis* and anaerobes (Mårdh & Weström, 1976; Sobel et al, 1981, 1982) can adhere to vaginal epithelial cells but whether adherence plays a part in the causation of the disease is not known. Moi, Danielsson & Schoenknecht (1984) analysed the effect of menstrual cycle and pH on the adherence of *Mobiluncus spp.* and *Bacteroides spp.* to vaginal epithelium. Haemagglutination has been used extensively as a model for studying bacterial adherence and Ison & Easmon (1984) and Mårdh & Svensson (1984) have used this approach with *G. vaginalis* and *Mobiluncus spp.*

TAXONOMY AND IDENTIFICATION OF *GARDNERELLA* AND *MOBILUNCUS*

Gardnerella

The controversy over the classification of *G. vaginalis* which continued for nearly twenty years undoubtedly added to the confusion about bacterial vaginosis.

Gardner & Dukes (1955) considered it to be a gram-negative bacillus, and finding blood containing media necessary for its cultivation names it *Haemophilus vaginalis*. Both Lapage (1961) and Dunkleberg & McVeigh (1969) showed that '*H. vaginalis*' required neither haemin, nicotinamide adenine dinucleotide nor indeed blood. *H. vaginalis* was serologically distinct from other members of the genus.

Zinneman & Turner (1963) described the organism as gram-positive, and suggested inclusion in the genus *Corynebacterium* as *C. vaginale*. However, *C. vaginale* did not readily fit this genus. It was catalse negative, contained neither cell arabinose nor teichoic acid and differed from other members of the genus in its DNA G:C content.

Although neither *H. vaginalis* nor *C. vaginale* were wholly satisfactory classifications, both terms were used throughout the 1970s. Park et al (1968) had suggested that the organism should be placed in a new genus. Greenwood & Pickett (1980) proposed a new genus, *Gardnerella*, with a single species, *G. vaginalis*. Their submission, based on cell wall chemistry, biochemical reactions, electron microscopy and DNA hybridisation, was supported by the taxonomic work of Piot et al (1980). This has proved a satisfactory solution.

G. vaginalis can be grown on a wide variety of solid media. It requires an increased carbon dioxide concentration but can be grown anaerobically (modern anaerobic culture methods providing a raised carbon dioxide tension). The identification method of Dunkleberg et al (1970) using peptone starch dextrose agar and colonial morphology is too time-consuming for general use.

Human blood agar (Greenwood et al, 1977) is the mainstay of the most recent studies on *G. vaginalis*. The use of a bilayer plate improves the diffuse beta haemolysis that is characteristic of the organism, as does the addition of tween 80 (Totten et al, 1982). Antibiotic supplements of amphotericin B, nalidixic acid and colistin or gentamicin, have been used in a number of studies (Spiegel et al, 1980; Ison et al, 1983).

G. vaginalis is beta haemolytic on human but not on horse or sheep blood agar. It is gram-variable or gram-negative, oxidase and catalase negative and sensitive to a 50 μg metronidazole disc. Most strains hydrolyse hippurate. Carbohydrate fermentation tests (starch, maltose, glucose) have been used but are difficult to perform reliably. There is no consensus as to minimum criteria for the identification of *G. vaginale*, but differential haemolysis, gram-reaction and metronidazole sensitivity will be sufficient for most clinical purposes.

Mobiluncus

Curtis (1913) isolated motile curved flagellated anaerobic gram-negative bacilli from the vagina in women with abnormal vaginal discharges. Moore (1954) described two types of curved anaerobic rods from the vagina. Three years ago there was a cluster of reports of such organisms associated with bacterial vaginosis (Skarin et al, 1981; Spiegel et al, 1981; Holst et al, 1982; Phillips & Taylor, 1982). Sprott et al (1983) characterised two type of curved rod, one short, one long. Spiegel & Roberts (1984) have proposed the creation of a new genus, *Mobiluncus*, for these organisms, the short rods being speciated as *M. curtisii*, the long as *M. mulieris*. *M. curtisii* has two subspecies, *curtisii* and *holmesii*. This proposal was approved by a working party set up during a conference on bacterial vaginosis held in Stockholm (Mårdh & Taylor-Robinson, 1984).

Both species are stimulated by the presence of serum, starch and glycogen in the culture medium. The two species can be distinguished by their sensitivity to metronidazole (*M. curtisii* is relatively resistant with an MIC of 16–1000 mg/l), by their hippurate, β galactosidase and arginine reactions (*M. curtisii*-positive) and leucine aminopeptidase (*M. mulieris*-positive). The isolation and characterisation of *Mobiluncus spp* is not something that most diagnostic laboratories will wish to undertake unless the bacteria are isolated from invasive infections (Glupczynski et al, 1984).

EPIDEMIOLOGY

While there is little doubt that bacterial vaginosis is associated with sexual activity, it is not clear whether it is sexually transmitted and whether male carriage is an important epidemiological factor. Most of the work on epidemiology concerns *G. vaginalis*, less being known about anaerobic species. The recurrence rate of vaginosis is high even after successful therapy. Is this due to reinfection or regrowth?

G. vaginalis is part of the normal vaginal flora in many women (McCormack et al, 1977; Spiegel et al, 1980; Amsel et al, 1983; Ison et al, 1983). Among an unselected group of men urethral carriage rates of 7–11% have been reported, carriage usually being asymptomatic (Dawson et al, 1982; Kinghorn et al, 1982). Both Gardner & Dukes (1955) and Pheifer et al (1978) found that 80–90% of male partners of women with vaginosis were colonised with *G. vaginalis* and that after successful therapy recurrence rates were lower among women whose sexual partners use barrier contraceptives or who refrained from sexual intercourse.

While this supports the idea of sexual transmission, it is not conclusive. Proof requires a typing system for *G. vaginalis* with good discrimination. The only system for typing *G. vaginalis* is that reported by Piot et al (1984). They used eight biotypes based on β galactosidase and lipase activity and hippurate hydrolysis. Whether the system has sufficient discrimination to be useful in studying sexual transmission remains to be seen. The development of complementary methods such as serotyping would be helpful. A high recurrence rate of bacterial vaginosis after successful initial therapy could result from regrowth of a small residual population of bacteria rather than from reinfection. High carriage rates among male partners could simply reflect repeated passive acquisition from the female, and taken alone would not prove conclusively that these men acted as reservoirs of infection.

If sexual transmission from male to female occurs, semen is the likely medium. Ison & Easmon (1984) found *G. vaginalis* in 38% of semen samples from men attending an infertility clinic. (There was no association between the presence of *G. vaginalis* and low sperm counts). Viable counts ranged from 10^3 to 10^7 colony forming units/ml of semen. Unfortunately we do not know the minimum infecting dose of *G. vaginalis*, but semen could act as a medium for its transmission. Ison & Easmon (1984) also found non-sporing anaerobes in 35% of semen samples and *G. vaginalis* and anaerobes in 15.5%.

The efficacy of treating male contacts of women with bacterial vaginosis would provide good evidence that the male reservoir was important in the spread of the condition. To date there are no good controlled studies that show therapy of the male partner to be of value. As male carriage of *G. vaginalis* is asymptomatic, this type of study is difficult to carry out, there being little incentive for male partners to comply. The alternative explanation for the high rate of recurrence of vaginosis among cured women is their growth of *G. vaginalis* and anaerobes. With sensitive cultural techniques it is clear that these organisms are part of the vaginal microflora. It may be that semen provides a suitable stimulus for regrowth by raising vaginal pH. The association between continued intercourse and recurrence of bacterial vaginosis (Pheifer et al, 1978) does not therefore necessarily imply reinfection. In the past little attention has been paid to the anaerobic flora of the male urethra. Fontaine et al (1982, 1984) isolated a small gram-negative bacillus from the male urethra. It was present in 60% of men with non-gonococcal urethritis who were culture-negative for chlamydiae and ureaplasmas. The organism resembled *Bacteroides ureolyticus*. They have now found these organisms in women with bacterial vaginosis. Boriello et al (1984), Holst et al (1984) also isolated *B. ureolyticus*-like organisms from the male urethra. Fourteen of the 37 men had urethritis. A smaller number of men carried *Mobiluncus curtisii*. However, no male contacts of women who carried *Mobiluncus spp.* were themselves colonised. Currently the epidemiology of the anaerobic species associated with vaginosis is as confused as that of *G. vaginalis*.

MANAGEMENT

Although local therapy with sulphonamide cream, povidone iodine, neomycin and hexitine gel has been used (Gardner & Dukes, 1959; Dattani et al, 1982), systemic therapy is now generally recommended. Tetracycline, ampicillin and cephalosporins have been used (Gardner, 1980), but the nitroimidazoles metronidazole and tinidazole are currently the antimicrobial agents of choice (Pheifer et al, 1978; Balsdon et al, 1980; Spiegel et al, 1980). Nitroimidazoles may work because of their activity against anaerobes. They do, however, also have moderate activity against *G. vaginalis* and their hydroxymetabolites, major breakdown products, are significantly more active against *G. vaginalis* (Ralph & Amatnieks, 1980; Easmon et al, 1982). Five to seven day regimens (500 mg b.d.) have been claimed to be more effective than a single dose of 2 g (Blackwell et al, 1983) but in some cases the study design has been weighted against the single dose by evaluating patients a fixed time after the start rather than the end of therapy. Jones et al (1985) avoided this and showed no significant difference between the two regimens. Balsdon (1983) also found a 2 g single dose to be effective. A single dose given at the time of diagnosis has the advantage of ensuring patient compliance. Nitro imidazoles although safe are not the most pleasant drugs to take and can have an antabuse-like effect when taken with alcohol.

Three problems still remain. First, the high recurrence rate with all therapies.

Second, whether or not to treat male contacts. Third, the fact that the nitroimidazoles can be contra-indicated during pregnancy and lactation. The recent report that bacterial vaginosis during pregnancy may have an adverse effect on its outcome will, if confirmed, increase the importance of treating vaginosis during pregnancy (Eschenbach et al, 1984).

CONCLUSIONS

Some of the uncertainties about bacterial vaginosis have been resolved satisfactorily. A clear definition of the syndrome and its diagnostic criteria exist on which future work can be standardised. The taxonomy of *Gardnerella* has been settled as has that of the curved anaerobic rods. The nitroimidazoles are successful in producing a short term cure.

However, even more questions remain. The aetiology and pathogenesis of bacterial vaginosis are unclear. It is not even certain that it is primarily an infection. We know little of the relationship between *Gardnerella*, *Mobiluncus* and other anaerobes and vaginal epithelium, the influence of hormones and the menstrual cycle. We know little of the surface structures of these organisms and their relation to pathogenicity. Clinically, the importance of sexual transmission and the male urethra as a reservoir for infection remains to be clarified, as does the importance of treating male partners. Even with the initial success rate of nitroimidazole treatment, early relapse or recurrence is still common. The bacterial species associated with bacterial vaginosis are of low virulence, but are capable of invasive infections such as bacteraemia, urinary tract infection, amnionitis and endometritis. Their interplay with host defence mechanisms in these situations has not been investigated. Particularly intriguing is the possibility that vaginosis during pregnancy may be associated with adverse outcomes such as prematurity or pre-term rupture of membranes. There is increasing interest in the importance of the vaginal flora in this problem, but few good studies have yet been done.

In the past decade bacterial vaginosis has come in from the cold. It is to be hoped that the microbiological and clinical research interest that it has attracted will be of benefit to the thousands who suffer from this condition.

ACKNOWLEDGEMENT

My work on *G. vaginalis* and vaginosis is supported by the Medical Research Council.

REFERENCES

Amsel R, Totten P A, Spiegel C A, Chen K C S, Eschenbach D, Holmes K K 1983 Non-specific vaginitis. Diagnostic criteria and microbial and epidemiologic associations. American Journal of Medicine 74: 14–22
Balsdon M J 1983 Treatment of the *Gardnerella vaginitis* syndrome with a single 2 g oral dosage of metronidazole. Scandinavian Journal of Infectious Disease (Supplement) 40: 101–102
Balsdon M J, Pead L, Taylor G E, Maskell R 1980 *Corynebacterium vaginale* and vaginitis: a controlled trial of treatment. Lancet i: 501–504
Blackwell A L, Phillips I, Fox A R, Barlow D 1983 Anaerobic vaginosis (non-specific vaginitis): clinical microbiological and therapeutic findings. Lancet ii: 1379–1382
Borriello S P, Fontaine E A, Hawkins D, Taylor-Robinson D 1984 Development and evaluation of a selective medium for an anaerobe associated with non-gonococcal urethritis. In: Mårdh P-A, Taylor-Robinson D (eds) Bacterial vaginosis. Almqvist & Wiksell Int, Stockholm, 167–171

Chen K C S, Forsyth P S, Buchanan T M, Holmes K K 1979 Amine content of vaginal fluid from untreated and treated patients with non-specific vaginitis. Journal of Clinical Investigation 63: 828–835

Criswell B S, Ladwig C L, Gardner H L, Dukes C D 1969 *Haemophilus vaginalis* vaginitis by inoculation from culture. Obstetrics and Gynecology 33: 195–199

Curtis A H 1913 A motile curved anaerobic bacillus in uterine discharge. Journal of Infectious Disease 12: 165–169

Dattani I M, Gerken A, Evans B A 1982 Aetiology and managment of non-specific vaginitis. British Journal of Venereal Diseases 58: 32–35

Dawson S G, Ison C A, Csonka G, Easmon C S F 1982 Male carriage of *Gardnerella vaginalis*. British Journal of Venereal Diseases 58: 243–245

de Louvois J, Hurley R, Stanley V C 1975 Microbial flora of the lower genital tract during pregnancy relationship to morbidity. Journal of Clinical Pathology 28: 740–745

Dunkleberg W E, McVeigh I 1969 Growth requirements of *Haemophilus vaginalis*. Antonie Van Leeuwenhock 35: 129–145

Dunkleberg W E, Kellogg D S, Skaggs R 1970 Method for isolation and identification of *Corynebacterium vaginale (Haemophilus vaginalis)*. Applied Microbiology 19: 47–52

Easmon C S F, Ison C A, Kaye C M, Timewell R M, Dawson S G 1982 Pharmacokinetics of metronidazole and its principal metabolites and their activity against *Gardnerella vaginalis* British Journal of Venereal Diseases 58: 246–249

Eschenbach D A, Gravett M G, Chen K C S, Hoyme U B, Holmes K K 1984 Bacterial vaginosis during pregnancy. An association with prematurity and postpartum complications. In: Mårdh P-A, Taylor-Robinson D (eds) Bacterial vaginosis. Almqvist & Wiksell Int, Stockholm, 213–222

Fontaine E A R, Borriello S P, Taylor-Robinson D, Davies H A 1984 Characteristics of a gram-negative anaerobe isolated from men with non-gonococcal urethritis. Journal of Medical Microbiology 17: 129–140

Fontaine E A R, Taylor-Robinson D, Hanna N F, Coufalik E D 1982 Anaerobes in men with urethritis. British Journal of Venereal Diseases 58: 321–326

Gardner H L 1980 *Haemophilus vaginalis* vaginitis after twenty-five years. American Journal of Obstetrics and Gynecology 137: 385–390

Gardner H L, Dukes C D 1955 A newly defined specific infection previously classified 'non-specific vaginitis'. American Journal of Obstetrics and Gynecology 69: 962–976

Gardner H L, Dukes C D 1959 *Haemophilus vaginalis* vaginitis. Annals of the New York Academy of Science 83: 280

Glupczynski Y, Labbe M, Crokaert F, Pepersack F, Van Der Auwera P, Yourassowsky E 1984 Isolation of *Mobiluncus* in four cases of extragenital infections in adult women. European Journal of Clinical Microbiology 5: 433–435

Greenwood J R, Pickett M J 1980 Transfer of *Haemophilus vaginalis* (Gardner & Dukes) to a new genus *Gardnerella*. International Journal of Systemic Bacteriology 30: 170–178

Greenwood J R, Pickett M J, Martin W J, Mack E G 1977 *Haemophilus vaginalis (Corynebacterium vaginale)* method for isolation and rapid biochemical identification. Health Laboratory Science 14: 102–106

Hjelm F, Forsum U, Wallin J 1982 Anaerobic curved rods in vaginitis. Lancet i: 1353–1354

Holst E, Mårdh P-A, Thelin I 1984 Recovery of anaerobic curved rods and *Gardnerella vaginalis* from the urethra of men, including male heterosexual consorts of female carriers. In Mårdh P-A, Taylor-Robinson D (eds) Bacterial vaginosis. Almqvist & Wiksell Int, Stockholm, 173–177

Ison C A, Easmon C S F 1984 Studies on the mechanism of adhesion of *Gardnerella vaginalis* to human erythrocytes. In Mårdh P-A, Taylor-Robinson D (eds) Bacterial vaginosis. Almqvist & Wiksell Int, Stockholm, 191–194

Ison C A, Easmon C S F 1985 Carriage of *Gardnerella vaginalis* and anaerobes in semen. British Journal of Venereal Diseases 61: 120–123

Ison C A, Easmon C S F, Dawson S G, Southerton G, Harris J W R 1983 Non-volatile fatty acids in the diagnosis of non-specific vaginitis. Journal of Clinical Pathology 36: 1367–1370

Johnson A P, Ison C A, Hetherington C M, Osborn M F, Southerton G, London W T, Easmon C S F, Taylor-Robinson D 1984 A study of the susceptibility of three species of primate to vaginal colonisation with *Gardnerella vaginalis*. British Journal of Experimental Pathology 65: 389–396

Jones B M, Geary I, Alawattagama A B, Kinghorn C R, Duerden B I 1985 *In vitro* and *in vivo* activity of metronidazole against *Gardnerella vaginalis* bacteroides organisms and anaerobic curved rods in non-specific vaginitis. Journal of Clinical Pathology (in press)

Kinghorn G R, Jones B M, Chowdhury F H, Geary I 1982 Balanoposthitis associated with *Gardnerella vaginalis* infection in men. British Journal of Venereal Diseases 58: 127–129

Lapage S P 1961 *Haemophilus vaginalis* and its role in vaginitis. Acta Pathologica et Microbiologica Scandinavica 52: 34–54

Leopold S 1954 Heretofore undescribed organism isolated from the genito-urinary system. United States Armed Forces Medical Journal 4: 263–266

Lutz A, Grootten O, Wurch T 1956 Etudes des charactères culturaux et biochemiques de bacilles du type '*Haemophilus hemolyticus vaginalis*'. Revues d'Immunologie 20: 132–138

Mårdh P-A, Svensson S 1984 Haemagglutination by vaginal anaerobic curved rods and its inhibition by oligosaccharides. In: Mårdh P-A, Taylor-Robinson D (eds) Bacterial vaginosis. Almqvist & Wiksell Int, Stockholm, 179–184

Mårdh P-A, Taylor-Robinson D (eds) 1984 Bacterial vaginosis. Almqvist & Wiksell Int, Stockholm

Mårdh P-A, Westrom L 1976 Adherence of bacteria to vaginal epithelium. Infection and Immunity 13: 661–666

Mårdh P-A, Holst E, Møller B R 1984 The grivet monkey as a model for study of vaginitis. Challenge with anaerobic curved rods and *Gardnerella vaginalis*. In: Mårdh P-A, Taylor-Robinson D (eds) Bacterial vaginosis. Almqvist & Wiksell Int, Stockholm, 201–205

McCormack W M, Hayes C H, Rosner B, Evrard J R, Crockett V A, Alpert S, Zinner S H 1977 Vaginal colonisation with *Corynebacterium vaginale* (*Haemophilus vaginalis*). Journal of Infectious Diseases 136: 740–745

Moi H, Danielsson D, Schoenknecht F 1984 An *in vitro* study of the attachment to vaginal epithelial cells of anaerobic curved rods *Bacteroides bivius* and *Bacteroides disiens*. In: Mårdh P-A, Taylor-Robinson D (eds) Bacterial vaginosis. Almqvist & Wiksell Int, Stockholm, 185–190

Moore B 1954 Observations on a group of anaerobic vaginal vibrios. Journal of Pathology and Bacteriology 67: 461–473

Park C H, Fauber M, Cook C B 1968 Identification of *Haemophilus vaginalis*. American Journal of Clinical Pathology 49: 590–593

Pheifer T A, Forsyth P S, Durfee M A, Pollock H M, Holmes K K 1978 Non-specific vaginitis: role of *Haemophilus vaginalis* and treatment with metronidazole. New England Journal of Medicine 298: 1429–1434

Piot P, Van Dyck E, Godts P, Vanderheyden J 1982 The vaginal microbial flora in non-specific vaginitis. European Journal of Clinical Microbiology 1: 301–306

Piot P, Van Dyck E, Goodfellow M, Falkow S 1980 A taxonomic study of *Gardnerella vaginalis* (*Haemophilus vaginalis*). Journal of General Microbiology 119: 373–396

Piot P, Van Dyck E, Peeters M, Hale J, Totten PA, Holmes KK 1984 Biotypes of *Gardnerella vaginalis*. Journal of Clinical Microbiology 20: 677–679

Ralph E D, Amatnieks Y E 1980 Relative susceptibilities of *Gardnerella vaginalis* (Haemophilus vaginalis), *Neisseria gonorrhoeae* and *Bacteroides fragilis* to metronidazole and its two major metabolites. Sexual Transmitted Diseases 7: 157–160

Skarin A, Mårdh P-A 1982 Comma shaped bacteria associated with vaginitis. Lancet i: 342–343

Skarin A, Spiegel C A, Weström L, Holmes K K, Mårdh P-A 1981 Demonstration of a strictly anaerobic gram-negative comma-shaped bacterium in females with symptoms of lower genital tract infection. In: Abstracts of 4th International Meeting on Sexually Transmitted Diseases (Heidelberg), 9

Sobel J D, Myers P, Levison M E, Kaye D 1982 Comparison of bacterial and fungal adherence to vaginal exfoliated epithelial cells and human vaginal epithelial tissue culture cells. Infection and Immunity 35: 697–701

Sobel J D, Schneider J, Kaye D, Levison M E 1981 Adherence of bacteria to vaginal epithelial cells at various times of menstrual cycle. Infection and Immunity 32: 194–197

Spiegel C A, Roberts M 1984 *Mobiluncus* gen nov *Mobiluncus curtisii* subsp *curtisii* sp nov *Mobiluncus curtisii* susbp *holmesii* nov and *Mobiluncus mulieris* sp nov, curved rods from the human vagina. International Journal of Systemic Bacteriology 34: 177–184

Spiegel C A, Skarin A, Mårdh P-A, Holmes K K 1981 Isolation and characterisation of a curved motile anaerobic organism associated with non-specific vaginitis. In: Abstracts of the 4th International Meeting on Sexually Transmitted Diseases (Heidelberg), 8

Spiegel C A, Amsel R, Eschenbach D, Schoenkneckt F, Holmes K K 1980 Anaerobic bacteria in non-specific vaginitis. New England Journal of Medicine 303: 601–606

Sprott M S, Pattman R S, Ingham H R, Eisenstadt R L, Short G R, Narang H K, Sisson P K, Selkon J B 1983 Characteristics of motile curved rods in vaginal secretions. Journal of Medical Microbiology 16P: 175–182

Taylor E, Phillips I 1982 Anaerobic curved rods in vaginitis. Lancet i: 221

Totten P A, Amsel R, Hale J, Piot P, Holmes K K 1982 Selective differential human blood bilayer medium for isolation of Gardnerella (*Haemophilus*) *vaginalis*. Journal of Clinical Microbiology 15: 141–147

Zinneman K, Turner G C 1963 The taxonomic position of *Haemophilus vaginalis* (*Corynebacterium vaginale*). Journal of Pathology and Bacteriology 85: 213–219

12. Reactive arthritis and Reiter's syndrome

Andrew Keat

It has been recognised for two centuries or more that genital-tract infections lead, in a small proportion of individuals, to arthritis. In such instances the joint lesion may be septic with replicating bacteria — usually gonococci — within the joints or a sterile self-limiting arthritis. This latter condition has been described as 'reactive'. Aseptic arthritis associated with genital-tract infection is probably the commonest form of acute arthritis affecting young adult males in the Western World.

Reactive arthritis may be defined as sterile synovitis occurring in association with a localised infection at a distant site. Two major sites of infection are recognised, the lower genito-urinary tract and the gastrointestinal tract. However, the clinical features of reactive arthritis are also seen in individuals in whom no evidence of initiating infection can be identified. Approximately one third of patients with reactive arthritis, irrespective of the type of initiating infection, have the characteristic triad of Reiter's syndrome- arthritis which predominently affects the lower limbs, genital-tract inflammation and ocular inflammation.

Many terms have been introduced to refer to patients with this form of arthritis. Each was coined to apply to a particular subgroup of patients, most are now redundant and none is entirely satisfactory. The term 'sexually acquired reactive arthritis' (SARA) refers specifically to disease precipitated by sexually transmitted infection (Keat et al, 1978a). The relationship between reactive arthritis and conditions described as 'post-infective' (Dumonde & Steward, 1978) remains uncertain; these conditions differ clinically and genetically from reactive arthritis, although it is possible that similar mechanisms operate in both instances.

Reactive arthritis shares important clinical features with other forms of sero-negative arthritis, in particular psoriatic arthritis and ankylosing spondylitis. Acute anterior uveitis (AAU) occurs in both reactive arthritis and spondylitis and psoriasiform skin and mucous membrane lesions occur in some patients with reactive arthritis, so that on occasion it is impossible to distinguish with certainty between reactive arthritis and psoriatic arthritis. In addition, within the families of probands with one condition, features of another within the group are not infrequently present. Lawrence (1974) showed that there is an excess of psoriasis within the family members of individuals with Reiter's syndrome. Because of these clinically apparent interrelationships and overlaps the term seronegative spondarthritides was coined (Wright, 1978) to include ankylosing spondylitis, reactive arthritis, psoriatic arthritis and enteropathic arthritis. Recent genetic studies have reinforced this concept by demonstrating the sharing of the same genetic marker, the histocompatibility antigen HLA-B27, by all members of the group and by isolated circinate balanitis and AAU in addition (Brewerton, 1976). This grouping is clinically useful and emphasises the common genetic, and therefore possibly aetiological, factors between the individual entities.

EPIDEMIOLOGY

Reactive arthritis occurs world-wide, in all racial groups. In Europe and North America, genital-tract infections appear to be the major precipitating causes whilst in North Africa and elsewhere, enteric infections are the principal aetiological factors. Individuals in the third decade of life are principally affected, although the disease is well documented from early childhood until at least the sixth decade. The age incidence of reactive arthritis associated with genital-tract infection closely mirrors that of uncomplicated non-gonococcal urethritis (NGU).

Arthritis develops in approximately 1% of men presenting with NGU at hospital clinics (Csonka, 1958) and in 2–3% of patients with certain bacterial enteric infections (Keat, 1983). Both of these figures are approximations, as individuals with mild short-lived disease may not present themselves for medical attention. Sexually acquired reactive arthritis is predominantly a male disease with a male to female ratio of 10:1. However, the apparent magnitude of the male predominance in this condition may be exaggerated as some large and important studies involved military personnel on active service, and genital-tract infection in women may be underdiagnosed. Recent reports suggest that this form of arthritis is being increasingly recognised in women (Smith, Bennett & Regan, 1980; Neuwelt, Borenstein & Jacobs, 1982).

CLINICAL FEATURES

Reactive arthritis ranges from a gross, disabling, multi-system disease to transient painless joint effusion associated with trivial or no symptoms. Therefore, a high index of suspicion is required; reactive arthritis should always be suspected in a young adult male presenting with joint symptoms. Although genito-urinary and joint lesions are prominent in reactive arthritis, lesions of entheses, eyes, skin and mucous membrane are highly characteristic. These lesions are easily overlooked, though their presence may confirm the diagnosis.

Presentation

People with reactive arthritis may present to a wide variety of specialities, including orthopaedic surgeons, dermatologists, accident and emergency departments, venereologists and rheumatologists. Many of those presenting with urinary symptoms fail to recognise the significance of minor rheumatic symptoms, attributing them to trivial injuries, or fail to mention them, assuming that they are unrelated to their more prominent symptoms. Conversely, in some patients symptoms of infection are trivial or absent, so that presentation is with an apparently isolated episode of arthritis. In patients with sexually acquired disease, urogenital symptoms generally develop 8–15 days after contact and in 90% arthritis follows within 30 days (mean 14 days). Joint and urogenital symptoms may, however, arise simultaneously. In a few individuals the interval between the acquisition of infection and the development of arthritis is much longer; in these, there may be persistent or subclinical infection which is allowed to recrudesce by changes in the patient's immune status; or the two events may be unrelated.

Knee synovitis is the commonest joint lesion, nearly 50% of patients presenting with swelling at one or both knees. Less commonly, the first symptoms arise at the metatarsophalangeal (MTP) or ankle joints, or as a result of extensor tendonitis or enthesopathy. Enthesopathies affecting the Achilles' tendon and plantar fascia insertions at the calcaneum are not uncommon and reactive arthritis should be considered as the most likely diagnosis in a young man presenting with heel pain. Occasionally, joint symptoms are absent or minimal in the presence of substantial joint effusion.

Peripheral arthritis

Joint involvement is typically oligoarticular, often involving two or three joints and usually less than six. In up to 10% of patients, arthritis is restricted to a single joint, usually the knee. Involvement of upper limb joints is unusual and should raise the possibility of psoriatic arthritis. When a group of joints such as MTP joints is affected, it is characteristic for only one or two of the group to be involved, in contrast to the typically symmetrical joint involvement of rheumatoid disease. The full clinical picture usually evolves over two to three weeks, it being unusual for new sites to become affected after this time. Large cystic extensions of the knee joint may form posteriorly (Baker's cysts); these occasionally rupture producing dramatic calf swelling simulating deep venous thrombosis.

Radiographic joint abnormalities are rarely demonstrated during the acute episode. When joint rupture is suspected, however, venography is the investigation of choice, as it is essential to exclude venous thrombosis as either the primary event or a secondary complication of joint rupture. Persistence of small joint synovitis however, especially in the feet, leads to non-specific changes of juxta-articular osteoporosis and may lead on to bony erosions resembling those seen in rheumatoid disease. In severe instances there may be destruction of the MTP joints with gross subluxation of the toes.

In the acute phase, synovial fuid is usually turbid and rich in polymorphonuclear leucocytes. Examination of joint fluid is important for the exclusion of bacterial infection and crystal synovitis, though it does not yield other specific diagnostic information. Synovial biopsy, similarly, usually reveals information of exclusory value only, appearances being indistinguishable from those seen in other acute or chronic forms of synovitis. Immunofluorescence studies of synovial biopsies obtained within the first few weeks of disease, may show the presence of immunoglobulin and complement deposits consistent with the deposition or local formation of immune complexes (Yates et al, 1975; Baldassare et al, 1981).

Spondylitis

Sacroiliitis and spondylitis both occur in some patients with reactive arthritis but estimates of their prevalence vary widely. Low back pain is common during the acute episode and studies using scintigraphic techniques have suggested that this is due to sacroiliitis (Russell et al, 1977). In patients with severe, chronic or recurrent disease persisting for five years or more, radiographic sacroiliac abnormalities have been noted in approximately 50% of patients (Sholkoff, Glickman & Steinbach, 1971; Steinbach & Jensen, 1976). Typical spondylitis has been observed in 23% of such individuals (Good, 1965) but in those with less severe disease of shorter duration it is likely that spondylitis develops in a far lower proportion. Since both spondylitis and reactive arthritis share a common genetic factor, it is not yet clear whether one condition genuinely leads to the other, or whether both may develop independently in the same individual. Radiographic non-marginal syndesmophytes or bony bridges have also been observed in patients with reactive arthritis (Cliff, 1971; Sunderam & Patton, 1975). These may occur in the absence of sacroiliitis or back symptoms but are also seen in psoriatic spondylitis and occasionally in asymptomatic, healthy individuals.

Enthesopathies

Enthesopathies are inflammatory lesions at junctional zones between tendon or fascia and bone (Niepel & Sit'aj, 1979; Resnick & Miwayama, 1983). They occur in approximately 30% of patients with reactive arthritis but may also be present in other forms of seronegative arthritis. The sites of attachment of the plantar fascia and Achilles' tendon at the calcaneum are most commonly involved, producing highly typical lesions with local pain and swelling which may be the major source of discomfort and disability. There may be associated Achilles' tendon bursitis producing posterior ankle swelling best seen from behind. Less commonly, muscle and tendon attachments at the pelvis, tibial tubercle and feet may be similarly affected. In the early stage, these lesions appear radiographically as localised osteoporotic areas or 'erosions, though later there is healing with the formation of wispy new bone which, at the calcaneum, leads to the formation of typical fluffy bony spurs. Similar exuberant new bone formation may also occur around affected joints such as the hip, leading to marked limitation of joint movement.

Eye lesions

Inflammatory eye lesions have received considerable attention and their presence in an individual with urethritis and arthritis completes the triad of Reiter's syndrome. However, clinically detectable ocular inflammation occurs in no more than one third of patients with reactive arthritis so that it should not be regarded as an essential diagnostic criterion. The chief lesion is unilateral or bilateral conjunctivitis; although symptoms may be severe, with secondary infection, complete resolution without sequelae is the rule. In contrast, AAU is uncommon during an acute episode, although a past history of this may be obtained. The distinction between conjunctivitis and AAU is usually impossible to make without slit-lamp examination by a specialist; in view of the risk of rapid impairment of vision associated with AAU, all patients with arthritis and painful red eyes should be examined urgently by an ophthalmologist. The causes of ocular inflammation in reactive arthritis remain poorly understood. Several other less common ocular lesions have been recorded; these include hypopyon secondary to AAU, intra-ocular haemorrhage, corneal ulceration, keratitis, optic neuritis and posterior uveitis.

Skin and mucous membrane lesions

Highly characteristic psoriasiform skin and mucous membrane lesions occur in up to a third of patients with sexually acquired reactive arthritis. Keratoderma blenorrhagica develops in 10% of patients as a scaling pustular rash on the soles of the feet and raised circinate lesions on the glans penis occur in approximately 20%. Similar psoriasiform lesions have been described on the female genitalia (Thambar et al, 1977). Histologically, these lesions closely resemble those of pustular psoriasis both light (Kulka, 1962) and electron (Kanerva et al, 1982) microscopic levels. Shallow painless ulcers on the buccal mucosa, tongue, palate or fauces may also be present.

These lesions contrast with the discreet and extremely painful lesions of Behçet's syndrome.

In reactive arthritis associated with gut infection, erythema nodosum has been well described, though this appears to be rare in sexually acquired disease. In contrast, circinate balanitis and keratoderma blenorrhagica appear rare in reactive arthritis associated with salmonella, campylobacter or yersinia infection.

Cardiovascular lesions

Electrocardiographic abnormalities occurring during the acute episode have been reported in around 10% of patients with Reiter's syndrome (Csonka, 1961; Leisisalo et al, 1982). Changes resemble those seen in acute rheumatic fever with conduction delay and flattening or inversion of the T-waves. Complete heart block has been described and myocarditis or pericarditis may also occur. Recent studies have suggested that chronic myocardial abnormalities may occur in a significant proportion of patients with Reiter's syndrome (Ribeiro et al, 1984). Aortic valve disease develops in 1–2% of patients and successful aortic valve replacement has been successfully carried out.

Other rare lesions

Numerous other abnormalities have been described in patients who have features of reactive arthritis, including pulmonary infiltrates, neurological defects, thrombophlebitis and thyroid disorders. At present, however, the significance of these features is uncertain.

COURSE OF DISEASE

In contrast to rheumatic fever and gonoccocal arthritis, joint involvement in reactive arthritis is additive rather than migratory. Erosive joint disease occurs in a minority, the small joints of the feet being those principally affected. Affected large joints usually recover fully, though long-standing joint disease may predispose to the late development of osteoarthritis. Approximately 70% of patients recover completely within six months. Up to 15%, however, have continuing symptoms for one year and some of these will continue to run a chronic relapsing and remitting course. In one Scandinavian study, 10% of patients developed chronic disease (Kousa 1978). Of those that recover fully, 50% will suffer one or more recurrences of arthritis or enthesopathy, with a few unfortunates having repeated episodes. Recurrence of rheumatic symptoms is not always associated with evidence of genital-tract inflammation or further sexual contact; conversely, individuals who have suffered from reactive arthritis in the past may develop undoubted venereal urethritis without recurrence of rheumatic symptoms. Recurrence appears to be less common in disease precipitated by gastro-intestinal infection. An American report that 26% of patients had had to change or give up their work (Fox et al, 1979) is certainly atypical of experience of reactive arthritis in Britain. It is likely that some studies have selected in favour of the most severely affected patients, so that although some patients become substantially disabled, estimates of the frequency of severe disability are spuriously high.

Life-threatening complications of reactive arthritis are rare. A few patients, however, principally those with severe acute episodes or recurrent disease, develop heart failure due to aortic valve disease or blindness following inadequately treated AAU. Significant amyloid deposition appears to be rare. Bad prognostic features include severe initial involvement progressing to rapid joint erosion, and the development of multiple extra-articular lesions. HLA-B27 positive patients tend to develop more severe disease than HLA-B27 negative individuals (Morris et al, 1974; Keat et al, 1979; Leirisalo et al, 1982).

INHERITED SUSCEPTIBILITY

The occurrence of reactive arthritis among members of the same family is well recognised, though uncommon. Similarly, features of reactive arthritis with or without evidence of precipitating infection may occur in close relatives of probands with other disorders within the seronegative spondarthritis group. The existence of inherited factors predisposing to reactive arthritis has been confirmed by the finding of the genetic marker HLA-B27 in 67–96% of patients (Brewerton et al, 1973; Woodrow, Treanor & Usher, 1974; Morris et al, 1974) compared with 7–14% of controls. No association with HLA-D locus or other inherited determinants has been demonstrated to date. An HLA-B27 positive man with NGU is approximately 40–50 times more likely to develop reactive arthritis than an HLA-B27 negative one. Moreover, it is now clear than HLA-B27 positivity also predisposes to seronegative peripheral arthritis without evidence of infection, isolated calcaneodynia, tendonitis and AAU irrespective of associated rheumatic disease. In contrast, however, HLA-B27 status does not appear to influence the development of arthritis in streptococcal (Falk et al, 1973; Caughey et al, 1975) meningococcal (Friis, 1975) or certain viral (Robitaille et al, 1976; Griffiths et al, 1977) infections, nor does it influence susceptibility to NGU itself (Keat et al, 1978b).

It is likely that the inherited basis of reactive arthritis is multigenic. Nevertheless, HLA-B27 holds the key. The structure and function of the HLA system is reviewed elsewhere (Bodmer & Bodmer, 1978; Festenstein & Demant, 1978; Svejgaard et al, 1981). Considerable controversy surrounds the possible mechanisms by which possession of this antigen predisposes to the development of arthritis (Keat, 1982). Two principal hypotheses exist. The B27 cell surface antigen may interact directly with microbial antigens and/or immunocompetent cells and thereby initiate or perpetuate the inflammatory reaction. Alternatively, the B27 gene may be an innocent marker, the principal culprits being other gene(s) within the major histocompatibility complex which are inherited together with it, in linkage disequilibrium. The involvement of linked genes is favoured by the mounting evidence that a substantial number of genes in the HLA region of the sixth chromosome are intricately involved in aspects of the immune response to infectious agents (McMichael et al, 1977; Zinkernagel & Doherty, 1977; Thorsby et al, 1981). However, recent in vitro studies have shown that HLA-B27 can act as a receptor for soluble antigens derived from certain gram negative bacteria, including those known to precipitate reactive arthritis (Ebringer et al, 1976; Seager et al, 1979; Geczy et al, 1980; Edmonds et al, 1981; Prendergast et al, 1983; Van Bohemen, Grumet & Zanan, 1984). Indirect evidence is accumulating that HLA antigens in general play important roles in cell interactions by acting as receptor sites for soluble transmitter molecules; it is possible, therefore, that both hypotheses are partially correct, the B27 antigen being one of a group of critical cell surface determinents involved in the recognition of microbial antigens and the establishment of an inappropriate inflammatory response. This is consistent with the clinical view that the development of overt disease is precipitated by infection in an already susceptible individual. The clinical overlaps and the sharing of the genetic marker HLA-B27 among members of the seronegative spondarthritis group suggests that similar mechanisms operate in each condition.

INITIATING INFECTIONS

Three major aetiological groups of reactive arthritis exist. Disease precipitated by genito-urinary and gastro-intestinal infection are well recognised. The third group consists of patients in whom characteristic clinical features of reactive arthritis are present, but in whom no evidence of infection can be found. Studies of possible sites of infection in these patients will be of particular importance.

In Europe and the United States, genital-tract infection is regarded as the most common initiator of reactive arthritis. Whereas the capacity of gastro-intestinal infection to initiate arthritis is clearly demonstrated by the occurrence of arthritis during outbreaks of bacterial diarrhoea, evidence implicating genital-tract infection is less clear. Sexually transmitted infection is implicated by a history of appropriate exposure in more than 80% of cases, the presence of signs of genital-tract inflammation in all patients and regular time intervals between exposure to infection, development of genital-tract disease and arthritis (Csonka, 1958; Ford & Rasmussen, 1964; Keat et al, 1979). The absence of a history of recent sexual contact, or exceptionally prolonged time intervals, may be explicable by spontaneous recurrence of urethritis which had previously been sexually acquired or by recent acquisition of infection by the regular sex partner. In these circumstances, since urethritis may also accompany gastrointestinal infection, it may not be possible to establish with certainty whether genital-tract infection is of aetiological significance, in which case the predisposing cause should be regarded as 'unknown'.

Harkness (1950) proposed that only non-gonococcal infections were important in the initiation of arthritis, demonstrating that even if gonococci were present, after treatment with penicillin a co-existing non-gonococcal infection was revealed. However, this traditional view has recently been questioned (Rosenthal & Danielson, 1978; Rosenthal, Olhagen & Ek, 1980) and the possibility that gonococci may induce aseptic arthritis in susceptible individuals should not be entirely discounted.

Present evidence suggests that no single micro-organism is responsible for the genital-tract and joint disease in all patients with sexually acquired reactive arthritis. All micro-organisms which have been implicated, however tenuously, in the aetiology of urethritis must be considered as possible triggers of arthritis.

Arthritis has also been reported in association with genital-tract infections other than acute urethritis. Oligoarticular arthritis is well described in lymphogranuloma venereum. This is rare in the UK but is of some interest as the causal micro-organism is known. Chronic prostatitis has been reported in a high proportion of men with sacroiliitis and spondylitis (Romanus, 1953; Mason et al, 1958; Domeij et al, 1958; Grainger & Nicol, 1959); however, similar findings have been observed in control individuals (Domeij, 1958) so that, in the absence of firm criteria for the diagnosis of prostatitis, the significance of these reports is uncertain. There is little evidence to suggest that men with chronic prostatitis are especially likely to develop spondylitis (Moller, Vinje & Fryjordet, 1980). However, Scandinavian work has indicated that a high proportion of women developing acute salpingitis subsequently progress to develop sacroiliitis (Julkunen & Pietila, 1964; Szanto & Hagenfeldt, 1979): further work is necessary to confirm these findings and to provide detailed microbiological analyses of such patients.

Reactive arthritis develops in 2–3% of individuals with acute enteric infections by *Shigella flexneri* and *dysenteriae*, *Salmonella enteritidis* and *typhimurium*, *Yersinia enterocolitica* and *Campylobacter jejuni* (Keat, 1983). The prevalence of arthritis in individual outbreaks varies considerably from one population to another; genetic factors are clearly important in this, though it is uncertain whether individual strains of bacteria vary in their capacity to produce arthritis. *Shigella sonnei* infections appear not to lead to arthritis. It is clear that, in many patients, gastro-intestinal symptoms are trivial or absent; this applies particularly to campylobacter infections which have recently been identified as a common cause of minor bowel upsets (Skirrow, 1979). Other gut infections including amoebic dysentery, non-specific 'traveller's' diarrhoea and giardiasis have also been associated with the development of reactive arthritis but these reports are unconfirmed.

Chlamydial infection

C. trachomatis causes approximately 50% of cases of NGU in men and is a common pathogen in the female genital tract (Taylor-Robinson & Thomas, 1980). Chlamydial infection in animals, notably cattle and sheep, is a well recognised cause of infective polyarthritis, and in these animal diseases it is likely that the genital tract is the portal of entry of the infection. Naturally, therefore, chlamydiae have been considered a likely cause of human arthritis.

Since the introduction of sensitive cell culture techniques for isolating chlamydiae, *C. trachomatis* has been isolated from the genital tract of 0% (Ford & McCandlish, 1969) to 69% (Kousa et al, 1978) of men presenting with Reiter's syndrome. A mean isolation rate of 35% hs been calculated from data from several major studies (Keat, Thomas & Taylor-Robinson, 1983). These data are difficult to collect as many patients have been treated with antibiotics by the time arthritis develops, while others present late, when shedding of micro-organisms in the genital tract may be reduced.

The question as to whether viable chlamydiae enter the joint is of critical importance but remains unresolved. In studies using culture in embryonated hens' eggs, some positive isolations from joint material were reported (Schachter, 1976). However, in studies using cell culture isolation techniques only two isolates have been reported (Shatkin, Popov & Scherbakova, 1976; Vilppula et al, 1981). In *C. psittaci* arthritis is calves, chlamydiae are demonstrable in the joints up until the 28th day. After this point, micro-organisms can no longer be detected although synovitis persists (Storz, 1971). It is possible, therefore, that some parallel situation exists in human *C. trachomatis* infection so that further studies of patients with very early disease, using highly sensitive techniques, are needed to explore this crucial issue.

Although non-trachomatous chlamydial eye disease, in the form of adult and neonatal inclusion conjunctivitis is well recognised, the extent to which chlamydiae may be involved in the ocular lesions of reactive arthritis is uncertain. As with cultures of joint material, early studies using isolation in eggs resulted in some positive isolates from conjunctivae of patients with Reiter's syndrome (Ostler, Dawson & Schachter, 1971; Schachter & Dawson, 1978). However, the introduction of cell culture techniques, which have increased the isolation rate in inclusion conjunctivitis to 90% (Darougar, 1977), has reduced the rate of recovery from patients with reactive arthritis to 4% (Keat, Thomas & Taylor-Robinson, 1983). Therefore, it is unlikely that conjunctivitis in these patients is caused by direct infection by chlamydiae.

Using modifications of the micro-immunofluorescence (mIF) test, studies from Finland (Kousa et al, 1978; Vilppula et al, 1981), the United Kingdom (Vaughan-Jackson et al, 1972; Keat et al, 1980) and the United States (Martin et al, 1984) have showed that chlamydial serum antibody is present in a high proportion of patients. Moreover, in these individuals, the geometric mean titre (GMT) of serum antibody is significantly higher than that found in individuals with uncomplicated NGU, other forms of arthritis or healthy controls. Unlike men with NGU, all isolate-positive patients with arthritis produced high titres of serum antibody, and sequential studies of a small number of patients showed high initial titres of chlamydial IgM which rapidly fell and rising titres of IgG antibody which peaked at around six weeks and thereafter slowly declined. Most of the patients studied in this way have been male but recently similar high titres of chlamydial antibody were found in females (Vilppula et al, 1981). Patients with reactive arthritis associated with enteric infection ('post diarrhoeal Reiter's syndrome') do not produce detectable chlamydial serum antibody (Martin et al, 1984).

Studies of cell-mediated immunity to chlamydia have in general been difficult to interpret. Skin testing has been used to a limited extent: Dunlop (1975) using extracts of oculogenital and LGV strains of C. trachomatis, found positive skin tests in nine of 13 patients with Reiter's syndrome compared with nine of 50 men with uncomplicated NGU. Increased lymphocyte transformation responses to chlamydial antigens have also been reported in a high proportion of patients with arthritis associated with genital-tract infection compared with patients with uncomplicated NGU or with post-diarrhoeal arthritis (Martin et al, 1984). Other workers, however, have not shown a difference between patients with uncomplicated NGU and those with arthritis (Amor et al, 1972).

It may be concluded that approximately 50% of patients with sexually acquired reactive arthritis yield isolates of C. trachomatis from the urethra and that, in the majority of these patients, specific humoral, and possibly cellular, immune responses to chlamydia are enhanced in comparison with uncomplicated chlamydial urethritis.

Mycoplasmas and ureaplasmas

Mycoplasmas are known to induce arthritis in some animals and M. pneumoniae has been associated with transient arthritis in man (Ponka, 1980). Both M. pneumoniae and Ureaplasma urealyticum have been isolated from inflamed joints of immunodeficient human hosts (Taylor-Robinson et al, 1978; Webster et al, 1978; Johnston et al, 1983). There is no evidence that large colony mycoplasmas are pathogenic in the genital tract or joints of immunologically normal individuals.

In contrast, U. urealyticum has been shown experimentally to induce urethritis in humans (Taylor-Robinson, Csonka & Prentice, 1977) as well as in non-human primates. Carriage of mycoplasmas and ureaplasmas in the lower genital tract appears to be of equal prevalence in men with reactive arthritis and in those with uncomplicated urethritis (Csonka, Williams & Corse, 1967; Ford, 1968) but no difference in antibody response between the two groups has been demonstrated (Taylor-Robinson et al, 1983). As with chlamydiae, eradication of mycoplasmas and ureaplasmas from the genital tract by antibiotic treatment does not influence the development or course of arthritis (Kleineberger-Nobel, 1959; Ford & Rasmussen, 1964). Attempts to isolate mycoplasmas and ureaplasmas from the eyes of men with reactive arthritis have produced almost uniformly negative results. Initial reports of the isolation of mycoplasmas from the joints of patients with Reiter's syndrome were almost certainly spurious, but further studies searching for ureaplasmas in the joint are needed. The role, if any, of the newly discovered mycoplasma *M. genitalium* in urethritis or reactive arthritis has yet to be evaluated.

Gonococci

Around 10% of patients presenting with sexually acquired reactive arthritis have gonorrhoea at presentation (Keat et al, 1979; Leirisalo et al, 1982), and the possibility that *N. gonorrhoeae* itself might trigger off arthritis has been raised by Swedish workers (Rosenthal & Danielson, 1978; Rosenthal, Olhagen & Ek, 1980). Evidence similar to that implicating *C. trachomatis* has been presented so that the possibility that this micro-organism is a genuine precipitating agent requires further clarification.

Other bacteria and viruses

Many other bacteria including *Staphylococcus epidermidis*, *Clostridium difficile* and *Gardnerella vaginalis* have been isolated from patients with NGU, but their pathogenicity under these circumstances has yet to be fully determined. Attempts to isolate viruses from the genital tract and joints of patients with reactive arthritis have yielded no firm evidence of the presence of virus at either site.

CONCLUSIONS

Reactive arthritis is a common sequel to sexually transmitted urogenital infection. The clinical spectrum of this condition is wide, with many patients having relatively trivial disease, and women may be affected more often than has been recognised. The prognosis for the great majority of patients is good. It appears unlikely that any one microorganism is the single cause of sexually acquired reactive arthritis but exaggerated humoral and cellular immune responses to *C. trachomatis* in such patients suggests that this microorganism may be one precipitating factor. However, a great deal of work remains to be done in order to establish the precise link between inherited predisposing factors and 'trigger' micro-organisms.

REFERENCES

Amor B, Kahan A, Lecoq F, Delbarre F 1972 Le test de transformation lymphoblastique par des antigenes bedsoniens (TTL Bedsonien). Revue de Rhumatisme 39: 671–676

Baldassare A R, Weiss T D, Tsai C C, Arthur R E, Moore T L, Zuckner J 1981 Immunoprotein deposition in synovial tissue in Reiter's syndrome. Annals of the Rheumatic Diseases 40: 281–285

Bodmer W F, Bodmer J G 1978 Evolution and function of the HLA system. British Medical Bulletin 34: 309–316

Brewerton D A 1976 HLA-B27 and the inheritance of susceptibility to rheumatic disease. Arthritis and Rheumatism 19: 656–668

Brewerton D A, Caffrey M, Nicholls A, Walters D, Oates J K, James D C O 1973 Reiter's disease and HL-A27. Lancet 2: 996–998

Caughey D E, Douglas R, Wilson W, Hassall I B 1975 HL-A antigens in Europeans and Maoris with rheumatic fever and rheumatic heart disease. Journal of Rheumatology 5: 319–322

Cliff J M 1971 Spinal bony bridging and carditis in Reiter's disease. Annals of Rheumatic Diseases 30: 171–179

Csonka G W 1958 The course of Reiter's syndrome. British Medical Journal 1: 1088–1090

Csonka G W, Litchfield J W, Oates J K, Willcox R R 1961 Cardiac lesions in Reiter's disease. British Medical Journal 1: 243–247

Csonka G W, Williams R E O, Corse J 1967 T-strain mycoplasmas in non-gonococcal urethritis. Annals of the New York Academy of Sciences 143: 794–798

Darougar S, Woodland R M, Forsey T, Cubitt S, Alani J, Jones B R 1977 Isolation of chlamydia from ocular infections. In: Hobson D, Holmes K K (eds) Non-Gonococcal urethritis and related infections, American Society of Microbiology, Washington DC 295–298

Domeij B, Giertz E, Olhagen B, Romanus R 1958 Genito-urinary focus in rheumatic disorders in the male. Acta Chirurgica Scandinavica 115: 1–10

Dumonde D C, Steward M W 1978 The role of microbial infection in rheumatic disease. In: Scott J T (ed) Copeman's textbook of the rheumatic diseases, 5th edn, Churchill Livingstone, Edinburgh 221–258

Dunlop E M C 1975 Non-specific genital infection. Laboratory aspects. In: Morton R S, Harris J R (eds) Recent advances in sexually transmitted diseases. Churchill Livingstone, 267–295

Ebringer A, Cowling P, Ngwa Suh N, James D C O, Ebringer R W 1976 Cross-reactivity between Klebsiella aerogenes species and B27 lymphocyte antigen as an aetiological factor in ankylosing spondylitis. Symposium HLA and Disease, Paris, abstract 1–15 INSERM

Edmonds J, Macauley S, Tyndall A, Liew M, Alexander K, Geczy A, Bashir H 1981 Lymphocytotoxicity of anti-klebsiella antibodies in ankylosing spondylitis and related arthropathies. Arthritis and Rheumatism 25: 1–7

Falk J A, Fleischman J L, Zabriskie J B, Falk R E 1973 A study of HL-A antigen phenotypes in rheumatic fever and rheumatic heart disease patients. Tissue Antigens 3: 173–178

Festenstein H, Demant P 1978 HLA and H-2. Basic immunogenetics. Biology and clinical relevance. Edward Arnold, London

Ford D K 1968 Non-gonococcal urethritis and Reiter's syndrome: personal experience with aetiological studies during fifteen years. Canadian Medical Association Journal 99: 900–910

Ford D K, McCandlish L 1969 Isolation of TRIC agents from the human genital tract. British Journal of Veneral Diseases 45: 44–46

Ford D K, Rasmussen G 1964 Relationships between genitourinary infection and complicating arthritis. Arthritis and Rheumatism 7: 220–227

Fox R, Calin A, Gerber R C, Gibson D 1979 The chronicity of symptoms and disability in Reiter's syndrome. An analysis of 131 consecutive patients. Annals of Internal Medicine 91: 190–193

Friis J 1975 HL-A27 in neisseria infected patients with arthritis. Scandinavian Journal of Rheumatology (suppl) 8: (abstract no 30–12)

Geczy A F, Alexander K, Bashir H V, Edmonds J P 1980 A factor(s) in Klebsiella culture filtrates specifically modifies an HLA-B27 associated cell-surface component. Nature 283: 782–784

Good A E 1965 Reiter's disease and ankylosing spondylitis. Acta Rheumatologica Scandinavica 11: 305–317

Grainger R G, Nicol C S 1959 Pelvic infection as a cause of bilateral sacroiliac arthritis and ankylosing spondylitis. British Journal of Venereal Diseases 35: 92–98

Griffiths M M, Spruance S L, Ogra P L, Thompson G R, De Witt C W 1977 HLA and recurrent episodic arthropathy associated with rubella vaccination. Arthritis and Rheumatism 20: 1192–1197

Harkness A H 1950 In: Non-gonococcal urethritis, Livingstone, Edinburgh 99–145

Johnston C L W, Webster A D B, Taylor-Robinson D, Rapaport D, Hughes G R V 1982 Primary late onset hypogammaglobulinaemia associated with inflammatory polyarthritis and septic arthritis due to *Mycoplasma pneumoniae*. Annals of The Rheumatic Diseases 42: 108–110

Julkunen H, Pietila K 1964 Chronic salpingo-oophoritis and rheumatoid spondylitis. Acta Rheumatologica Scandinavica 10: 209–214

Kanerva L, Kousa M, Niemi K M, Lassus A, Juvakoski T, Lauharanta J 1982 Ultrahistopathology of balanitis circinata. British Journal of Venereal Diseases 58: 188–195

Keat A 1982 HLA-linked disease susceptibility and reactive arthritis. Journal of Infection 5: 227–239

Keat A C 1983 Reiter's syndrome and reactive arthritis in perspective. New England Journal of Medicine 309: 1606–1615

Keat A C, Maini R N, Nkwazi G C, Pegrum G D, Ridgway G L, Scott J T 1978a Role of *Chlamydia trachomatis* and HLA-B27 in sexually acquired reactive arthritis. British Medical Journal 1: 605–607

Keat A C, Pegrum G D, Maini R N, Scott J T, Nkwazi G C, Ridgway G L 1978b HLA antigens, *Chlamydia trachomatis* infection and reactive arthritis. Tissue Antigens 12: 63–64

Keat A C, Maini R N, Pegrum G D, Scott J T 1979 The clinical features and HLA associations of reactive arthritis associated with non-gonococcal urethritis. Quarterly Journal of Medicine 48: 323–342

Keat A C, Thomas B J, Taylor-Robinson D, Pegrum G D, Maini R N, Scott J T 1980 Evidence of *Chlamydia trachomatis* infection in sexually acquired reactive arthritis. Annals of The Rheumatic Diseases 39: 431–437

Keat A C, Thomas B J, Taylor-Robinson D 1983 Chlamydial infection in the aetiology of arthritis. British Medical Bulletin 39: 168–174

Kleineberger-Nobel E 1959 Pleuropneumonia-like organisms in genital infections. British Medical Journal 1: 19–23

Kousa M 1978 Clinical observations on Reiter's disease with special reference to the venereal and non-venereal aetiology. Acta Dermatovenerologica 58: suppl 81

Kousa M, Saikku P, Richmond S, Lassus A 1978 Frequent association of chlamydial infection with Reiter's syndrome. Sexually Transmitted Diseases 5: 57–61

Kulka J P 1962 The lesions of Reiter's syndrome. British Journal of Venereal Diseases 53: 260–262

Laitinen O, Leirisalo M, Skylv G 1977 Relation between HLA-B27 and clinical features in patients with yersinia arthritis. Arthritis and Rheumatism 20: 1121–1124

Lawrence J S 1974 Family survey of Reiter's disease. British Journal of Venereal Diseases 50: 140–145

Leirisalo M, Skylv G, Kousa M, Voipio-Pulkki L M, Suoranti H, Nissila M, Hvidman L, Damm Nielsen E, Svejgaard A, Tiilikainen A, Laitinen O 1982 Follow up study of patients with Reiter's disease and reactive arthritis with special reference to HLA-B27. Arthritis and Rheumatism 25: 249–259

Martin D H, Pollock S, Kuo C-C, Wang S P, Brunham R C, Holmes K K 1984 *Chlamydia trachomatis* infections in men with Reiter's syndrome. Annals of Internal Medicine 100: 207–213

Mason R M, Murray R S, Oates J K, Young A C 1958 Prostatitis in ankylosing spondylitis. British Medical Journal 1: 748–751

McMichael A, Ting A, Zweerink H J, Askonas B A 1977 Major transplantation antigens, viruses and specificity of surveillance T cells. Contemporary Topics in Immunobiology 7, Plenum Press, New York 779–986

Moller P, Vinje O, Fryjordet A 1980 HLA antigens and sacroiliitis in chronic prostatitis. Scandinavian Journal of Rheumatology 9: 138–140

Morris R, Metzger A L, Bluestone R, Terasaki P I 1974 HL-A W27 — a clue to the diagnosis and pathogenesis of Reiter's syndrome. New England Journal of Medicine 290: 554–556

Neuwelt C M, Borenstein D G, Jacobs R P 1982 Reiter's syndrome: a male and female disease. Journal of Rheumatology 9: 268–272

Niepel G A, Sit'aj S 1979 Enthesopathy. Clinics in Rheumatic Diseases. 5: 857–872

Ostler H B, Dawson C R, Schachter J, Engleman E P 1971 Reiter's syndrome. American Journal of Ophthalmology 71: 986–991

Ponka A 1979 Arthritis associated with *Mycoplasma pneumoniae* infection. Scandinavian Journal of Rheumatology 8: 27–32

Prendergast J K, Sullivan J S, Geczy A, Uphold L I, Edmonds J P, Bashir H V, Reiss-Levy E 1983 Possible role of enteric organisms in the pathogenesis of ankylosing spondylitis and other seronegative arthropathies. Infection and Immunity 41: 935–941

Resnick D, Niwayama G 1983 Entheses and enthesopathy. Radiology 146: 1–9

Riberio K, Morley K D, Shapiro L M, Garnett R A F, Hughest G R V, Goodwin J F 1984 Left ventricular function in patients with ankylosing spondylitis and Reiter's disease. European Heart Journal 5: 419–422

Robitaille A, Cockburn C, James D C G, Ansell B M 1976 HLA frequencies in less common arthropathies. Annals of the Rheumatic Diseases 35: 271–273

Romanus R 1953 Pelvo-spondylitis ossificans in the male and genito-urinary infection. Acta Medica Scandinavica (suppl) 280: 172–178

Rosenthal L, Danielsson D 1978 Induction of DNA synthesis in lymphocytes, in vitro, by various bacteria, with special reference to *Neisseria gonorrhoeae* in patients with uro-arthritis (Reiter's disease). Scandinavian Journal of Rheumatology 7: 101–108

Rosenthal L, Olhagen B, Ek S 1980 Aseptic arthritis after gonorroea. Annals of the Rheumatic Diseases 39: 141–146

Russell A S, Davis P, Percy J S, Lentle B C 1977 The sacroiliitis of acute Reiter's syndrome. Journal of Rheumatology 4: 293–296

Schachter J 1976 Can chlamydial infections cause rheumatic disease? In: Dumonde D C (ed) Infection and immunology in the rheumatic diseases. Blackwell, Oxford 151–157

Schachter J, Dawson C R 1978 Human chlamydial infections. PSG publishing company, Littleton, MA 141–146

Seager K, Bashir H V, Geczy A F, Edmonds J, De Vere Tyndall A 1979 Evidence for a specific B27-associated marker on the lymphocytes of patients with ankylosing spondylitis. Nature 277: 68–70

Shatkin A A, Popov N L, Scherbakova N I 1976 Morphology of Halprowia (chlamydia) isolated in Reiter's syndrome. Zhurnal Mikrobiologii Epidemiologii I Immunobiologii 4: 60–64

Sholkoff S D, Glickman M D, Steinbach H L 1971 The radiographic pattern of polyarthritis in Reiter's syndrome. Arthritis and Rheumatism 14: 551–565

Skirrow M B 1977 Campylobacter enteritis: a new disease. British Medical Journal 2: 9–11

Smith D L, Bennett R M, Regan M G 1980 Reiter's disease in women. Arthritis and Rheumatism 23: 335–340

Steinbach H L, Jensen P S 1976 Roentgenographic changes in the arthritides (Part II). (Reiter's syndrome, gout, osteoarthrosis, chondrocalcinosis, sarcoidosis, haemochromatosis, systemic lupus erythematosus, progressive systemic sclerosis). Seminars in Arthritis and Rheumatism 5: 203–246

Storz J 1971 Chlamydial polyarthritis In: Thomas C C, Chlamydia and chlamydia-induced diseases, Springfield, Illinois 216–232

Sundaram M, Patton J T 1975 Paravertebral ossification in psoriasis and Reiter's disease. British Journal of Radiology 48: 628–633

Svejgaard A, Morling N, Platz P, Ryder L P, Thomsen N 1981 HLA and disease associations with special reference to mechanisms. Transplantation Proceedings 13: 913–917

Szanto E, Hagenfeldt K 1979 Sacroiliitis and salpingitis: quantitative 99mTc pertechnetate scanning in the study of sacroiliitis in women. Scandinavian Journal of Rheumatology 8: 129–135

Taylor-Robinson D, Csonka G W, Prentice M J 1977 Human intra-urethral inoculation of ureaplasmas. Quarterly Journal of Medicine 46: 309–326

Taylor-Robinson D, Gumpel J M, Hill A, Swannell A J 1978 Isolation of *Mycoplasma pneumoniae* from the synovial fluid of a hypogammaglobulinaemic patient in a survey of patients with inflammatory polyarthritis. Annals of the Rheumatic Diseases 37: 180–182

Taylor-Robinson D, Thomas B J 1980 The role of *Chlamydia trachomatis* in genital-tract and associated diseases. Journal of Clinical Pathology 33: 205–233

Taylor-Robinson D, Thomas B J, Furr P M, Keat A C 1983 The association of *Mycoplasma hominis* with arthritis. Sexually Transmitted Diseases 10: suppl 341–344

Thambar I V, Dunlop R, Thin R N, Huskisson E C 1977 Circinate vulvitis in Reiter's syndrome. British Journal of Venereal Diseases 53: 260–262

Thorsby E, Bergholtz B, Berle E, Braathen L, Hirschbirg H 1981 Involvement of HLA in T-cell immune responses. Transplantation Proceedings 13: 903–908

Van Bohemen C G, Grumet F C, Zanan H C 1984 Identification of HLA-B27 M1 and M2 cross-reactive antigens in Klebsiella, Shigella and Yersinia. Immunology 52: 607–610

Vaughan-Jackson J D, Dunlop E M C, Darougar S, Dwyer R, Jones B R 1972 Chlamydial infection. Results of tests for *Chlamydia* in patients suffering from acute Reiter's disease compared with results of tests from the genital tract and rectum in patients with ocular infection due to TRIC agents. British Journal of Venereology 48: 445–451

Vilppula A H, Yli-Kerttula U I, Ahlroos A K, Terho P E 1981 Chlamydia isolation and serology in Reiter's syndrome. Scandinavian Journal of Rheumatology 10: 181–185

Webster A D B, Taylor-Robinson D, Furr P M, Asherson G L 1978 Mycoplasmal (ureaplasma) septic arthritis in hypogammaglobulinaemia. British Medical Journal 1: 478–479

Woodrow J C, Treanor B, Usher N 1974 The HL-A system in Reiter's syndrome. Tissue Antigens 4: 533–540

Wright V 1978 Seronegative polyarthritis. A unified concept. Arthritis and Rheumatism 21: 619–633

Yates D B, Maini R N, Scott J T, Sloper J C 1975 Complement activation in Reiter's syndrome. Annals of the Rheumatic Diseases 34: 468 (abstract)

Zinkernagel R M, Doherty P C 1977 Major transplantation antigens, viruses and specificity of surveillance T cells. Contemporary topics in immunobiology 7. Plenum Press, New York 13: 903–908

13. Epidemiology and prevention of the acquired immunodeficiency syndrome (AIDS)

D. Peter Drotman   John W. Ward   James W. Curran

INTRODUCTION

Acquired immunodeficiency syndrome (AIDS) is a disease first recognised in 1981, when homosexual men in the United States were noted to have opportunistic diseases and evidence of immunosuppression (CDC, 1981a, CDC, 1981b, Hymes et al, 1981, Gottlieb et al, 1981). This outbreak has raised considerable public health concern because of the rapidly increasing number of persons being diagnosed, high case-fatality rate, and lack of effective therapy. There is now convincing evidence that AIDS is caused by infection with a human retrovirus variously termed human T-cell lympho-tropic virus, type III (HTLV-III), lymphadenopathy-associated virus (LAV), or AIDS-related virus (ARV). AIDS has been defined by the Centers for Disease Control (CDC) for surveillance purposes (Table 13.1). This definition continues to be useful

Table 13.1 AIDS case definition

For the limited purposes of epidemiologic surveillance, CDC defines a case of the acquired immunodeficiency syndrome (AIDS) as an illness characterised by:

I. one or more opportunistic diseases*, diagnosed by methods considered reliable, that are at least moder-ately indicative of underlying cellular immunodeficiency, and

II. absence of all known underlying causes of cellular immunodeficiency (other than infection with the virus presumed to cause AIDS) and absence of all other causes of reduced resistance† reported to be associated with at least one of those opportunistic diseases.

* These diseases include cryptosporidiosis; *Pneumocystis carinii* pneumonia; toxoplasmosis causing infection in internal organs other than liver, spleen or lymph nodes; disseminated strongyloidosis; candidiasis causing esophagitis; cryptococcosis causing central nervous system or disseminated infection; disseminated atypical mycobacterial infection; cytomegalovirus causing infection in internal organs other than liver, spleen, or lymph nodes; mucocutaneous herpes simplex virus infection with ulcers persisting more than a month or pulmonary, gastrointestinal, or disseminated infection; progressive multifocal leukoencephalopathy; Kaposi's sarcoma; lymphoma limited to the brain.
† These known causes of reduced resistance include: systemic corticosteroid therapy within 1 month before diagnosis, systemic cytotoxic chemotherapy within 1 year before diagnosis, Hodgkin's disease or non-Hodgkin's lymphoma, lympho-cytic leukemia, multiple myeloma, or any other cancer of lymphoreticular or histiocytic tissue. Additional conditions need to be excluded in pediatric patients, such as diagnoses of neonatal toxoplasmosis or herpes simplex virus infection (in those less than 28 days of age at diagnosis) or cytomegalovirus infection (in those less than 6 months of age at diagnosis); an immunodeficiency atypical of AIDS, such as one involving hypogammaglobulinemia, or an immunodeficiency of which the cause appears to be a genetic or developmental defect; or exogenous malnutrition (starvation).

in monitoring trends and comparing morbidity between countries. Cases have been identified retrospectively in the United States (CDC, 1985c) as early as 1978. By May 1985, 10 000 cases were reported in the United States, and the cumulative case count is projected to approach 20 000 by mid-1986. Two areas of the United States, the New York metropolitan area and California, have reported more then 60% of the cases, but at least one AIDS case has been diagnosed in residents of all but four of the 50 states. Subsequent to AIDS being recorded in the United States, the syndrome has been recognised in many other Western countries, where it has epidemio-logic features similar to those in the United States. Cases from Haiti and central

African countries have also been reported, but the epidemiologic pattern appears quite different in those regions (Pape et al 1983, Clumeck et al, 1984).

As is so often the case with newly discovered illnesses, epidemiologists described the basic modes of transmission of AIDS prior to the discovery of the agent that gives rise to the syndrome. However, interrupting the transmission of AIDS has proven considerably more difficult than removing the handle from the Broad Street pump, as John Snow did to end the cholera epidemic in London in the 1850s, well before the *Vibrio cholerae* was isolated.

By discerning that the main modes of transmission of AIDS were sexual and blood-borne, epidemiologists provided direction for laboratory investigators. Ultimately, laboratory researchers at the National Cancer Institute and the Institut Pasteur isolated the causal retrovirus. Screening and diagnostic tests are now being developed, but the basic knowledge necessary to launch preventive programmes has been available for some time. However, AIDS is a unique public health problem with special obstacles to its control, including biomedical, public health, and social barriers. Diverse challenges remain, such as defining the precise mechanisms of transmission, detecting what specific exposures potentially result in transmission, devising appropriate prevention messages and delivering these to populations that may be socially isolated, overcoming concerns for the safety of medical and laboratory workers, and educating health professionals about the health, social, and sexual concerns of populations at risk for AIDS.

THE CASE DEFINITION AND ITS IMPLICATIONS

Much of what has been published on AIDS is based on data derived from patients who fit the CDC surveillance definition. This case definition was designed to be strict (with high specificity and less regard for sensitivity), because data collected on the early cases were used to formulate public policy, prevention recommendations, research priorities, and other equally important considerations. The definition is used worldwide for surveillance and is officially recognised by the World Health Organisation. The case definition includes only two criteria, encompassing selected opportunistic diseases and known causes of cellular immunodeficiency that fulfil these criteria (Table 13.1).

The case definition was designed for use in epidemiologic surveillance, and it suits that purpose quite well. It may not be the best definition for purposes of clinical investigation, disability determination, or sexual counselling. Nonetheless, it has become the most well-recognised definition for AIDS in its short but intense history. This is somewhat ironic, because it does not truly define the spectrum of illness. Ultimately, a definition that includes evidence of infection with HTLV-III/LAV will be combined with other criteria, probably not as rigorous as those in the current definition, to delineate AIDS cases.

Because the goal has been to keep abreast of the AIDS epidemic by keeping track of time, place, and person, the particular definition is likely to be less consequential than its consistent application. In the United States, CDC has stressed this issue, and, as a result, epidemiologic surveillance has been reasonably consistent since it commenced in mid-1981.

The cases CDC has tracked clearly represent the tip of a large clinical 'iceberg'.

With newly developed serologic tests for antibody to HTLV-III/LAV, the full breadth and depth of this iceberg are becoming much more clear. The clinical spectrum is analogous to that of hepatitis B, with some severe cases, but many asymptomatic infections (Alter & Francis, 1984). The portion of the iceberg below the surface of the water includes other cancers, lymphadenopathy syndrome, idiopathic thrombocy-topenic purpura, and asymptomatic infections (Jaffe HW et al, 1985a). These issues, as well as defining the full natural history of HTLV-III/LAV infection, are current topics of active research.

Incidence of AIDS in the United States, By Quarter of Diagnosis

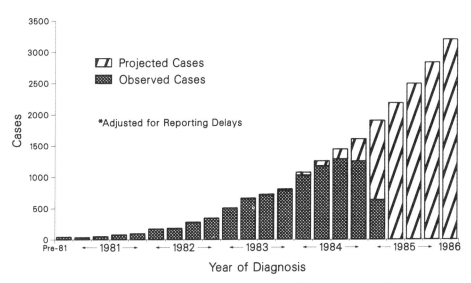

Fig. 13.1   Epidemic curve depicting actual and projected cases of AIDS, based on the 9214 cases reported to CDC as of April 1, 1985.

THE EPIDEMIOLOGY AND SEXUAL TRANSMISSION OF AIDS

Since its discovery in 1981, AIDS has demonstrated a strikingly relentless pattern. Cases reported to CDC from the United States have increased exponentially with time, as the epidemic curve shows (Fig. 13.1). The epidemic curves for other industrialised nations have similar shapes, although the time scale lags somewhat.

As with any infectious disease, the epidemiologic patterns reflect the modes of transmission of the aetiologic agent. The modes of transmission of the virus that causes AIDS are limited: sexual transmission, exposure to transfused blood or certain blood products (mainly clotting factor concentrates), exposure to blood by needle-sharing among IV drug users or, perhaps in developing countries, other unsterile needles, and from mother to unborn or newborn child. Nearly all patients have fallen into one or more high-incidence groups (Table 13.2). For the United States, these groups are listed with trends in group composition over time (Table 13.3).

Table 13.2   Adult and pediatric AIDS cases, as of May 1, 1985. Demographic characteristics of patient groups

Adult/adolescent hierarchical patient category	Cases N	Median Age Yrs	Sex %		Race %			Other/ Unk
			M	F	W	B	Hisp	
Homosexual/ bisexual men	7220	35	100.0	0.0	72.6	15.2	10.7	1.5
IV drug users	1684	33	79.4	20.6	19.3	48.8	31.2	0.8
Hemophiliacs	65	33	95.4	4.6	78.5	9.2	10.8	1.5
Sexual contacts of above group members	81	31	11.1	88.9	18.5	46.9	34.6	0.0
Transfusion recipients	133	57	58.7	41.4	75.2	15.0	6.8	3.0
Others*	661	33	75.6	24.4	19.1	68.8	10.1	2.0
Total	9844	35	93.5	6.5	59.5	24.7	14.3	1.4

* Includes 292 persons born in countries in which most AIDS cases have not been associated with known risk factors.

Pediatric (<13 yrs) hierarchical Patient category	Cases N	Median Age Yrs	Sex %		Race %			Unk
			M	F	W	B	Hisp	
Hemophiliacs	6	10	100.0	0.0	33.3	33.3	33.3	0.0
Parent with AIDS or at increased risk	79	<1	53.2	46.8	11.4	65.8	21.5	1.3
Transfusion recipients	14	1	85.7	14.3	71.4	14.3	7.1	7.1
Others	10	<1	70.0	30.0	30.0	40.0	30.0	0.0
Total	109	<1	61.5	38.5	22.0	55.1	21.1	1.8

The primary route of transmission of the virus that causes AIDS is sexual. This seemed likely early in the outbreak investigation, because most of the first cases were in gay men. Auerbach et al (1984) provided support for this conclusion by establishing that nine of the first 13 AIDS patients in Southern California from whom they obtained sexual histories could be linked together by sexual contact. They were able to extend this cluster and thereby link sexually 40 patients in 10 cities. This cluster accounted for more than 16% of the total number of reported cases in gay men in the United States at the time of investigation.

In the first national case-control study of gay men with AIDS, Jaffe H W et al (1983) found several measures of sexual activity to be the variables that best distinguished cases from controls. Indeed, the main risk associated with the development of AIDS is homosexual or bisexual contact. Over 72% of the cases reported to CDC have this sexual history. The precise mechanism of transmission is not known, but sexual contact clearly is implicated. Specific factors, such as having a sexual partner with AIDS, frequent sexual contact with anonymous partners, and a history of other sexually transmitted diseases, including hepatitis B and syphilis, are associated with increased risk of developing AIDS (Jaffe H W et al, 1983). Specific sexual practices that may facilitate transmission of HTLV-III/LAV infection are difficult to define, although receptive anal intercourse and 'fisting' (inserting hand or fist into partner's rectum) may facilitate transmission by exposing partners to infected semen or blood or by traumatising the rectal mucosa, facilitating a portal of entry for the virus (Darrow

Table 13.3 Adult and pediatric AIDS cases, as of May 1, 1985 Distribution (%) by patient group for each report year

Adult/adolescent hierarchical patient category	Year of Report				May 1 1985	Total Cases
	1981 N = 202	1982 N = 742	1983 N = 2384	1984 N = 4672	N = 1844	N = 9844
Homosexual/bisexual men	84.7	70.1	71.4	73.9	74.5	73.3
IV drug users	9.9	17.1	18.4	16.9	16.9	17.1
Hemophiliacs	0.0	0.8	0.5	0.8	0.5	0.7
Sexual contacts of above group members	0.5	1.1	0.8	0.8	0.9	0.8
Transfusion recipients	0.0	0.8	1.2	1.4	2.1	1.3
Others	4.9	10.1	7.8	6.3	5.3	6.7
	100.0	100.0	100.0	100.0	100.0	100.0

Pediatric (<13 yrs) Hierarchical patient category	Year of Report			May 1 1985	Total Cases
	1982 N = 13	1983 N = 45	1984 N = 45	N = 6	N = 109
Hemophiliacs	7.7	4.4	4.4	16.7	5.5
Parent with AIDS or at increased risk	53.8	71.1	80.0	66.7	72.5
Transfusion recipients	15.4	15.6	11.1	0.0	12.8
Others	23.1	8.9	4.4	16.7	9.2
	100.0	100.0	100.0	100.0	100.0

et al, 1985). No single sexual activity has been shown to be safe with an infected person, although activities that reduce the exchange of body fluids are recommended. On theoretical grounds, condoms are recommended as a barrier to body fluid exposure, although there is not yet evidence for their efficacy (CDC, 1985a).

SEROEPIDEMIOLOGY

Identification of HTLV-III/LAV and the ability to culture this virus resulted in efforts to produce serologic tests to detect antibody to viral antigens. These tests include electrophoretic blotting (Western blot), radioimmunoprecipitation techniques, and enzyme-linked immunosorbent assay (ELISA).

Serologic tests have been used to support the etiologic role of HTLV-III/LAV in AIDS and to identify the extent of this infection in populations known to be at risk for AIDS. The prevalence of antibody is high in AIDS patients. In their initial study, Sarngadharan et al (1984) found 43 (88%) of 49 AIDS patients to have antibody by ELISA. Other investigators have confirmed these results, with 88 to 100% of AIDS patients tested being seropositive (Levy et al, 1984; Safai et al, 1984). Prevalence of antibody is also increased in persons with AIDS-related conditions (84–100%) but, in contrast, less than 1% of controls are seropositive. Levy et al (1984) and Safai et al (1984) found 21–57% of asymptomatic gay men to be positive for antibody. Whether this prevalence is representative of all gay men is not known, but it clearly demonstrates that many more persons have been infected than have developed AIDS. The fraction of those with positive antibody tests who actually are infected remains unknown.

Currently, persons capable of shedding virus can be identified only by culturing peripheral blood lymphocytes. Virus has been recovered from the peripheral blood, semen, and saliva (Barre-Sinoussi et al, 1983; Gallo et al, 1984; Zagury et al, 1984; Groopman et al, 1984a; Ho et al, 1984). In a study of high-risk group members who had donated blood to persons who subsequently developed AIDS, nearly 90% of seropositive donors had virus recovered from blood specimens collected as long as 4 years after donation (Feorino et al, 1985). Whether this high degree of infectivity holds true for all seropositive persons remains to be established. However, a significant proportion of asymptomatic persons with antibody appears to be persistently infected and capable of transmitting infection to others.

The prognosis for seropositive individuals is unknown. The incubation period of AIDS is long, ranging from a few months to at least 5 years. In a large cohort of gay men from San Francisco, a subgroup of 31 men has been positive for antibody for a median duration of 5 years since 1978. Of these, two (6%) have developed AIDS, eight (25%) have developed a related condition, and the others are without symptoms (Jaffe H W et al, 1985b). The larger studies now under way are necessary to determine the natural history of HTLV-III/LAV infection. What is clear is that large fractions of many populations at risk for HTLV-III/LAV infection have developed antibody. By the time the first AIDS cases appear in a population, many individuals already are infected. This situation presents special challenges to disease control programmes.

THE NATURAL HISTORY OF HTLV-III/LAV INFECTION (Table 13.4)

The San Francisco Health Department and CDC have followed a cohort of 6875 gay men since 1978 to study incidence, risk factors, and prevention of hepatitis B. Originally recruited from the city's sexually transmitted disease clinic, these men have been shown to be at very high risk for HTLV-III/LAV infection; about two-thirds of those tested showed evidence of antibody by the end of 1984. Over the same time, 2.7% of this group had been diagnosed with AIDS (Jaffe H W et al, 1985b). Antibody levels in stored sera from this group were found to have risen dramatically since 1978, when only 4.5% of stored samples were found positive for antibody. This figure rose to 24% of those tested from 1980, one year before the first case of AIDS was reported. An epidemic of infection with HTLV-III/LAV preceded the AIDS epidemic in this population by several years, and some of these men have remained asymptomatic for years without developing AIDS.

Heterosexual transmission of HTLV-III/LAV is suggested by the fact that female contacts of male intravenous drug users, and sexual contacts of other risk-group members represent about 1% of all cases reported to CDC. Furthermore, heterosexual activity, mainly having large numbers of sexual partners, is an emerging risk factor for AIDS in the United States (CDC, 1984e).

Many AIDS cases have been related to exposure to blood or blood products. First, 17% of the reported cases in the United States have been diagnosed in heterosexual men and women with histories of intravenous drug abuse. (About 15% of gay men with AIDS also have this history.) Over 80% of these live in the New York metropolitan area, where sharing needles and other injection materials in 'shooting galleries' is common and implicated as the mode of transmission (Guinan et al, 1984). Sexual contacts of these persons also are at risk of infection (Harris et al, 1983).

Approximately 2% of the reported cases are in persons with haemophilia (CDC, 1984d) and in those with no other risk factor than having received blood transfusions since 1978 (Curran et al, 1984). Persons with haemophilia are exposed through their use of concentrated clotting factor. Transfusion-associated AIDS cases frequently have been found to have donors who were gay or IV drug users and/or were positive for HTLV-III/LAV antibody (Peterman et al, 1985).

Table 13.4   Estimates of incidence rates* of AIDS in selected population groups, June 1983–May 1984, United States

Population group and selected characteristics	Incidence rate*
Single men: United States	8.9
Manhattan	175.5
San Francisco	204.5
IV drug users: United States	113.3
New York City	203.2
New Jersey	268.9
Haitian entrants: Entry after 1977	82.0
Entry before 1978	1.8
Persons with hemophilia: Type A	198.8
Type B	34.5
Female sexual contacts of male IV drug users	
United States	3.1
New York City	9.4
New Jersey	8.5
Recipients of blood transfusions	
Adult patients	0.40
Pediatric patients	2.43
Persons not in above groups	0.1

* Rate per 100 000 population in specified group
Data from Hardy et al, 1985

The remaining 7% of reported AIDS cases in the United States includes 3% in persons born in Haiti or central Africa. This population encompasses a larger number of cases in females; 15% of the Haitian patients are female compared with 6% for all reported cases. This suggests that heterosexual contact may have a larger role in the transmission of HTLV-III/LAV infection in this group. Early investigations in several African countries have also implicated heterosexual transmission; the number of cases in females closely approaches that in males (Van De Perre et al, 1984; Piot et al, 1984). Of the men who have been reported to CDC with no identified risk, 17 (26%) of 65 had a history of sexual contact with prostitutes (CDC, 1984e). The true magnitude of this potential risk factor for AIDS remains to be established.

Children of risk group members are at increased risk of developing AIDS themselves (CDC, 1982b; Oleske, 1983). Of the more than one hundred children reported to CDC by mid-1985, 72% have a parent who is an intravenous drug user, Haitian, or bisexual; 19% have received transfusions of blood or blood products. The remaining 10% could not be investigated completely. Older children in the same families and sociocultural environments are not at risk for the syndrome. This supports the theory that exposure occurs in utero or perinatally, but not as a result of household contact (Redfield et al, 1985).

CLINICAL ASPECTS: IMMUNE DYSFUNCTION

AIDS primarily affects cell-mediated immunity, but the entire immune system may show evidence of abnormalities. Two types of T-lymphocytes compose the cellular immune system and may be identified by specific antigens on the cell membrane, T4 (Leu-3) and T8 (Leu-2). Generally, the T4 (Leu-3) cells, which augment immune response, are known as helper T-cells, while the T8 (Leu-2) cells have cytotoxic and suppressor functions and are termed suppressor T-cells (Benacerraf & Unanue, 1984). In AIDS patients, the number of T-helper cells is profoundly decreased, both in terms of the ratios to suppressor T-cells and in absolute number (Fahey et al, 1984). AIDS patients consistently show a decrease in cutaneous hypersensitivity reaction and have decreased mitogen response when lymphocytes are stimulated in vitro (Seligmann et al, 1984). It has been hypothesised that this reflects the inability to mount a cell-mediated immune response due to a loss of absolute number and function of T-helper cells, as well as a reduction in lymphokines, such as gamma interferon, which stimulate macrophage proliferation (Murray H W et al, 1984).

Immunoglobulin levels are often normal or elevated in AIDS patients. The ability of B-cells to produce antibody to 'new' antigens may be diminished, especially in the terminal stages of AIDS. The exact mechanism of this is not known, but it may either reflect direct stimulation of this cell population by agents such as cytomegalovirus or result from interaction with specific subsets within the T-cell population (Lane et al, 1983) The T-cells responsible for augmenting B-cell proliferation and production of antibody are not reduced in persons with AIDS-related conditions (Nicholson et al, 1984).

The cause of this cellular immunodeficiency is infection with the lymphocytotropic retrovirus variously known as HTLV-III or LAV. Retroviruses are so named because of their use of a reverse transcriptase enzyme to transcribe genetic information from single-stranded RNA diploid genomes to the DNA of the host cell (Bishop, 1978). Retroviruses cause malignancies and immunosuppression in a number of animal species, the most well-documented example being feline leukaemia virus in cats (Essex 1982). HTLV-III/LAV is noted to have tropism for T-helper cells (Popovic et al, 1983) and to destroy these cells following infection (Mitsuya et al 1984). HTLV-III/LAV is similar to previously described human retroviruses, HTLV-I and HTLV-II, in several ways: tropism for T4-cells, antigenic determinants of similar molecular weight, a reverse transcriptase similar in biologic properties, and the induction of multinucleated giant cells in vitro (Broder & Gallo 1984). HTLV-III/LAV, however, has a cytopathic effect on infected cells, whereas HTLV-I and II tend to immortalise them (Popovic et al, 1984). In the first AIDS patients cultured, 36–49% had evidence of HTLV-III/LAV virus, and over 85% of persons with conditions related to AIDS were viremic (Gallo et al, 1984). Presently, viral cultures remain a research technique, not readily available for clinical purposes.

CLINICAL ASPECTS: MANIFESTATIONS AND MANAGEMENT

The clinical presentation of AIDS is variable, depending on the presenting opportunistic disease. *Pneumocystis carinii* pneumonia, which is the most common serious infection, is diagnosed in at least 60% of AIDS patients (CDC, 1985c). The time between the onset of respiratory symptoms and diagnosis (median, 28 days) is longer than with cases of PCP not related to AIDS (Walzer et al, 1974). Symptoms may include nonproductive cough, low-grade fever, mild to severe dyspnoea, and generalised chest pain (Murray J F et al, 1984). Diagnosis cannot be made on the basis of sputum examination, but requires bronchoscopy, open lung biopsy, transbronchial biopsy, or other biopsy procedure (Wong, 1984). Sulfa/trimethoprim compounds have been used as an effective therapy, but the development of side effects ranging from thrombo-cytopenia to skin reactions in over 50% of treated patients complicates management (Jaffe H S et al, 1983). Pentamidine isethionate may be used, but demonstrates even greater toxicity in some patients. Adverse reactions have prohibited prophylactic ther-apy with either of these compounds. Consequently, recurrent PCP is very common among AIDS patients who survive the initial episode (Haverkos et al, 1984).

Kaposi's sarcoma (KS) is diagnosed in slightly more than 25% of all AIDS patients in the United States (CDC, 1985c); with about 95% of these patients being gay men (CDC, 1983b). Blue-black or red-brown skin lesions are the characteristic presenting manifestations (Templeton, 1976). The tumour may be multicentric and can spread rapidly to involve the extremities, the trunk, and internal organs, such as lymph nodes, lungs, and gastrointestinal tract (Friedman-Kien et al, 1982). Genetic studies performed in homosexual men with KS show a higher prevalence of the DR5 human leukocyte antigen (HLA) type, compared with a group of heterosexual controls (Prince et al, 1984), but the implications of this are not clear. Haverkos et al (1985) suggested that heavy use of inhalant nitrites used as sexual stimulants or another factor correlated with such use might help explain the greater incidence of KS in gay men. Interferon has shown some promise in treatment of KS in AIDS patients (Groopman et al, 1984b).

The other opportunistic infections included in the case definition each occur in less than 10% of reported cases at the time of initial report (CDC, 1985c), but most patients with AIDS eventually experience several opportunistic infections throughout their clinical course. *Toxoplasma gondii* usually represents a reactivation of previous infection and presents as meningitis or focal lesions in the grey matter of the brain, resulting in seizures or peripheral neurologic defects (Wong et al, 1984).

Cryptosporidiosis, an infection very rarely seen in humans before AIDS was recog-nised, is now the presenting disease in 3% of cases at the time of diagnosis. The infection results in a debilitating form of diarrhoea for which there is no satisfactory treatment (Soave et al, 1984), although trials of spiramycin, a macrolide antibiotic, have had limited success (CDC, 1984a). Disseminated mycobacterial infections, par-ticularly with *Mycobacterium avium-intracellulare*, are commonly diagnosed in AIDS patients, but these tend to occur later in the clinical course and not as a presenting problem (unpublished CDC data, 1985).

The type of opportunistic disease diagnosed influences mortality. Persons diagnosed with KS alone have a better prognosis (32% crude case-fatality rate) than persons with PCP (51% crude case-fatality rate) or the remaining opportunistic diseases (56% crude case-fatality rate). Overall, the 1 year mortality rate for AIDS is 45%, rising to 85% 3 years following diagnosis. None of those diagnosed have had their underlying immunologic defect corrected. The various investigational therapies, including gamma interferon, bone marrow transplant, and thymic transplant, have not proven effective. Some agents such as ribavirin, suramin, ansamycin, antimoniotungstate, and others show promise in laboratory systems by inhibiting viral activity, but this has yet to be translated into clinical success. Newer avenues for clinical investigations will include multiple interventions, such as combinations of antivirals, immunomodulators, transplants, and white cell infusions. Much progress remains to be made in this area.

CLINICAL ASPECTS: PRECAUTIONS FOR STAFF

Recommendations for infection control have been published about providing services and care to patients known to have or suspected of having AIDS (CDC, 1982a; CDC, 1983c) and for handling specimens from them (CDC & NIH, 1984). These are quite similar to safety precautions used for hepatitis B patients or specimens.

The most common percutaneous health care-related exposures to AIDS patients have been needlestick injuries resulting from attempts to replace plastic caps over hypodermic needles (CDC, 1985b; McCray et al, 1985). These injuries are completely preventable, as CDC recommends that such caps not be replaced at all, but that disposable needles and syringes be discarded as a unit into puncture-resistant containers designated for that purpose.

Preliminary interim results from the largest survey of health care workers exposed to AIDS patients percutaneously or through mucous membranes or open wounds reveal that none of the 502 health care workers followed for a mean interval of about one year has developed AIDS. None of those tested has developed antibody to HTLV-III/LAV (McCray et al, 1985). There has been a single report of a nurse who developed antibody 4–7 weeks after a needlestick injury sustained in caring for an African AIDS patient (anonymous, 1984). These findings suggest that HTLV-III/LAV transmission is possible in health care settings but is not common. Therefore, none of the precautions previously made for inpatient care have been rescinded, and consideration should be given to adopting or adapting at least some of these for outpatient areas, such as sexually transmitted diseases clinics.

PREVENTION STRATEGIES FOR THE FUTURE

The continuing and spreading worldwide outbreak of AIDS, its severe clinical course, and the lack of adequate treatment methods and biologic means of prevention all underscore the importance of public health education, information dissemination, and prevention activities. Although gay men have demonstrated willingness and ability to change some high-risk behaviours (CDC, 1984b), the incidence of HTLV-III/LAV infection seems to be quite high in at least some geographic areas (CDC, 1984c). This suggests that prevention strategies, to be effective, must adopt a long-term posture and aim at targets in more distant future than those usually dealt with in sexually transmitted diseases control programmes.

Guidelines for safer sexual practices have been promulgated and disseminated by many groups, and they have been endorsed and adopted widely (CDC, 1983a; Safer Sex Committee of New York, 1984), but much more will be necessary. However, it is unclear whether any sexual encounter with an infected person can truly be considered 'safe.' Fundamental changes in knowledge, attitudes, and beliefs must occur before infection with HTLV-III/LAV becomes as widespread as are other sexually transmitted viruses in gay communities: histories of and evidence for infections with hepatitis A and B viruses, cytomegalovirus, Epstein-Barr virus, and herpes simplex virus types I and II are almost universal (Rogers et al, 1983). Without radical changes, HTLV-III/LAV will be added to the list, but with even more severe consequences.

Public health professionals should prepare themselves to work with gay professionals as well as community organisations and patients to develop solutions that are viewed as acceptable, useful, advantageous, economic, and appealing to the groups and communities they serve. The changes must evolve from within gay communities if sexual behaviours are to be significantly modified. If this requires another 'sexual revolution,' then so be it. Radical problems demand radical solutions.

Consideration should be given to including safer sexual practices in the curriculum of sex education classes of young people. Clinicians concerned with AIDS should be prepared to consult with health educators on this topic or seek out the programmes in their areas and help to evaluate them. Similarly, drug abuse prevention and education programmes should not be omitted from consideration.

The AIDS outbreak shows no sign of waning. Although it may become endemic in the future, even if effective, safe, economical early intervention methods were to become available soon, AIDS will be part of the spectrum of sexually transmitted diseases for the forseeable future. It behoves every reader of this text to learn about it, become committed to its prevention, and to take action to inform patients, educate the community, and plan for the future.

REFERENCES

Alter M J, Francis D P 1984 Hepatitis B transmission between homosexual men: A model for the acquired immune deficiency syndrome (AIDS). In: Ma P, Armstrong D (eds) The acquired immune deficiency syndrome and infections of homosexual men. Yorke Medical Books, New York, p 97–106

Anonymous 1984 Needlestick transmission of HTLV-III from a patient infected in Africa. Lancet 2: 1376–1377

Auerbach D M, Darrow W W, Jaffe H W, Curran J W 1984 Cluster of cases of acquired immune deficiency syndrome: patients linked by sexual contact. American Journal of Medicine 76: 487–492

Barre-Sinoussi F, Chermann J C, Rey F, et al 1983 Isolation of a T-lymphotropic retrovirus from a patient at risk for acquired immune deficiency syndrome (AIDS). Science 220: 868–871

Benacerraf B, Unanue E R 1984 Regulation of Immune Responses by T-lymphocytes. Stamathis G (ed) Textbook of immunology, 2nd edn. Williams and Wilkins, Baltimore, Chapter 8, p 167–189

Bishop J M 1978 Retroviruses. Annual Review of Biochemistry 47: 35–88

Broader S, Gallo R C 1984 A pathogenic retrovirus (HTLV-III) linked to AIDS. New England Journal of Medicine 311: 1292–1297

CDC 1981a *Pneumocystis* pneumonia — Los Angeles. MMWR 30: 250–2

CDC 1981b Kaposi's sarcoma and Pneumocystis pneumonia among homosexual men — New York City and California. MMWR 30: 305–308

CDC 1982a Acquired immune deficiency syndrome (AIDS): precautions for clinical and laboratory staffs. MMWR 31: 577–580

CDC 1982b Unexplained immunodeficiency and opportunistic infections in infants — New York, New Jersey, California. MMWR 31: 665–667

CDC 1983a Prevention of acquired immunodeficiency syndrome (AIDS): report of inter-agency recommendations. MMWR 32: 101–104

CDC 1983b Update: Acquired immunodeficiency syndrome (AIDS) — United States. MMWR 32: 389–391

CDC 1983c Acquired immunodeficiency syndrome (AIDS): precautions for health-care workers and allied professionals. MMWR 32: 450–451

CDC 1984a Update: The treatment of cryptosporidiosis in patients with acquired immunodeficiency syndrome (AIDS) MMWR 33: 117–119

CDC 1984b Declining rates of rectal and pharyngeal gonorrhea among males — New York City. MMWR 33: 295–297

CDC 1984c Antibodies to a retrovirus etiologically associated with acquired immunodeficiency syndrome (AIDS) in populations with increased incidences of the syndrome. MMWR 33: 377–379

CDC 1984d Update: Acquired immunodeficiency syndrome (AIDS) in persons with hemophilia. MMWR 33: 589–591

CDC 1984e Update: acquired immunodeficiency syndrome (AIDS) — United States. MMWR 33: 661–664

CDC 1985a Provisional Public Health Service inter-agency recommendations for screening donated blood and plasma for antibody to the virus causing acquired immunodeficiency syndrome. MMWR 34: 1–5

CDC 1985b Update: prospective evaluation of health-care workers exposed via the parenteral or mucous-membrane route to blood or body fluids from patients with acquired immunodeficiency syndrome — United States. MMWR 34: 101–103

CDC 1985c Update: Acquired immunodeficiency syndrome — United States. MMWR 34: 245–248

CDC and National Institutes of Health 1984 Biosafety in Microbiological and Biomedical Laboratories. U.S. Government Printing Office, Washington

Clumeck N, Sonnet J, Taelman H 1984 Acquired immunodeficiency syndrome in African patients. New England Journal of Medicine 310: 492–497

Curran J W, Lawrence D L, Jaffe H W 1984 Acquired immunodeficiency syndrome (AIDS) associated with transfusions. New England Journal of Medicine 310: 69–75

Darrow W W, O'Malley P, Jaffe H W, et al 1985 Risk factors for HTLV-III/LAV seroconversion in a cohort of homosexual male clinic patients. Presented at: International Conference on Acquired Immunodeficiency Syndrome, Atlanta

Essex M E 1982 Feline leukemia: a naturally occurring cancer of infectious origin. Epidemiologic Review 4: 189–203

Fahey J L, et al 1984 Quantitative changes in T-helper or T-suppressor/cytotoxic lymphocyte subsets that distinguish acquired immune deficiency syndrome from other immune subset disorders. The American Journal of Medicine 76: 95–100

Feorino P M, Jaffe H W, Palmer E, et al 1985 Transfusion-associated acquired immunodeficiency syndrome (AIDS): evidence for persistent infection in blood donors. New England Journal of Medicine 312: 1293–1296

Friedman-Kien A L, et al 1982 Disseminated Kaposi's sarcoma in homosexual men. Annals of Internal Medicine 96: 693–700

Gallo R C, Salahuddin S Z, Popovic M 1984 Frequent detection and isolation of cytopathic retroviruses (HTLV-III) from patients with AIDS and at risk for AIDS. Science 224: 500–503

Gottlieb M S, Schroff R, Schanker H M 1981 *Pneumocystis carinii* pneumonia and mucosal candidiasis in previously healthy homosexual men. New England Journal of Medicine 305: 1425–1431

Groopman J E, Salahuddin S Z, Sarngadharan M G 1984a HTLV-III in saliva of people with AIDS-related complex and healthy homosexual men at risk for AIDS. Science 226: 447–449

Groopman J E, et al 1984b Recombinant alpha-2 interferon therapy for Kaposi's sarcoma associated with the acquired immunodeficiency syndrome. Annals of Internal Medicine 100: 671–676

Guinan M E, Thomas P A, Pinsky P F, et al 1984 Heterosexual and homosexual cases of acquired immune deficiency syndrome: a comparison of surveillance, interview, and laboratory data. Annals of Internal Medicine 100: 213–218

Hardy A M, Allen J R, Morgan W M, Curran J W 1985 The incidence rate of acquired immunodeficiency syndrome in selected populations. Journal of the American Medical Association 253: 215–220

Harris L, Small C B, Klein R S, et al, 1983 Immunodeficiency in female sexual partners of men with the acquired immunodeficiency syndrome. New England Journal of Medicine 308: 1181–1184

Haverkos H W, PCP Therapy Project Group 1984 Assessment of therapy for *Pneumocystis carinii* pneumonia. American Journal of Medicine 76: 501–508

Haverkos H W, Pinsky P F, Drotman D P, Bregman D J 1985 Disease manifestation among homosexual men with acquired immunodeficiency syndrome (AIDS): a possible role of nitrites in Kaposi's sarcoma. Sexually Transmitted Diseases (in press)

Ho D D, Schooley R T, Rota T R 1984 HTLV-III in the semen and blood of a healthy homosexual man. Science 226: 451–453

Hymes K, Cheung T, Greene J B 1981 Kaposi's sarcoma in homosexual men. Lancet 2: 598–600

Jaffe H S, Abrams D I, Ammann A J, Lewis B J, Golden J A 1983 Complications of co-trimoxazole in treatment of AIDS — associated *Pneumocystis carinii* pneumonia in homosexual men. Lancet 2: 1109–1111

Jaffe H W, Choi K, Thomas P et al 1983 National case-control study of Kaposi's sarcoma and *Pneumocystis carinii* pneumonia in homosexual men: Part 1, epidemiologic results. Annals of Internal Medicine 99: 145–151

Jaffe H W, Feorino P M, Darrow W W, et al 1985a Persistent Infection with HTLV-III/LAV in apparently healthy homosexual men. Annals of Internal Medicine 102: 627–628

Jaffe H W, et al 1985b AIDS, AIDS-related conditions and infection with HTLV-III/LAV in a cohort of homosexual men: A 6-year follow-up study. (Submitted for publication)

Lane H C, Masur H, Edgar L C, Whalen G, Rook A H, Fauci A S 1983 Abnormalities of B-cell activation and immunoregulation in patients with the acquired immunodeficiency syndrome. New England Journal of Medicine 309: 453–458

Levy J A, Hoffman A D, Kramer S M, Landis J A, Shimabukuro J M, Oshiro L S 1984 Isolation of lymphocytopathic retroviruses from San Francisco patients with AIDS. Science 225: 840–842

McCray E, Winslow N, Solomon S L, et al 1985 Prospective evaluation of health-care workers with parenteral or mucous-membrane exposure to blood from patients with acquired immunodeficiency syndrome, United States: an update. Presented at: International Conference on Acquired Immunodeficiency Syndrome (AIDS), Atlanta

Mitsuya H, Guo H-G, Messon M, Trainor C, Reitz M S Jr, Broder S 1984 Transformation and cytopathogenic effect in an immune human T-cell clone infected by HTLV-I. Science 223: 1293–1296

Murray H W, Rubin B Y, Masur H, Roberts H B 1984 Impaired production of lymphokines and immune (gamma) interferon in the acquired immunodeficiency syndrome. New England Journal of Medicine 310: 833–839

Murray J F, Felton C P, Garay S M, et al 1984 Pulmonary complications of the acquired immunodeficiency syndrome: report of a National Heart, Lung, and Blood Institute workshop. New England Journal of Medicine 310: 1682–1688

Nicholson J K, McDougal J S, Spira T J, Cross G D, Jones B M, Reinherz E L 1984 Immunoregulatory subsets of the T-helper and T-suppressor cell populations in homosexual men with chronic unexplained lymphadenopathy. Journal of Clinical Investigation 73: 191–201

Oleske J, Minnefor A, Cooper R Jr 1983 Immune deficiency in children. Journal of the American Medical Association 249: 2345–2349

Pape J W, Liautaud B, Thomas F et al 1983 Characteristics of the acquired immunodeficiency syndrome (AIDS) in Haiti. New England Journal of Medicine 306: 945–950

Peterman T, Jaffe H W, Feorino P M, et al 1985 Transfusion-associated AIDS in the United States. presented at: International Conference on Acquired Immunodeficiency Syndrome (AIDS), Atlanta

Piot P, Quinn T C, Taelman H et al 1984 Acquired immunodeficiency syndrome in a heterosexual population in Zaire. Lancet 2: 65–69

Popovic M, et al 1983 Isolation and transmission of human retrovirus (human T-cell leukemia virus). Science 219: 856–859

Popovic M, Sarngadharan M G, Read E 1984 Detection, isolation, and continuous production of cytopathic retroviruses (HTLV-III) from patients with AIDS and pre-AIDS. Science 224: 497–500

Prince H E, Schroff R W, Aroub G, Han S, Gottlieb M S, Fahey J L 1984 HLA studies in acquired immune deficiency syndrome patients with Kaposi's sarcoma. Journal of Clinical Immunology 403: 242–245

Redfield R R, Markham P D, Salahuddin S Z, et al 1985 Frequent transmission of HTLV-III among spouses of patients with AIDS-related complex and AIDS. Journal of the American Medical Association 253: 1571–1573

Rogers M F, Morens D M, Stewart J A, et al 1983 National case-control study of Kaposi's sarcoma and *Pneumocystis carinii* pneumonia in homosexual men: Part 2, laboratory results. Annals of Internal Medicine 99: 151–158

Safai B, et al 1984 Seroepidemiological studies of human T-lymphotropic retrovirus type III in acquired immunodeficiency syndrome. Lancet 1: 1438–1440

Safer Sex Committee of New York 1984 Healthy sex is great sex. Gay Men's Health Crisis, New York

Sarngadharan M G, Popovic M, Bruch L 1984 Antibodies reactive with human T-lymphotropic retroviruses (HTLV-III) in the serum of patients with AIDS. Science 224: 506–508

Seligmann M, Chess L, Fahey J L, et al 1984 AIDS-an immunologic reevaluation. New England Journal of Medicine 311: 1286–1292

Soave R, Donner R L, Honis C L, et al 1984 Cryptosporidiosis in homosexual men. Annals of Internal Medicine 100: 504–511

Templeton A C 1976 Kaposi's Sarcoma. In: Andrade R (ed) Cancer of the skin, W B Saunders, Philadelphia 1183–1225

Van de Perre P, Rouvroy D, Lepage P 1984 Acquired immunodeficiency syndrome in Rwanda. Lancet 2: 62–65

Walzer P D, Perl D P, Krogstad D J, Rawson P G, Schultz M G, 1974 *Pneumocystis carinii* pneumonia in the United States. Annals of Internal Medicine 80: 83–93

Wong B, et al 1984 Central-nervous system Toxoplasmosis in homosexual men and parenteral drug abusers. Annals of Internal Medicine 100: 36–42

Wong B 1984 Parasitic diseases in immunocompromised hosts. American Journal of Medicine 76: 479–486

Zagury D, Bernard J, Leibowitch J, et al 1984 HTLV-III in cells cultured from semen of two patients with AIDS. Science 226: 449–451

14. Clinical aspects of AIDS and other HTLV-III related conditions

Anthony J. Pinching

INTRODUCTION

The emergence of the acquired immune deficiency syndrome (AIDS) as a new sexually transmitted disease has been rapid and dramatic. Its clinical consequences have been devastating but the pursuit of its aetiology and pathogenesis has been one of the most exciting chapters in the study of human pathology (reviewed for example by Gottlieb et al, 1983; Fauci et al, 1984; Pinching, 1984a; Pinching & Weiss, 1986). As with many infectious diseases, the recognition of the clinical spectrum of disease produced by the infectious agent has taken some time and remains incomplete; nevertheless we have come to regard the clinical disorder known as AIDS as but the most severe manifestation of infection by a novel retrovirus, designated Human T-Lymphotropic Virus/Lymphadenopathy Associated Virus (HTLV-III/LAV) (Barre-Sinoussi et al, 1983; Montagnier et al, 1984a; Vilmer et al, 1984; Brun-Vezinet et al, 1984; Gallo et al, 1984; Sarngadharan et al, 1984; Popovic et al, 1984; Safai et al, 1984a; Cheingsong-Popov et al, 1984; Pinching, 1984b; Pinching & Weiss, 1986). AIDS was the first recognisable consequence of infection by this virus and was already well documented by the time the aetiological agent was identified. Because of this, our current perception of this infectious disease tends to be rather distorted. To take an analogy, if we were to regard fulminant fatal hepatitis as the primary clinical disorder caused by Hepatitis B, out view of the spectrum of possible outcomes of infection by that virus would be very incomplete. The appropriateness of such a model remains to be determined by the long-term study of infected individuals, but as the focus of our attention moves from AIDS to HTLV-III/LAV we must appreciate that these terms are not freely interchangable (Cheingsong-Popov et al, 1984). While it is reasonable for the clinician to concentrate on the more severe consequences of the infection, it is crucial to appreciate the full spectrum, not least for the interpretation of laboratory tests and for the effective counselling of all patients.

This chapter aims.to help physicians to recognise the presenting features of the very diverse clinical manifestations of AIDS and related conditions, which are generally unfamiliar. While patients may present to a wide variety of specialists, subjects at risk (especially homosexual males) may seek advice first from a sexually transmitted disease clinic, because of their knowledge of and concern about AIDS. Aspects of management and specific therapy are also considered.

AIDS and opportunist infection

AIDS has always been, and is likely to remain, a clinical diagnosis based upon the framework provided by the Centers for Disease Control (CDC) surveillance definition (see previous chapter). In effect AIDS is thus defined as opportunist infection or

223

opportunist tumours indicative of cellular immunodeficiency occurring in previously normal persons who have no known cause for immunosuppression. For clinical practice however the strict surveillance criteria for diagnosis of individual manifestations may be more flexibly interpreted and B cell lymphomas in at risk patients can usefully be incorporated.

Opportunist infection results when an organism takes advantage of an opportunity provided by a defect in host response (in this case cellular immunity) to cause disease. This includes organisms that are not normally pathogenic (e.g. Pneumocystis carinii, Mycobacterium avium-intracellulare) or ones which cause mild, self-limiting disease in normal subjects but which cause more severe or more disseminated disease which may not be self-limiting in the compromised host (e.g. Herpes simplex, Cytomegalo-virus-CMV, Toxoplasma gondii). Even conventional pathogens can act as opportunists in the latter sense (e.g. Mycobacterium tuberculosis). I use the term opportunist tumours to describe the very particular group of tumours which are seen in the immu-nocompromised host — Kaposi's sarcoma and B cell lymphoma. Interestingly, these are tumours in which herpesviruses may play a pathogenetic role and against which some form of immune surveillance, such as that mediated by natural killer cells, probably operates in the normal host.

The opportunist diseases seen in AIDS patients not only reflect the underlying immune defect but are also determined by the range of organisms prevalent in the environment or latent in the host. This means that patterns of disease differ according to geographical location, past travel, age, life style and medical history. Furthermore the profound defect of cellular immunity in AIDS modifies the clinical and laboratory features of many of the infections, even compared with other immunosuppressed hosts, so that diagnostic criteria may need to be revised.

The clinical spectrum of AIDS

AIDS itself is a susceptibility; its clinical consequences not only reflect the type but also the degree of immunodeficiency. Thus Kaposi's sarcoma alone is the mildest form with less evidence of immunosuppression on testing and patients with this form have a correspondingly better prognosis (2 year survival about 50%). Even within this entity, patients whose Kaposi's sarcoma is limited to skin and/or lymph nodes have a more benign course than those in whom it is disseminated to other organs. Patients with opportunist infections have a generally worse outlook (2 year survival being less than 5%), although patients with Pneumocystis pneumonia or oesophageal candidiasis alone fare better in the short term than those with other opportunists. Those with mixed opportunist diseases generally have a worse prognosis. The acknow-ledgement of such a spectrum within AIDS is important for the counselling and management of patients.

Prodromes and variants of AIDS

For a disorder to be prodromal it has reliably to precede the development of frank AIDS. Good evidence exists that this is true for patients with prolonged and unex-plained wasting, fever, diarrhoea, oral candidiasis and lymphopenia, with or without lymphadenopathy (Mathur & Mildvan, 1984). 77% of such patients developed AIDS at a mean of 4 months. The emergence of persistent generalised lymphadenopathy (PGL) at the same time as AIDS in the same epidemiological risk groups led to an association between AIDS and PGL (Mildvan et al, 1982a). This has been confirmed by evidence of the same retrovirus infection in PGL patients. The earlier presumption that PGL was prodromal may only be true for a proportion, even a minority (between 5 and 20% at 2 years — Abrams et al, 1984; Mathur-Wagh et al, 1984). In some of the remainder it may be an end point in itself, a different phenotypic response to the same retrovirus. Idiopathic thrombocytopenic purpura is similarly associated (Morris et al, 1982; Walsh et al, 1984). Subtler subclinical events may occur following infection with HTLV-III/LAV, such as transient and asymptomatic alterations in T cell subsets.

CLINICAL SYNDROMES IN AIDS

The development of frank AIDS may be accompanied by a number of non-specific clinical features, including fever, profuse night sweats, unexplained diarrhoea and

Table 14.1   Principal infections in AIDS by site

Lung	Gut	CNS	Systemic
Pneumocystis	Candida	Cryptococcus	Cytomegalovirus
Cytomegalovirus	Cryptosporidium	Toxoplasma	Mycobacteria
Mycobacterium a-i	Isospora	Cytomegalovirus	Salmonella
Mycobacterium tb	Cytomegalovirus	PML* (JC Virus)	Candida
Candida	Herpes simplex	Other viruses	Cryptococcus
Cryptococcus	Salmonella		Herpes zoster
Legionella	Shigella		
Nocardia			
IIP†			

* PML = Progressive multifocal leucoencephalopathy
† IIP = Idiopathic interstitial pneumonitis

wasting. It has hitherto been hard to determine an infective cause for these symptoms, although it seems likely that they too represent early opportunist infection. Oral candidiasis frequently accompanies these symptoms but may occur in isolation. Although it may respond to topical treatment with antifungals such as nystatin or amphotericin, recurrences are common. It is an early clue to immunodeficiency (Klein et al, 1984) and such patients should always be followed carefully for evidence of other more serious opportunist infections, especially oesophageal candidiasis. Skin lesions are common and include folliculitis, painless white comedones, vasculitis and a generalised seborrhoeic dermatitis (Eisenstat & Wormser, 1984). In some instances this may be a resurgence of atopic eczema, often silent since childhood, and may be accompanied by asthma or other allergic manifestations. In PGL patients who develop AIDS, the lymph nodes and spleen may regress (Mathur-Wagh et al, 1984). Some patients however, develop frank AIDS without any prodromal illness. The commonest specific opportunist infections affect three major organ systems: the lungs, the gut and the central nervous system; in some instances these are accompanied by wide dissemination of infection to other sites (Table 14.1).

Pulmonary infections

Patients typically present with gradually increasing dyspnoea on exertion and dry cough; often they have associated fever and malaise. The onset may be very insidious. Pulmonary function testing shows a reduction in the transfer factor for carbon monoxide (Coleman et al, 1983) and this seems to be the most sensitive indicator of disease, especially if monitored serially (Weber, Holt, Keal & Pinching, unpublished observations). Chest X-ray may be normal in the early stages of infection, but later shows diffuse interstitial shadowing; this is especially notable in the perihilar regions but may be patchy. Mycobacterial lesions may be more focal but do not show the typical appearances seen in normal hosts; a miliary pattern may be seen. Gallium scanning may be normal in early infection and, although recommended by some (Murray et al, 1984), appears to be a relatively insensitive test. The presence of pulmonary symptoms and decreased transfer factor in a patient likely to have AIDS are sufficient indication for fibreoptic bronchoscopy with transbronchial biopsy and bronchoalveolar lavage. Histology, cytology and culture must be undertaken with particular attention to the type of pathogens normally seen in AIDS; it is essential to recognise that host response, such as the capacity to form granulomas, is profoundly reduced. It should also be remembered that multiple infections commonly occur and care must be taken to seek all relevant pathogens. Serology is almost valueless, because of the defect in humoral immunity (Lane et al, 1983).

Pneumocystis carinii is certainly the most common pathogen (Gottlieb et al, 1981; Masur et al, 1981; Follansbee et al, 1982; Mildvan et al, 1982b; Coleman et al, 1983; Kovacs et al, 1984), although its frequency may vary in different countries. It is a more slowly progressive disorder than the same infection in other immunocompromised hosts such as those on long term immunosuppression (Kovacs et al, 1984). The symptoms may take several weeks before reaching the point of severe hypoxia compared with a few days in other settings. CMV pneumonitis may be relatively mild without causing hypoxia. Patients with severe pulmonary disease from whom CMV has been isolated commonly harbour another pathogen, commonly Pneumocystis, perhaps because of a local or systemic immunosuppressive effect of CMV (Gottleib et al, 1981; Follansbee et al, 1982). Atypical mycobacterial disease has been common in the US cases (Greene et al, 1982; Zakowski et al, 1982; Macher et al, 1983) and M tuberculosis is particularly seen among the Haitian population (Vieira et al, 1983; Pitchenik et al, 1983); both are being seen increasingly in the UK. Legionella and Nocardia infections are surprisingly infrequent. In the USA, histoplasmosis, blastomycosis and coccidiomycosis have also been seen. In a number of patients a rapidly progressive clinical course is seen but no definite organism can be identified despite adequate sampling (Weber et al, 1984; Gellene et al, 1984). This may represent a form of idiopathic interstitial pneumonitis; it may be of infective (?viral) origin and resembles that seen in other compromised patients. Such patients do not respond to broad empirical antimicrobial therapy but may paradoxically benefit from steroid therapy.

Gastrointestinal infections

Extensive plaques of oral candidiasis are commonly evident in AIDS patients with infection. These are commonly accompanied by oesophageal candidiasis (Gottlieb et al, 1981; Masur et al, 1981; Weber et al, 1984), although not all patients have dysphagia. The lesions may be readily demonstrated by barium swallow or endoscopy. Oesophageal candidiasis is not seen in the immunocompetent host. Candidal infection may extend throughout the gastrointestinal tract with substantial small bowel colonisation. Perianal lesions are also common. Many patients have latent Herpes simplex (labial or genital). This is commonly reactivated, but instead of the normal self-limiting course the lesions show slow and progressive ulceration, which may be extensive (Siegal et al, 1981). The early perianal lesions may present as 'piles' but are typically more painful than haemorrhoids. Tender inguinal lymphadenopathy may give a clue to an infective cause for 'piles'. Some lesions may resemble pressure sores. Biopsy, culture and/or electron microscopy may be helpful in diagnosis.

Many AIDS patients suffer chronic diarrhoea and wasting, even in the face of adequate calorie intake. The diarrhoea is often steatorrhoeic and accompanied by evidence of malabsorption. It is not always possible to define a causative pathogen but a number have now been characterised. Two coccidian protozoa, cryptosporidium and isospora belli, are responsible for severe diarrhoeal disease in AIDS patients, with pronounced malabsorption (Goldfarb et al, 1982; Pitchenik et al, 1983; Male-branche et al, 1983; Pape et al, 1983; Soave et al, 1984). The diarrhoea may have a secretory component and can be of cholera-like proportions. These infections tend to run a slowly progressive course to a cachectic death and there is no effective therapy. However patients' symptoms may be considerably ameliorated and further weight loss averted by judicious use of elemental or short peptide based enteral nutrition. Some patients have achlorydria and upper gastrointestinal overgrowth with gram-positive organisms and Candida; their symptoms may be reduced by appropriate narrow spectrum antimicrobial therapy (Weber & Pinching, unpublished observations). In European and African patients troublesome infection with Salmonella spp. has been seen (Clumeck et al, 1984; Piot et al, 1984; van de Perre, 1984; Weber et al, 1984). In some, the infection becomes systemic and Salmonella septicaemia may be hard to eradicate. Small bowel infiltration with Mycobacterium avium intracellulare has been described as a cause of diarrhoea and malabsorption in US patients (Zakowski et al, 1982); the appearances may resemble Whipple's disease (Strom & Gruninger, 1983) and granulomas are absent or poorly formed. CMV infection of the small bowel may lead to malabsorption but CMV may also cause severe colitis or proctitis. Herpes simplex is another cause of proctitis, especially in homosexual men, and may coexist with CMV. Pathogenic amoebae may be seen in the stools of AIDS patients, but many amoebic isolates in homosexual men, whether or not they have AIDS, are of non-pathogenic strains strains and symptoms do not resolve on metronidazole therapy, casting some doubt on their proposed role as opportunist infections. It seems likely that a number of other opportunist gut pathogens will be identified to account for the many other currently unexplained gut manifestations.

Central nervous system infections

Meningitis due to cryptococcus (Masur et al, 1981; Mildvan et al, 1982b; Follansbee et al, 1982; Snider et al, 1983a; Vieira et al, 1983; Pitchenik et al, 1983; Pape et al, 1983; Clumeck et al, 1984; Piot et al, 1984; van de Perre, 1984) may present with non-specific features such as fever, malaise, poor concentration, headache and ataxia. Physical signs may be minimal, and photophobia and neck stiffness are unusual. Lumbar puncture is essential for diagnosis but should usually be performed after computed tomography (CT scanning) as similar symptoms may be the presenting features of mass lesions. Cerebrospinal fluid examination should include cell count (although lymphocytosis may be minimal), protein, sugar (with simultaneous blood sugar), gram and Ziehl Neelsen stains and examination for cryptococci with India

Ink or latex agglutination tests. Cultures should include those for mycobacteria, fungi and viruses.

Focal brain lesions may be seen in cerebral toxoplasmosis, fungal abscesses and progressive multifocal leucoencephalopathy. These may present with non-specific symptoms like those of meningitis, but focal neurological symptoms and signs, fits, and loss of higher functions are usual. CT scanning is obligatory. In toxoplasmosis (Anderson et al, 1983; Snider et al, 1983a; Horowitz et al, 1983; Wong et al, 1984) the irregular enhancing ring shadows (often multiple) are typically surrounded by pronounced areas of low density indicating oedema. Fungal lesions may lack this latter feature. PML lesions are more diffusely distributed through the white matter, and are characteristically irregular low density areas which do not enhance (Miller et al, 1982; Bedri et al, 1983). An important differential diagnosis is cerebral lymphoma (Ziegler et al, 1982, Snider et al, 1983b; Levine et al, 1984). Other patients have a more slowly progressive deterioration of higher function, sometimes with epilepsy, but they lack focal lesions and show diffuse cerebral atrophy on CT scanning. These patients may have elevated CSF proteins and a few lymphocytes but culture is generally negative. They show relentless progression over many months to a vegetative state. Some instances appear to be due to CMV but HTLV-III/LAV itself may be responsible for this diffuse encephalopathy (Snider et al, 1983). Brain biopsy has been undertaken in patients with cerebral parenchymal lesions but diagnostic yield is not high and some patients deteriorate acutely following such procedures. Empirical anti-toxoplasma therapy may be necessary. Serological diagnosis of toxoplasmosis is highly unreliable owing to the abnormal humoral responses of AIDS patients (Lane et al, 1983; Luft et al, 1983; McCabe et al, 1983).

Retinal lesions are common in AIDS patients and may be of diagnostic value. Cotton-wool spots are seen in some patients during active Pneumocystis infections but may also be seen in Kaposi's sarcoma patients without infection, especially during alpha interferon therapy. In some cases these may be due to immune complex mediated vasculitis. CMV retinitis is common and may be extensive and progressive. The lesions can result in vascular occlusions with major visual loss. Toxoplasma may also affect the retina or choroid but the appearances are atypical. Fungal abscesses may also be seen. Anterior uveitis may accompany the retinal lesions.

Systemic infections

The symptoms and signs of systemic infections are generally non-specific with fever, malaise and weight loss. In some instances a major target organ is also involved and in others there are skin, mucosal or fundal signs of infection. A generally mild form of vasculitis may be seen especially in the skin of AIDS patients. CMV infection is frequently generalised and in addition to the major organ systems above it may affect the liver, adrenals and (rarely) other viscera. Mycobacterial infection may present with widespread lymphadenopathy, miliary disease or with bacteraemic dissemination to many tissues. Salmonella septicaemia may be accompanied by signs of chronic gram-negative septicaemia. Candidiasis may rarely be seen as a disseminated infection with haematogenous spread. Other mycoses seen mainly in the USA may be systemic. Herpes zoster presenting as shingles is unexpectedly uncommon in frank AIDS, although it may be seen in prodromal disease. Disseminated zoster has been described.

Kaposi's sarcoma

Most commonly Kaposi's sarcoma presents with skin or mucosal lesions (Hymes et al, 1981; Friedman-Kien et al, 1982; Volberding, 1984). These are generally multiple reddish or purplish macules or papules. They are indurated and may be palpable before they are visible. Lesions may be raised and sessile, and others pigmented. Some authors have divided them into patch, plaque and nodular lesions but the distinctions are often blurred. Kaposi's sarcoma in AIDS may resemble a wide variety of common and more benign skin lesions so that in at risk patients a biopsy is rarely avoidable. Many patients have similar plaques of Kaposi's sarcoma in the buccal mucosa, generally on the hard palate, but similar lesions may be seen on any mucosal surface, e.g. pharynx, bronchial tree and gut. In the gut lesions may be nodular and only evident on endoscopy (Friedman-Kien et al, 1982), but other patients have more diffuse involvement of gut with bowel symptoms of diarrhoea, sometimes with mucus and blood (Weber et al, 1985). Lymph node and spleen involvement is common, manifested as enlargement. Virtually any vascularised site may be affected by this tumour of probable endothelial origin. Histological diagnosis may be difficult, especially in early lesions, and the appearances are often more subtle than seen in the classical form of the disease (Safai et al, 1984b). Some evidence suggests that lymphatic endothelium may be a major site of early disease. There is serological and molecular biological evidence that Kaposi's sarcoma may be a manifestation of CMV oncogenesis in the compromised host (Giraldo et al, 1978, Hymes et al, 1981; Safai et al, 1984b). CMV may normally be latent in endothelial cells. A number of patients may present with lymphadenopathy, which on histology shows hypervascular follicular hyperplasia (Castleman's disease) with small foci of Kaposi's sarcoma (Harris, 1984). These two conditions have been shown to coexist before in other settings, and the former may be a precursor of Kaposi's sarcoma.

B cell lymphoma

Although B cell lymphoma is, with the exception of isolated central nervous system lymphoma, excluded from the surveillance definition of AIDS, it is clearly a part of the AIDS epidemic, being newly seen to a major extent in homosexual men (Ziegler et al, 1982; 1984; Snider et al, 1983; Levine et al, 1984). It is also a tumour which has been strongly associated with immunosuppression in other settings. Epstein Barr virus latency in B cells is a possible background and the tumour may arise, like Kaposi's sarcoma, by viral oncogenesis (Ziegler, 1981; Ziegler et al, 1982; Hochberg et al, 1983; Levine et al, 1984) following the failure of natural killer or other immune surveillance mechanisms. The tumour may be multifocal, and AIDS-related B cell lymphoma is unusual in having a high frequency of extranodal involvement (Levine et al, 1984; Ziegler et al, 1984). The cells appear to be monoclonal, at least at any one site, and they may represent malignant change at one of several stages of B lymphocyte differentiation. Diagnosis is based on histology of relevant lesions, which may present with lymphadenopathy or local symptoms depending on the site affected. The lesions are generally of the diffuse undifferentiated non-Hodgkin's or Burkitt-like type. A few patients have been described with angioblastic lymphadenopathy or with preleukaemic lymphoblastic neoplasia, which may have a similar pathogenetic background to B cell lymphoma in such patients.

Other tumours

Although an increased incidence of other tumours has been noted in homosexual men, it is less certain whether these are truly part of the AIDS spectrum. These tumours include cloacogenic carcinoma of the rectum (Cooper et al, 1979) and squamous carcinoma of the oral cavity. In some instances they have been documented in homosexual men before the beginnings of the AIDS epidemic (Daling et al, 1982). However the development of 'hairy leucoplakia' of the tongue in AIDS or AIDS risk patients, as a possible consequence of papova or herpesvirus infection, does suggest a pathogenetic link (Greespan et al, 1984).

THERAPY

Since no effective means of reconstituting cellular immunity has yet emerged, the mainstay of the management of AIDS patients is treatment of the secondary diseases. In general, this is most effective if begun early, emphasising the need for prompt, accurate and complete diagnosis. There is rarely any justification for empirical therapy without first attempting appropriate diagnostic manoeuvres; when used, it is usually regretted. In some instances prophylaxis is indicated. However it is also important to note that general measures are also of great importance in the management of these patients. The most important of these is to ensure appropriate nutrition that is sufficient to enable the patient to become anabolic.

While patients are encouraged to avoid obvious sources of opportunist infection, they are as far as possible encouraged to lead a normal life. Apart from the absolute proscription of blood donation, the only major restriction is on sexual activity. This either has to cease altogether or has to be severely restricted; the patient should restrict himself exclusively to those regular partners with whom he has already been in sexual contact prior to diagnosis and to whom the patient may present little or no additional risk. The other potential benefit from absolute or relative celibacy is that the patients will not be exposed to a range of sexually transmitted infections. These could not only act as opportunists but may also promote dissemination of the causative retrovirus throughout the cells of the immune system, hence rendering the patient more immunodeficient (Montagnier et al, 1984; Pinching, 1984b). For this and for the patient's general psychological rehabilitation, considerable counselling is required, for himself, his partners, close contacts and family. These general considerations are at least as important as the specific antimicrobial or antineoplastic measures in the management of the patients during their remaining life span.

High dose contrimoxazole is the treatment of choice for Pneumocystis carinii pneumonia and a three week course is usually adequate (Murray et al, 1984; Kovacs & Masur, 1984). AIDS patients characteristically have a high incidence (c70%) of reactions to the suphonamide component, with rash, fevers and/or leucopenia, which may curtail therapy (Jaffe et al, 1983; Gordin et al, 1984). For these patients, Pentamidine isethionate is a valuable alternative (Murray et al, 1984), although it has a high incidence of toxicity, including sterile muscle abscesses. The risk of sensitisation is one reason why prophylaxis with cotrimoxazole is usually avoided. However in situations where recurrence is common, prophylactic Fansidar (pyrimethamine and sulphadoxine) has apparently been effective without unduly frequent drug reactions (Gottlieb et al, 1984). Toxoplasma infections respond well to Pyrimethamine and

Sulphadiazine) used in high dose initially i.v. (combined with folinic acid) (Kovacs & Masur, 1984). After about a month of treatment, most treatment schedules reduce the dose to one or two tablets of Fansidar weekly for at least six months. Attempts to stop therapy are commonly promptly followed by relapse (Wong et al, 1984; Kovacs & Masur, 1984), so prophylaxis with one tablet weekly is usual. Cryptosporidiosis and Isospora infection are not clearly affected by any known antibiotic (Goldfarb et al, 1982; Soave et al, 1984), although some limited success has been reported in the former with spiramycin (Whiteside et al, 1984). Associated bacterial overgrowth with gram-positive organisms and candida may respond to vancomycin and nystatin orally (Weber & Pinching, unpublished observations).

Mucosal candidiasis is generally well controlled by oral ketoconazole but most patients will relapse if it is discontinued (Kovacs & Masur, 1984). Long-term prophylaxis is therefore usually necessary. In the rare instances when candidiasis is disseminated, amphotericin B and 5-flucytosine are the agents of choice; there is no evidence that miconazole or any other antifungals are effective. Cryptococcal meningitis is also best managed with intravenous amphotericin B and 5-flucytosine (Kovacs & Masur, 1984). Therapy should last at least one month but prophylaxis does not appear to be necessary. Other systemic mycoses merit a similar regime which may need to be continued for longer.

Mycobacteria should be treated with conventional antituberculous drugs if they are sensitive. Atypical mycobacterial infections respond poorly, and third line drugs may be needed. Ansamycin and clofazimine have been used with limited success for M avium-intracellulare (Kovacs & Masur, 1984). Salmonella spp may be treated with chloramphenicol, ampicillin, mecillinam, gentamicin or colomycin according to sensitivities, but in the face of poor host defence the response may be negligible, even to combination therapy (Weber et al, 1984). Legionella infection should be treated with erythromycin or rifampicin, and nocardia with doxycycline.

Herpes simplex ulceration responds well to acyclovir therapy (oral or intravenous) but again long term prophylaxis using a low dose regime is necessary to prevent relapse (Kovacs & Masur, 1984). Disseminated Herpes zoster may however be readily controlled by acyclovir. CMV did not respond to any previously available antiviral therapy but newer forms of treatment such as DHPG show promise. There is no known therapy effective against PML.

The most limited forms of Kaposi's sarcoma may not require therapy, although excision biopsy is sometimes helpful. Local radiotherapy in the few patients with very localised lesions may be an alternative to excision biopsy; however the cosmetic result may be poor, from residual skin staining. As patients with Kaposi's sarcoma are in the best prognostic group of AIDS but are already mildly immunodeficient it is important to avoid if possible the use of therapies that may further immunosuppress the patient. The use of recombinant alpha interferon is valuable in this sense as it appears to act by stimulating residual immune defence against such tumours. Daily intramuscular injection of about 20 megaunits per M2 daily for 3 months induces partial or complete remission in about 40% of cases (Krown et al, 1983a,b; Groopman et al, 1984; Volberding, 1984), mainly those with disease restricted to skin and/or lymph nodes. Relapse on dose reduction or cessation of therapy is not uncommon however. Patients with severe visceral disease or more profoundly depressed immunity may not respond however and these patients require more aggressive chemotherapy.

The optimal regime for this is yet to be established but vinblastine, epidophyllotoxin and combination adriamycin, bleomycin and vinblastine have all shown some efficacy (Volberding, 1984). Considerable problems with opportunist infections are to be expected following such treatment, and the pulmonary fibrosis caused by bleomycin may pose additional diagnostic problems.

B cell lymphomas have generally been treated with conventional regimes such as CHOP (cyclophosphamide, adriamycin, vinblastine and prednisolone) with central nervous system irradiation or intrathecal chemotherapy and these appear to be effective in some cases (Ziegler et al, 1982; Levine et al, 1984). Recurrence is common and early mortality is high, however. The use of prednisolone in this particular context must be viewed with some concern and regimes tailored to the particular setting of AIDS-related B cell lymphoma may need to be developed.

The use of antiviral therapy against HTLV-III/LAV is now being investigated. It is most likely to be useful early in infection and against the HTLV-III/LAV encephalopathy.

OTHER HTLV-III/LAV-RELATED DISORDERS

Persistent generalised lymphadenopathy

The emergence of AIDS has been accompanied by or just preceded by a similar exponential rise in cases of unexplained persistent generalised lymphadenopathy (PGL) in the same epidemiological risk groups (Mildvan et al, 1982a; Ioachim et al, 1983; Metroka et al, 1983; Mathur-Wagh et al, 1984; Abrams et al, 1984). This, and the fact that some patients clearly have had lymphadenopathy before developing AIDS, led to the idea that PGL could be a prodromal disorder. However, it has become apparent that this may not be the case for all such patients. More recently it has been shown that the great majority of PGL cases are seropositive for HTLV-III/LAV and virus may be isolated from many of them, strongly indicating that PGL is indeed caused by the same agent as AIDS (Barre-Sinoussi et al, 1983; Montagnier et al, 1984a; Brun-Vezinet et al, 1984; Gallo et al, 1984; Sarngadharan et al, 1984; Safai et al, 1984a, Cheingsong-Popov et al, 1984).

PGL is currently defined as lymphadenopathy of more than 3 months' duration affecting two or more extrainguinal sites and for which no other cause may be found. Many of these patients have general malaise and fatigue and 10–20% have night sweats, fevers, unexplained diarrhoea, weight loss and/or oral candidiasis. Some of these patients show similar immunological abnormalities to those seen in AIDS (see below), but they are generally lesser in degree. In a substantial proportion, however, T helper cells are normal but T suppressor cells increased. On histology the features of most lymph nodes are an explosive follicular hyperplasia, but a minority show follicular involution (Metroka et al, 1984).

It has become clear by longitudinal follow up of PGL patients that many of them do not progress to AIDS over 2–3 years and while some do progress, other regress (Mathur-Wagh et al, 1984; Abrams et al, 1984). This suggests a heterogeneity within the bland definition of PGL; it seems likely that progression is restricted to a subset of PGL patients, while uncomplicated PGL may be a more benign response to infection by HTLV-III/LAV. Using immunohistological techniques it has been possible to subdivide PGL patients into those who show germinal centre destruction as judged by changes in the staining of follicular dendritic reticular cells and those in whom these structures are preserved, albeit expanded (Janossy et al, 1985). From preliminary data it would seem that the germinal centre destruction, which in its most several form may be evident on conventional histology as follicular involution, is associated with progression to AIDS or with features which have been described as part of prodromal AIDS. The ability to make the distinction on clinical or (immuno-)histological grounds is important not only for counselling patients but also for planning of possible therapy (see below).

Prodromal AIDS
Mathur & Mildvan (1984) have defined a group of patients who have a combination of weight loss, diarrhoea, fever, oral candidiasis and T helper cell depletion, with or without lymphadenopathy, in whom progression to AIDS was frequent (77% at a mean of 4 months). This seems to characterise a truly prodromal disorder, and many of the individual clinical and laboratory features are also seen in the PGL patients who progress. Others have used the term 'AIDS-related complex', with varying clinical definitions, but generally incorporating lymphadenopathy and some of the associated symptoms to characterise this type of disorder (Quinn, 1984; Klein et al, 1984). The delineation of the spectrum of 'lesser' AIDS in relation to prognosis is critically important.

Other variants
A number of other minor clinical disorders have been seen which may represent other mild phenotypic variants of or possible prodromes for AIDS. These include idiopathic thrombocytopenia (Morris et al, 1982), herpes zoster (Kovacs & Masur, 1984) and possibly transient immunological abnormalities in symptom-free subjects. As HTLV-III/LAV serology becomes more widely available, it seems likely that a number of other conditions will come to be included within the widening spectrum of possible clinical outcomes of infection with HTLV-III/LAV. It is important to appreciate the possibility that some of these are not necessarily an early stage of an inevitable progression to AIDS.

THE IMMUNOLOGY OF AIDS

The characteristic pattern of opportunist infections and tumours seen in AIDS is the principal evidence of a predominantly cellular immunodeficiency in AIDS, using the ultimate bioassay: man in his environment. However the laboratory features of patients with the disease provide confirmation of the clinical impression (reviewed in Gottlieb et al, 1983; Fauci et al, 1984; Pinching, 1984a, Bowen et al, 1984; Seligmann et al, 1984; Pinching & Weiss, 1986). Although the diagnosis of AIDS still rests on its clinical features, the laboratory investigations may be of some value in supporting that diagnosis. In a number of apparently related disorders, the finding of a similar pattern of immunological abnormalities may assist in diagnosis. However, many of the tests are non-specific and similar findings may be seen in a wide variety of unrelated disorders, including for example during active pyogenic infection. It is important to recognise that no single immunological test can make the diagnosis and any combination of tests still has to be interpreted in a defined clinical setting.

Characteristic features of AIDS

Patients are generally lymphopenic, and this is due to a reduction in the numbers of T lymphocytes (responsible with macrophages and related cells for cellular immune mechanisms and immune regulation), the numbers of B cells (responsible for antibody production) being unaffected. In particular, AIDS patients typically have a reduction in the absolute numbers of so called T helper cells (T4+ cells). It is important to recognise that the designation 'helper' for T4+ cells is a phenotypic one and only loosely correlated with helper function. These cells are also involved in delayed type hypersensitivity responses, in some cytotoxic effector functions and in regulating the activity of suppressor cells. The numbers of T suppressor/cytotoxic cells (T8+ cells) in AIDS patients may be slightly elevated, normal or reduced; as the disease progresses there is a tendency for a reduction in these cells. Although the alterations in the T cell subsets generally lead to a reduction in the so called T helper/T suppressor ratio, there is no diagnostic advantage in this formulation. This is because the ratio will also incorporate patients with an absolute increase in T suppressor cells; such an increase is commonly seen following a wide variety of events, including many other viral infections. Furthermore the ratio in blood has no evident biological significance. In AIDS it is the absolute T helper decrease that is important.

Proliferative responses of lymphocytes to mitogens (e.g. phyohaemagglutinin, pokeweed mitogen) and antigens in vitro are abnormal. These may be the consequence of alterations in cell numbers and in the relative proportions of different effectors or of changes in lymphokine production or responsiveness. Patients also have abnormalities of natural killer cell function. These are cells that are apparently important in the non-specific elimination of virus-infected and possibly certain tumour cells, and may be relevant to the emergence of opportunist tumours in AIDS. Specific cytotoxic T cell functional defects may also occur in AIDS (Rook et al, 1983) but these are less well documented.

Monocyte function (phagocytosis and chemotaxis) may also be abnormal in AIDS patients. The macrophages that derive from monocytes show defects in intracellular killing which may be relevant to the development of some opportunist infections, such as those due to Toxoplasma, Salmonella and Mycobacteria. Some data suggests that this defect is only present in the context of collaboration with patients' T cells and that the macrophages are intrinsically normal (Murray et al, 1984), but our own data do not entirely support this (Eales & Pinching, unpublished observations). Antigen presenting cells, such as the Langerhans cells of skin, show reduced expression of HLA antigens (Belsito et al, 1984), which may modify their capacity to function normally in antigen presentation, the induction phase in the immune response. It is not yet clear whether this is a primary defect or is secondary to the effects of immune complexes. The failure of T cell cooperation with macrophages leads to defective delayed type hypersensitivity responses such as skin test reactions to tuberculin and candida; it also causes defective granuloma formation, for example in the tissue response to mycobacteria. The HLA type DR5 has been associated with the development of Kaposi's sarcoma, both in its classical form and in AIDS (Friedman-Kien et al, 1982; Pollack et al, 1983), and has also been associated with PGL (Enlow et al, 1983). In the case of Kaposi's sarcoma this appears to apply only to patients of Mediterranean or Ashenazy Jewish extraction.

Humoral responses in AIDS are also abnormal, with raised levels of immunoglobulins in a non-specific, polyclonal manner. This is the result of polyclonal B cell activation (Lane et al, 1983). This means that antibody responses to antigens that have previously been encountered by the host are raised while there is no response to newly encountered antigens. This underlies the unreliability of diagnostic serology in AIDS patients. Immune complexes are commonly found and this may also be a secondary effect of the functional B cell alterations. A wide variety of immunologically important molecules such as interferons, interleukins and other lymphokines, thymic hormones and other factors such as beta-2 microglobulin have been shown to be altered in AIDS (Zolla-Pazner, 1984); their specificity and primary relevance have yet to be established. They may well be consequent upon the primary cellular defects. Their potential utility as surrogate markers for AIDS and related disorders may be undermined by the possibility of HTLV-III/LAV serology, but this too will need careful interpretation.

Thus the typical profile of AIDS comprises lymphopenia, T helper cell depletion, polyclonally raised immunoglobulins (G ± A) and cutaneous anergy (Seligmann et al, 1984). Patients with Kaposi's sarcoma generally have similar defects but they are less pronounced, which fits with their immune deficiency being less severe and their prognosis correspondingly better. Although this pattern is frequently found in AIDS patients defined clinically and can be used to support a clinical diagnosis, it cannot at present be used as the sole evidence for making that diagnosis.

The immunopathogenesis of AIDS

The compelling evidence that a novel human retrovirus (HTLV-III/LAV) is the aetiological agent of AIDS, and the special properties of that virus, now begin to allow the characteristic immunological defects to be linked to the pathogenesis of the immunodeficiency (Pinching, 1984b; Pinching & Weiss, 1986). The family of human T lymphotropic retroviruses is typified by a tropism for T cells, specifically for T4+ ('helper') cells (Klatzmann et al, 1984). While HTLV I and II are transforming viruses associated with epidemic T cell leukaemia/lymphoma (Broder et al, 1984), HTLV III appears to be cytopathic (Montagnier et al 1984a; Popovic et al, 1984). There is in vitro evidence that some Epstein-Barr virus transformed B cells can also be infected by HTLV-III (Montagnier et al, 1984b) and possibly also monocytes. There is now evidence that the T4 surface antigen may be the 'receptor' for HTLV-III/LAV (Dagleish et al, 1984). The direct in vivo infection of T4+ cells, and possibly of these other cells, could account for their numerical and functional abnormalities in AIDS patients. Abnormalities of one or more of these cells could have knock-on consequences for the rest of the immune system and its regulators, leading to the ultimate profile seen in full-blown AIDS. Work is now under way to try to dissect which are the primary events and which are secondary. The concept that HTLV-III/LAV requires some cofactor(s) for inducing clinical disease and indeed for primary infection is now receiving much attention.

Possible treatment for AIDS and related disorders

Clearly, once patients have been infected and their T4+ and possibly other cells rendered defective, any treatment of the underlying immunodeficiency should be aimed either at restoring the cells or their normal products. Attempts to restore the cells, by bone marrow transplantation or lymphocyte transfusions, or to enhance the maturation of precursor T cells, by thymic hormones or transplants, have hitherto been largely unsuccessful (Volberding, 1984; Lane et al, 1984). This may be because the new cells or newly matured cells are susceptible to infection by virus still present in the patients. For this reason much effort has been concentrated on the application of therapy based on reconstituting the normal products of T4+ cells. The major T4 cell products include interleukin 2, also known as T cell growth factor, and gamma interferon, which is one of the main macrophage activating lymphokines. So far little success had been achieved, but the optimal dose and regime may not have been found. It may be that a 'cocktail' of several mediators of immune responses is needed to replace the defective T4+ cell function. On the other hand, as these cells and their humoral mediators normally act in small lymphoid microenvironments, there may be more fundamental reasons why systemic administration of these agents fails to provide clinically effective reconstitution. This is a major area of current research and it may take some time for clear efficacy of any therapeutic regime to be established. The application of alpha interferon in the treatment of Kaposi's sarcoma, where it is probably acting to stimulate the function of the remaining natural killer cells, is another example of attempted reconstitution for which limited, but clinically useful, success has been achieved (Krown et al 1983a,b; Groopman et al, 1984; Volberding, 1984).

Obviously the best time to intervene therapeutically is likely to be long before the immune defect is clinically evident. It is therefore crucial to determine which patients can be reliably diagnosed as having a state that leads inevitably to AIDS (i.e. a truly prodromal disorder), so that therapy can be instituted while a major part of the immune system remains normal. For this reason much interest has been expressed in the treatment of PGL and other prodromal disorders. While similar regimes of immune reconstitution as those used for AIDS may be appropriate, the objectives at such an early stage may be quite different (Pinching, 1984b). This could be with the aim of preventing the spread of HTLV-III/LAV to other cells, by enhancing any protective immune response against it, or by acting directly against the virus or its products. There is in vitro evidence that T4+ cells are more readily infected, and that viral replication in infected cells is enhanced, if these cells are activated (Montagnier et al, 1984a). If this is true in vivo, it is important to avoid therapeutic measures which may activate T4+ cells. Some of the agents which are appropriate to reconstituting AIDS patients, who have lost all T4+ function, may cause T4 cell activation in patients who still have functioning T4 cells, thus potentially enhancing the spread of virus through the cells of the immune system. A number of treatment regimes are being studied or considered, but insufficient data are available to allow comment. However the question of activation of T cells as a possible cofactor does suggest that measures taken to reduce the likelihood of T cell activation in vivo (such as that occurring during intercurrent viral infection) may be helpful in patients with latent virus infection. Reduction of casual sexual encounters may reduce the risk of such infections and may thus offer a means for infected patients to minimise the chances of HTLV-III/LAV replication and spread within their immune system.

Idiopathic thrombocytopenia has been treated with intravenous immunoglobulin, splenectomy and/or steroids with varying degrees of success; again the optimal regime to avoid compounding the immunodeficiency has yet to be established and, in the absence of bleeding, thrombocytopenia may be best left untreated.

SCREENING

The enormous concern that has been generated by AIDS has led to demands for screening programmes in various settings. Until recently, the focus was on surrogate markers or on the non-specific tests of immune function. Now that HTLV-III/LAV serology is available a more specific screening test would appear to be available. What should be clear from the foregoing is that we have yet to establish the full spectrum of responses to this new infectious agent. To find evidence of seroconversion in a member of an at risk group is not diagnostic of anything except prior exposure to and infection with HTLV-III/LAV (Cheingsong-Popov et al, 1984). It cannot be used at present to predict the subsequent clinical course. In subjects known to be seropositive, it may be of value to examine lymphocyte subsets serially, to document alterations in relation to possible clinical outcomes, but insufficient evidence exists as to the predictive value of such screening. For patients or well subjects who seek medical help because they are concerned about AIDS, retrovirus serology combined with immunological test (most simply a lymphocyte count) may assist in counselling the patient, but cannot be regarded as definitive. As a marker for potential infectivity, for example in the blood transfusion setting, HTLV-III/LAV antibody testing may be of value, but it may be that some seropositive patients are not infectious (cf. Hepatitis B antibodies), while others who are seronegative could be so. The role of HTLV-III/LAV serology outside the transfusion service has yet to be established. Its role in clinical diagnosis or in limiting the spread of the rotrovirus in the community is probably less than one might at first suspect. The indiscriminate testing of patients at this stage raises complex medical and ethical problems, given the current limitations on interpretation. The decision to test for HTLV-III/LAV antibodies should not be taken lightly; to inform a person, especially a well subject, of a positive test requires considerable resources for counselling, and consent to testing should be obtained first.

SAFETY CONSIDERATIONS

Because AIDS has occurred in an epidemiological pattern similar to that of Hepatitis B, the question of contracting the infection occupationally has inevitably arisen. Furthermore, as AIDS is seen to be a severe and generally fatal disease this has been a matter for great individual concern among health care workers. Nevertheless, there are no satisfactorily documented cases occurring among health care personnel who are not in known high risk groups. It is obviously prudent to take great care to avoid inoculation injury, and major exposure to blood or faeces, and to a lesser extent other body fluids, from AIDS, PGL and other HTLV-III/LAV seropositive patients. Guidelines on this matter have been provided (Centers for Disease Control, 1982, 1983; Conte et al, 1983; and from the Advisory Committee on Dangerous Pathogens (UK).

It should be recognised however that many persons who pose a potential biohazard will not be known to do so when being seen clinically or tested in the laboratory. The best way to avoid occupational infection is by good clinical and laboratory practice with *all* patients. The application of excessive measures that could reduce the level of clinical care needed for the proper management of such individuals is not only unnecessary but unethical; such an attitude ill befits our profession. People involved in the delivery of health care, at whatever level and in whatever role, should appreciate and accept the fact that such work involves many potential hazards. While sensible precautions appropriate to the hazard should be taken, we should still be able to look after our patients to the best of our ability.

CONCLUSIONS

AIDS and the related consequences of HTLV-III/LAV infection have posed a major challenge to clinical and basic sciences and have provided us with new insights in many areas. Although the acquisition of knowledge about the subject has been explosive, much remains to be established about the interaction between this new agent and its human host. For some of this we shall have to await the passage of time. Similarly it will take a great deal of patient research to indicate suitable therapy and prevention. In the meantime increasingly large numbers of physicians will have to care for AIDS patients and for those with the related conditions. All of us have much to learn about AIDS and even more to learn from it.

REFERENCES

Abrams D I, Lewis B J, Beckstead J H, Casavant C A, Drew W L 1984 Persistent diffuse lymphadenopathy in homosexual men: endpoint or prodrome? Annals of Internal Medicine 100: 801–808
Anderson K P, Atlas E, Ahern M J, Weisbrot I M 1983 Central nervous system toxoplasmosis in homosexual men. American Journal of Medicine 75: 877–881
Barre-Sinoussi F et al 1983 Isolation of a T-lymphotropic retrovirus from a patient at risk for acquired immune deficiency syndrome. Science 220: 868–871
Bedri J, Weinstein W, DeGregorio P, Verity M A 1983 Progressive multifocal leukoencephalopathy in acquired immunodeficiency syndrome. New England Journal of Medicine 309: 492–3
Belsito D V, Sanchez M R, Baer R L, Valentine F, Thorbecke G J 1984 Reduced Langerhans' cell Ia antigen and ATPase activity in patients with the acquired immunodeficiency syndrome. New England Journal of Medicine 310: 1279–1282
Bowen D L, Lane H C, Fauci A S 1984 Cellular immunity. In: Ebbesen P, Biggar R J Melbye M (eds) AIDS, Munksgaard, Copenhagen, ch 10, p 135–150
Broder S et al 1984 T-cell lymphoproliferative syndrome associated with human T-cell leukemia/lymphoma virus. Annals of Internal Medicine 100: 543–557
Brun-Vezinet F et al 1984 Detection of IgG antibodies to lymphadenopathy associated virus in patients with AIDS or lymphadenopathy syndrome. Lancet i: 1253–1256
Centers for Disease Control 1982 Acquired immune deficiency syndrome: precautions for clinical and laboratory staffs. Morbidity and Mortality Weekly Report 31: 577–580
Centers for Disease Control 1983 Acquired immunodeficiency syndrome: precautions for health-care workers and allied professionals. Morbidity and Mortality Weekly Report 32: 450–451
Cheingsong-Popov R et al 1984 Prevalence of antibody to human T-lymphotropic virus type III in AIDS and AIDS-risk patients in Britain Lancet ii: 466–480
Clumeck N et al 1984 Acquired immunodeficiency syndrome in African patients. New England Journal of Medicine 310: 492–497
Coleman D L, Dodek P M, Luce J M, Golden J A, Gold W M, Murray J F 1983 Diagnostic utility of fiberoptic bronchoscopy in patients with Pneumocystis carinii pneumonia and the acquired immune deficiency syndrome. American Review of Respiratory Disease 128: 795–799
Conte J E Jr et al 1983 Infection control guidelines for patients with the acquired immunodeficiency syndrome. New England Journal of Medicine 309: 740–744
Cooper H S, Patchefsky A S, Marko G 1979 Cloacogenic carcinoma of the anorectum in homosexual men: an observation of four cases. Diseases of the Colon and Rectum 22: 557–558

Dalgleish A G, Beverley P C L, Clapham P R, Crawford D H, Greaves M F, Weiss R A 1984 The CD4 (T4) antigen is an essential component of the receptor for the AIDS retrovirus (HTLV-III). Nature 312: 763–6

Daling J R et al 1982 Correlates of homosexual behaviour and the incidence of anal cancer. Journal of the American Medical Association 247: 1988–1990

Eisenstat B A, Wormser G P 1984 Seborrheic dermatitis and butterfly rash in AIDS. New England Journal of Medicine 311: 189

Enlow R W, Roldan A N, LoGalbo P, Mildvan D, Mathur U, Winchester R J 1983 Increased frequency of HLA-DR5 in lymphadenopathy stage of AIDS. Lancet ii: 51–52

Fauci A S et al 1984 Acquired immunodeficiency syndrome: epidemilogic, clinical, immunologic and therapeutic considerations. Annals of Internal Medicine 100: 92–106

Follansbee S E et al 1982 An outbreak of Pneumocystis carinii pneumonia in homosexual men. Annals of Internal Medicine 96: 705–713

Friedman-Kien A E et al 1982 Disseminated Kaposi's sarcoma in homosexual men. Annals of Internal Medicine 96: 673–700

Gallo R et al 1984 Frequent detection and isolation of cytopathic retroviruses (HTLV-III) from patients with AIDS and at risk for AIDS. Science 224: 500–503

Gellene R A, Stover D E, Gebhard D, Evans R L, Cunningham-Rundles C 1984 Lymphocyte alveolitis in acquired immune deficiency syndrome. Clinical and Experimental Immunology (in press)

Giraldo G, Beth E, Huang E S 1980 Kaposi's sarcoma and its relationship to cytomegalovirus (CMV). III CMV DNA and CMV early antigens in Kaposi's sarcoma. International Journal of Cancer 26: 23–29

Goldfarb J et al Cryptosporidiosis: assessment of chemotherapy of males with acquired immune deficiency syndrome. Morbidity and Mortality Weekly Report 32: 589–592

Gordin F M, Simon G L, Wofsy C B, Mills J 1984 Adverse reactions to trimethoprim-sulfamethoxazole in patients with the acquired immunodeficiency syndrome. Annals of Internal Medicine 100: 495–499

Gottlieb M S et al 1981 Pneumocystis carnii pneumonia and mucosal candidiasis in previously healthy homosexual men. New England Journal of Medicine 305: 1425–1431

Goittlieb M S, Groopman J E, Weinstein W M, Fahey J L, Detels R 1983 The acquired immunodeficiency syndrome. Annals of Internal Medicine 99: 208–220

Gottlieb M S, Knight S, Mitsuyasu R, Weisman J, Roth M, Young L S 1984 Prophylaxis of Pneumocystis carinii infection in AIDS with pyrimethamine-sulfadoxine. Lancet ii: 398–399

Greene J B et al 1982 Mycobacterium avium-intracellulare: a cause of disseminated life-threatening infection in homosexuals and drug abusers. Annals of Internal Medicine 97: 539–546

Greenspan D, Greenspan J S, Conant M, Petersen V, Silverman S Jr, de Souza Y 1984 Oral 'hairy' leucoplakia in male homosexuals: evidence of association with both papilloma virus and a herpes-group virus. Lancet ii: 831–834

Groopman J et al 1984 Recombinant alpha-2 interferon therapy for Kaposi's sarcoma associated with the acquired immunodeficiency syndrome. Annals of Internal Medicine 100: 671–676

Harris N 1984 Hypervascular follicular hyperplasia and Kaposi's sarcoma in patients at risk for AIDS. New England Journal of Medicine 310: 462–463

Hochberg F H, Miller G, Schooley R T, Hirsch M S, Feorino P, Henle W 1983 Central nervous system lymphoma related to Epstein-Barr virus. New England Journal of Medicine 309: 745–748

Horowitz S L, Bentson J R, Benson D F, Davos I, Pressman B, Gottlieb M S 1983 CNS toxoplasmosis in acquired immunodeficiency syndrome. Archives of Neurology 40: 649–652

Hymes K B et al 1981 Kaposi's sarcoma in homosexual men — a report of eight cases. Lancet ii: 598–600

Ioachim H L, Lerner C W, Tapper M L 1983 Lymphadenopathies in homosexual men; relationships with the acquired immune deficiency syndrome. Journal of the American Medical Association 250: 1306–1309

Jaffe H S, Abrams D I, Ammann A J, Lewis B J, Golden J A 1983 Complications of co-trimoxazole treatment of AIDS-associated Pneumocystis carinii penumonia in homosexual men. Lancet ii: 1109–1111

Janossy G et al 1985 An immunohistological approach to persistent lymphadenopathy and its relevance to acquired immune deficiency syndrome. Clinical and Experimental Immunology 59: 257–266

Klatzman D et al 1984 Selective tropism of lymphadenopathy associated virus (LAV) for helper-inducer T lymphocytes. Science 225: 59–63

Klein R S, Harris C A, Small C B, Moll B, Lesser M, Friedland G H 1984 Oral candidiasis in high-risk patients as the initial manifestation of the acquired immunodeficiency syndrome. New England Journal of Medicine 311: 354–358

Kovacs J A, Masur H 1984 Treatment of opportunistic infections. In: Ebbesen P, Biggar R J, Melbye M (eds) AIDS Munksgaard, Copenhagen, ch 6, p 84–98

Kovacs J A et al 1984 Pneumocystis carinii pneumonia: a comparison between patients with the acquired immunodeficiency syndrome and patients with other immunodeficiencies. Annals of Internal Medicine 100: 663–671

Krown S E et al 1983a Preliminary observations on the effect or recombinant leukocyte A interferon in homosexual men with Kaposi's sarcoma. New England Journal of Medicine 308: 1071–1076

Krown S E et al 1983b Interferon in the treatment of Kaposi's sarcoma. New England Journal of Medicine 309: 923–924

Lane H C, Masur H, Edgar L C, Whalen G, Fauci A S 1983 Abnormalities of B lymphocyte activation and immunoregulation in patients with the acquired immunodeficiency syndrome. New England Journal of Medicine 309: 453–458

Lane H C et al 1984 Partial immune reconstitution in a patient with the acquired immunodeficiency syndrome. New England Journal of Medicine 311: 1099–1103

Levine A M et al 1984 Development of B-cell lymphoma in homosexual men. Annals of Internal Medicine 100: 7–13

Luft B J et al 1983 Outbreak of central nervous system toxoplasmosis in Western Europe and North America. Lancet i: 781–783

Macher A M et al 1983 Bacteremia due to Mycobacterium avium-intracellulare in the acquired immunodeficiency syndrome. Annals of Internal Medicine 99: 782–785

Malebranche R et al 1983 Acquired immunodeficiency syndrome with severe gastrointestinal manifestations in Haiti. Lancet ii: 873–878

Masur H et al 1981 An outbreak of community-acquired Pneumocystis carinii pneumonia. New England Journal of Medicine 305: 1431–1438

Mathur U, Mildvan D 1984 Prodromal syndromes in AIDS Annals of the New York Academy of Sciences 437: 184–191

Mathur-Wagh U et al 1984 Longitudinal study of persistent generalised lymphadenopathy in homosexual men: relations to acquired immunodeficiency syndrome. Lancet i: 1033–1038

McCabe R E, Gibbons D, Brooks R G, Luft B J, Remington J S 1983 Agglutination test for diagnosis of toxoplasmosis in AIDS. Lancet i: 680

Metroka C E et al 1983 Generalised lymphadenopathy in homosexual men. Annals of Internal Medicine 99: 585–591

Mildvan D et al 1982a Persistent generalised lymphadenopathy among homosexual males. Morbidity and Mortality Weekly Report 31: 249–251

Mildvan D et al 1982b Opportunistic infections and immune deficiency in homosexual men. Annals of Internal Medicine 96: 700–704

Miller J R et al 1982 Progressive multifocal leukoencephalopathy in a male homosexual with T-cell immune deficiency. New England Journal of Medicine 307: 1436–1438

Montagnier L, Barre-Sinoussi F, Chermann J C 1984a Possible role of a new type of human T lymphotropic virus in the pathology of AIDS and related syndromes. In: Griscelli C, Vossen J (eds) Progress in immunodeficiency research and therapy I. Excerpta Medica, Amsterdam, p 367–372

Montagnier L et al 1984b Adaptation of lymphadenopathy associated virus (LAV) to replication in EBV-transformed lymphoblastoid cell lines. Science 225: 63–66

Morris L, Distenfeld A, Amorosi E, Karpatkin S 1982 Autoimmune thrombocytopenic purpura in homosexual men. Annals of Internal Medicine 96: 714–717

Murray H W, Rubin B Y, Masur H, Roberts R B 1984 Impaired production of lymphokines and immune (gamma) interferon in the acquired immunodeficiency syndrome. New England Journal of Medicine 310: 883–889

Murray J F et al 1984 Pulmonary complications of the acquired immunodeficiency syndrome. New England Journal of Medicine 310: 1682–1688

Pape J W et al 1983 Characteristics of the acquired immunodeficiency syndrome in Haiti. New England Journal of Medicine 309: 945–950

Pinching A J 1984a The acquired immune deficiency syndrome. Clinical and Experimental Immunology 56: 1–13

Pinching A J 1984b The probable cause of AIDS. Immunology Today 5: 196–199

Pinching A J, Weiss R A 1986 The spectrum of HTLV-III/LAV infection. International Review of Experimental Pathology. 281 (in press)

Piot P et al 1984 Acquired immunodeficiency syndrome in a heterosexual population in Zaire. Lancet ii: 65–69

Pitchenik A E et al 1983 Opportunistic infections and Kaposi's sarcoma among Haitians: evidence of a new acquired immunodeficiency state. Annals of Internal Medicine 98: 277–284

Pollack M S, Safai B, Myskowski P L, Gold J W M, Pandey J, Dupont B 1983 Frequencies of HLA and Gm immunogenetic markers in Kaposi's sarcoma. Tissue antigens 21: 1–8

Popovic M, Sarngadharan M G, Read E, Gallo R C 1984 Detection, isolation and continuous production of cytopathic retroviruses (HTLV-III) from patients with AIDS and pre-AIDS. Science 224: 497–500

Quinn T C 1984 Early symptoms and signs of AIDS and the AIDS-related complex. In: Ebbesen P, Biggar R J, Melbye M (eds) AIDS. Munksgaard, Copenhagen, ch 5, p 69–83

Rook A H et al 1983 Interleukin-2 enhances the depressed natural killer and cytomegalovirus-specific cytotoxic activities of lymphocytes from patients with the acquired immune deficiency syndrome. Journal of Clinical Investigation 72: 398–403

Safai B et al 1984a Seroepidemiological studies of human T-lymphotropic retrovirus type III in acquired immunodeficiency syndrome. Lancet i: 1438–1440

Safai B, Parris A, Urmacher C 1984b Histopathology of Kaposi's sarcoma and other neoplasms. In: Ebbesen P, Biggar R J, Melbye M (eds) AIDS, Munksgaard, Copenhagen, ch 9, p 123–131

Sarngadharan M G, Popovic M, Bruch L, Schupbach J, Gallo R C 1984 Antibodies reactive with human T-lymphotropic retroviruses (HTLV-III) in the serum of patients with AIDS. Science 224: 506–508

Seligmann M et al 1984 AIDS: an immunologic reevaluation. New England Journal of Medicine 311: 1286–1292

Siegal F P et al 1981 Severe acquired immunodeficiency in male homosexuals, manifested by chronic perianal ulcerative herpes simplex lesions. New England Journal of Medicine 305: 1439–1444

Snider W D, Simpson D M, Nielsen S, Gold J W M, Metroka C E, Posner J B 1983 Neurological complications of the acquired immune deficiency syndrome: analysis of 50 patients. Annals of Neurology 14: 403–418

Snider W D, Simpson D M, Aronyk K E, Nielsen S L 1983 Primary lymphoma of the nervous system associated with the acquired immune deficiency syndrome. New England Journal of Medicine 308: 45

Soave R 1984 Cryptosporidiosis in homosexual men. Annals of Internal Medicine 100: 504–511

Van de Perre P et al 1984 Acquired immunodeficiency syndrome in Rwanda. Lancet ii: 62–65

Vieira J, Frank E, Spira T J, Landesman S H 1983 Acquired immune deficiency in Haitians. New England Journal of Medicine 308: 125–129

Vilmer E et al 1984 Isolation of new lymphotropic retrovirus from two siblings with Haemophilia B, one with AIDS. Lancet i: 753–757

Volberding P 1984 Kaposi's sarcoma. In: Ebbesen P, Biggar R J, Melbye M (eds) AIDS. Munksgaard, Copenhagen, ch 7, p 99–110

Walsh C M, Nardi M A, Karpatkin S 1984 On the mechanism of thrombocytopenic purpura in sexually active homosexual men. New England Journal of Medicine 311: 635–639

Weber J N, Carmichael D J, Sawyer N, Pinching A J, Harris J R W 1984 Clinical aspects of the acquired immune deficiency in the United Kingdom. British Journal of Venereal Diseases 60: 253–257

Weber J N, Carmichael D J, Boylston A, Munro A, Whitear W P, Pinching A J 1985 Kaposi's sarcoma of the bowel — presenting as apparent ulcerative colitis. Gut 26: 295–300

Whiteside M et al 1984 Update: treatment of cryptosporidiosis in patients with acquired immunodeficiency syndrome. Morbidity and Mortality Weekly Report 33: 117–119

Wong B et al 1984 Central nervous system toxoplasmosis in homosexual men and parenteral drug abusers. Annals of Internal Medicine 100: 36–42

Zakowski P, Fligiel S, Berlin G W, Johnson L Jr 1982 Disseminated Mycobacterium avium-intracellulare infection in homosexual men dying of acquired immunodeficiency. Journal of the American Medical Association 248: 2980–2982

Ziegler J L 1981 Burkitt's lymphoma. New England Journal of Medicine 305: 735–745

Ziegler J L et al 1982 Outbreak of Burkitt's-like lymphoma in homosexual men. Lancet ii: 631–633

Ziegler J L et al 1984 Non-Hodgkin's lymphoma in 90 homosexual men. New England Journal of Medicine 311: 565–570

Zolla-Pazner S 1984 Serology. In: Ebbesen P, Biggar R J, Melbye M (eds) AIDS. Munksgaard, Copenhagen, ch 11, p 151–172

.

15. Proctocolitis in homosexual men

A. McMillan

Over the past decade the number of men attending genitourinary medicine clinics and giving a history of homosexual contact has increased. As a result of anal intercourse and oral-anal sexual contact with multiple partners, the prevalence of intestinal infection in this group is higher than in heterosexual patients, hence it is important for the clinican to take into account the research in recent years on proctocolitis in homosexual men.

The introductory section is an outline of the histological changes in infectious proctocolitis and is followed by a review of the methods used for the diagnosis of proctitis. The last section is an account of the various organisms found in association with proctocolitis.

HISTOPATHOLOGY OF PROCTITIS AND PROCTOCOLITIS

The epithelial surface of the rectum consists of a single layer of columnar epithelial cells with interspersed mucus producing goblet cells. Straight tubular glands, the crypts of Lieberkuhn, which are lined mainly with goblet cells, open on to the surface. Within the epithelial layer of the surface and crypts are lymphocytes, the majority of which are of the T8 phenotype (Selby et al, 1981): some of these cells contain granules and stain as mucosal mast cells. Supporting the surface epithelium and the glands and connecting it with the third and outermost layer of the mucosa, the muscularis mucosa, is the lamina propria, connective tissue containing unmyelinated nerve fibres, capillaries, lymphocytes (mainly of the T4 phenotype), plasma cells (principally IgA-producing), macrophages, fibroblasts, an occasional eosinophil and a few mast cells. Aggregates of lymphocytes are found commonly within the lamina propria.

Inflammation of the rectum can be induced by a variety of stimuli including infection with pathogens (bacterial, viral, protozoal and helminthic), chemicals, drugs, trauma and radiation. In addition there are the idiopathic inflammatory bowel diseases — ulcerative colitis and Crohn's disease — from which other causes of proctocolitis must be distinguished. As physicians working in genito-urinary medicine clinics are more likely to see cases of infective proctitis than other types this review concentrates on the former.

Generally the histology of rectal biopsies from patients with infective proctitis is not specific, the appearances being related to the time since the onset (Day et al, 1978; Dickinson et al, 1979; Mandal et al, 1982). In the acute stage of the disease there is mucosal oedema with dilatation and congestion of the capillaries of the lamina propria. Focal collections of polymorphonuclear leucocytes are found in the mucosa and submucosa and individual polymorphs may be found between the epithelial cells of the crypts and mucosal surface; in severe cases there may be crypt abscess formation with or without focal erosion of the epithelium. In contrast to active ulcerative colitis, there is no derangement of crypt architecture (although there may be reactive or degenerative changes in the epithelium) and there is little mucus depletion of the goblet cells. Also in comparison to chronic inflammatory bowel disease, there is only a slight increase in the numbers of mononuclear cells in the lamina propria. Although in the majority of cases, the histological appearances of infective and ulcerative proctocolitis are sufficiently distinct to allow a firm diagnosis to be made, in some their differentiation is not possible. During resolution of proctocolitis mucosal oedema becomes inapparent, there are regenerative changes in the surface and crypt epithelium, and there is a mild increase in the numbers of lymphocytes and plasma cells within the lamina propria (Kumar et al, 1982).

In many patients presenting with acute diarrhoea, the only histological abnormality will be a mild to moderate increase in the numbers of chronic inflammatory cells in the lamina propria (chronic proctitis) (Dickinson et al, 1979), findings which are difficult to interpret in the absence of studies with suitable controls.

DIAGNOSIS OF PROCTITIS

Although symptoms such as anorectal pain, anal discharge, bleeding, tenesmus and a change in bowel habit may suggest a diagnosis of proctitis and proctocolitis, objective criteria are necessary to reach a firm diagnosis.

The most sensitive method for the diagnosis of proctitis is the histological examination of rectal biopsies (Watts et al, 1966). The taking of a biopsy has, however, in rare instances, been complicated by haemorrhage or intestinal perforation and for this reason other diagnostic criteria have been adopted by many genito-urinary physicians. In a survey of clinical practices in England and Wales, Adler (1978) reported that 77% of consultants working in 98 clinics used only one criterion (most commonly the number of polymorphonuclear leucocytes in a Gram-stained smear of rectal exudate) for the diagnosis of non-specific proctitis. In such an examination however, in which an indefinite area of rectal mucosa is sampled with a cotton wool-tipped swab, the author found little correlation between the number of polymorphs per unit area of a stained smear and the histology of the rectal mucosa. Quinn et al (1983), on the other hand, found that the mean number of polymorphonuclear leucocytes per oil immersion microscopic field was greater in those with an abnormal proctoscopic appearance than in those whose rectal mucosa appeared normal. In comparing the results of sigmoidoscopy, cytology of rectal exudate and rectal histology in the diagnosis of ulcerative colitis, Watts et al (1966) found good correlation between the presence or absence of inflammatory cells in stained impression smears and the histological grade. The author and his colleagues (1983a) found that cytological examination of impression smears of rectal mucosa was helpful in the diagnosis of acute infective proctitis, but the technique failed to identify the majority of cases of chronic proctitis.

Adler (1978) reported that the second most commonly used criterion for the diagnosis of proctitis in genito-urinary clinics was that of the 'clinical findings'. Since there is marked variation between observers in the description of the mucosal appearances of the rectum (Baron et al, 1964), only certain criteria (Watts et al, 1966) could be relied upon for the identification of acute proctitis, viz:

(i) the presence of a normal vascular pattern usually excludes mucosal disease (the corollary is not necessarily true);

(ii) contact bleeding does not occur and oedema is not present when the histology is normal.

It is clear, however, that microscopic disease is often present when the mucosa appears normal at sigmoidoscopy (Watts et al, 1966; McMillan et al, 1983a).

The microscopical examination of stained impression smears is a useful corroborative test (McMillan et al, 1983a) but is time consuming. In the diagnosis of chronic proctitis, neither sigmoidoscopic nor cytological findings are helpful and rectal biopsy is indicated in patients with anorectal symptoms when appropriate microbiological investigations have failed to detect infection. The author and his colleagues (1983a) concluded that histological examination of rectal tissue is essential when research work on any aspect of rectal disease is undertaken.

Table 15.1   Enteric pathogens transmissible by anal intercourse or by the faecal-oral route

Organisms acquired during penoreceptive anal intercourse	Organisms acquired by the faecal-oral route
Neisseria gonorrhoeae	*Shigella spp*
Neisseria meningitidis	*Salmonella spp*
Treponema pallidum	*Campylobacter spp*
? Brachyspira spp	
Chlamydia trachomatis	Enteroviruses (Echovirus 11)
? Mycoplasma hominis	Hepatitis A
? Ureaplasma urealyticum	*Entamoeba histolytica*
Herpes simplex virus	*Giardia lamblia*
? Cryptosporidium spp	*Cryptosporidium spp*
	Enterobius vermicularis
	Strongyloides stercoralis

ORGANISMAL CAUSES OF PROCTITIS AND PROCTOCOLITIS

Homosexual men may acquire rectal or intestinal infection by penoreceptive anal intercourse or by oral-anal sexual contact with an infected partner. Table 15.1 shows the enteric organisms which may be transmitted amongst homosexual men. As both types of sexual contact are often practised by the same individual with different partners, infection with more than one organism is common. For example, in a study of intestinal infection in homosexual men who attended a sexually-transmitted disease clinic in Seattle, USA, Quinn et al (1983) found that 22% of 119 men with symptoms of proctitis were infected with two or more pathogenic organisms. It is therefore difficult to determine with certainty the role of a particular organism in the aetiology of proctitis, and this should be borne in mind when ascribing pathogenicity to the organisms considered below. Trauma to the rectal mucosa is common during anal intercourse and may play a part in causing the inflammatory reaction seen in those also infected with organisms (Kreutzer & Hansbrough, 1979). Enemas are being used with increasing frequency by homosexual men as a prelude to anal intercourse and it is recognised that their use can produce changes in the rectal mucosa viz., oedema, goblet cell mucus depletion, disruption of the surface epithelium and the finding of occasional polymorphs within the lamina propria (Meisel et al, 1977).

Giardia lamblia

In infection with *Giardia lamblia* there may be diarrhoea but as this is associated with small intestinal disease proctocolitis does not result.

Neisseria gonorrhoeae

Neisseria gonorrhoeae is the most prevalent pathogenic microorganism isolated from the rectum of homosexual men; in studies on the aetiology of proctitis in homosexual men attending sexually transmitted disease clinics in the UK, Munday et al (1981a) and McMillan et al (1983a) cultured the organisms from rectal material from 14.4% of 180 men and 12.5% of 176 men respectively.

It is well recognised that less than 50% of homosexual men with rectal gonorrhoea have anorectal symptoms. Mild pruritus ani and mucoid anal discharge were the commonest symptoms in the series reported by McMillan & Young (1978) and Fluker et al (1980). The author and his colleagues (1983b) found that the macroscopic appearance of the rectal mucosa was normal in 48 of 57 infected men; when the mucosa appeared abnormal, the inflammatory changes were found within 8 cm of the anal margin. This contrasts with the findings of Lebedeff & Hochman (1980) who reported that the proctoscopic appearance of the mucosa was normal in only 21% of 554 men with rectal gonorrhoea; however these authors selected their study population from men with anorectal symptoms and this may explain the differences from the author's study. Munday et al (1981a) noted that there was no correlation between proctitis (as defined by clinical features and the number of pus cells in a Gram-stained smear of rectal exudate) and the isolation of any microorganism, including *N. gonorrhoeae*.

Although Harkness (1948) reported on the histopathology of rectal gonorrhoea in nine men the methods which were used for the diagnosis of gonorrhoea lacked specificity and laboratory methods for the exclusion of other causes of proctitis were not well developed at that time. McMillan et al (1983b) described the histopathology of rectal gonorrhoea in 57 homosexual men in whom other microbial causes of proctocolitis had been excluded; the findings were compared with those of a matched group of non-infected homosexuals. They found that non-specific inflammatory changes in the rectal mucosa were more prevalent in infected (40% of 57) than in non-infected men (19% of 57). In most patients (37%) with rectal gonorrhoea the proctitis was mild, with a moderate increase in the numbers of lymphocytes and plasma cells within the lamina propria; only three (5%) men had an acute proctitis with a predominantly polymorpho-nuclear leucocyte infiltration of the mucosa. Using an immunoperoxidase method, they showed that the mean numbers of plasma cells containing IgA, IgG and IgM in the rectal lamina propria were increased in cases of both gonococcal and non-gonococcal infection only when there was proctitis diagnosed on histological grounds. In individual cases of rectal gonorrhoea there was no correlation between the predominant class of immunoglobulin-containing plasma cell and the duration of the infection.

Culture of the organism from rectal material is the most sensitive and specific diagnostic procedure. Microscopic examination of Gram-stained smears lacks sensitivity; McMillan & Young (1978) showed that only 57% of 47 infected men would have been identified if microscopy had been the only diagnostic method used. Although the majority of rectal gonococcal infections will be detected by sampling once, McMillan & Young (1978) found that 7% of 114 infections would not have been diagnosed if tested only on one occasion. Similar results were noted by Deheragoda (1977).

Recently there has been debate on whether rectal material for microbiological examination should be obtained under direct vision through a proctoscope or, blindly, by the passage of a swab through the anal canal. Deheragoda (1977) diagnosed rectal gonorrhoea in 99 and 96 of 100 infected men whose samples had been taken at proctoscopy and through the anal canal respectively. In a smaller study William et al (1981) showed that 47% of 19 men with culturally-proven rectal gonorrhoea would not have been identified if the samples had been obtained through the anal canal.

Ncisseria meningitidis

Neisseria meningitidis with a broad representation of serogroups can be isolated from the rectum of between 2% and 31% of homosexual men (Judson et al, 1978; Carlson et al, 1980; Janda et al, 1980; Salit & Frasch, 1982). The significance of infection at this site is uncertain. Janda et al (1980) did not show any correlation between anorectal clinical features and culture of the organism and McMillan et al (1983b) found mild inflammatory changes in the lamina propria of one of two men from whose rectums *N. meningitidis* had been cultured.

Treponema pallidum

Although primary syphilis, in the form of a chancre or a fissure, is most frequently found at the anal margin, rectal ulceration, which may be confused with neoplasia, may occur (Marino, 1964; Gluckman et al, 1974; Drusin et al, 1977; Voinchet & Guivarc'h, 1980). The proctitis associated with the secondry stage of the disease is sometimes diffuse (Akdamar et al, 1977; McMillan & Lee, 1981) but it may be seen as localised irregular thickened mucosal lesions with or without ulceration (Nazemi et al, 1975; Akdamar et al, 1977).

Histologically there is an intense lymphocyte, histiocyte and plasma cell infiltration of the lamina propria with the formation of epithelioid cell granulomas, near to dilated blood vessels, which show endothelial swelling. *Treponema pallidum* can be demonstrated by silver staining (Akdamar et al, 1977) and by immunofluorescence (Quinn et al, 1982). From a clinical point of view such investigations are not necessary as a routine and demand special care.

Rectal spirochaetosis

On epithelial surfaces of the large intestine of man and other animals such as monkeys, treponemes of the genus Brachyspira (Hovind-Hougen 1982) and flagellated bacteria (family Spirillaceae) may be found; this situation has been referred to as intestinal spirochaetosis (Harland & Lee, 1967; Takeuchi et al, 1974). Although electron microscopy is necessary to distinguish these organisms, their presence in haematoxylin-eosin stained sections is indicated by a basophilic zone about 3 μm in width on the surface of the epithelium. As it is uncertain whether the entire mucosal surface of the intestine is occupied by these organisms, a more appropriate term may be rectal spirochaetosis (RS). The incidence of RS appears to vary geographically but generally it is found in under 10% of human rectal biopsies. Lee et al (1971), working in Glasgow and Takeuchi et al (1974) from Washington DC, reported prevalence rates of 6.9% and 2% respectively. In a series of rectal biopsies taken from 100 men who had had anal homosexual contact McMillan & Lee (1981) recorded RS in 36%; this finding had not been reported previously. The significance of RS is not clear. For about a century a role for intestinal spirochaetes in the aetiology of dysenteric-like illnesses has been proposed (Parr, 1923; Shera, 1962). The species of spirochaete observed by earlier workers may have differed from those described in rectal spirochaetosis first recognised and described by Harland & Lee in 1967.

Of 14 patients in whom RS had been detected in a rectal biopsy all had ano-rectal symptoms, but some other cause may have been responsible for the symptoms in all but two (Lee et al, 1971). Kaplan & Takeuchi (1979) cultured organisms resembling *T. vincenti* from a homosexual with anal discharge but, as in the case of treponemes isolated from the rectum of three asymptomatic homosexual men (Tompkins et al, 1981) it is doubtful that these organisms were the same species as those of RS.

Douglas & Crucioli (1981) recently described two male patients who had RS, diarrhoea and rectal bleeding. Following treatment with metronidazole the symptoms resolved and RS could not be detected in rectal biopsies taken some two months later. They suggested that spirochaetosis may be a readily treatable cause of acute diarrhoea or rectal bleeding, but as the anti-organismal effects of metronidazole cover a wide spectrum of species it is difficult to reach a definite conclusion. Gilmour & McMillan (1984) (unpublished data) were unable to confirm the association between the presence of RS and gastro-intestinal symptoms in homosexual men. When patients with some known intestinal disorder were excluded from consideration, symptoms were not more frequent in patients with RS than in those without: histologically, however, it was found that numbers of lymphocytes and plasma cells in the lamina propria were significantly more frequently increased in men with RS than in those without. Electron microscope studies (Takeuchi et al, 1974) have shown that the treponemes and flagellates are embedded side by side in the brush border of the colonic epithelial cells. Rarely the organisms are found in the cytoplasm of the cells, either enclosed by a single membrane or in an autophagic vesicle. They have been found also in the lamina propria (usually contained within macrophages) and in the cytoplasm of the Schwann cells of the unmyelinated nerves of the lamina propria (Antonakopoulos et al, 1982). The columnar cells appeared unaltered by the organisms and an inflammatory response was not found in the lamina propria. The inflammatory reaction seen in the rectal mucosa of Gilmour & McMillan's patients may, however, have been caused by some other undetected infection and the presence of RS may have been coincidental.

Further studies, in which microbiological and histological findings are compared, may lead to a better understanding of the condition of RS in homosexual men.

Chlamydia trachomatis
By micro-immunofluorescence, isolates of *C. trachomatis* can be separated into 15 serotypes. Serotypes D, E, F, G, H, I and J are associated with genital infection and paratrachoma and L_1, L_2 and L_3 with lymphogranuloma venereum. Although chlamydial infection is established as an important cause of non-gonococcal urethritis in the heterosexual male, there are conflicting data on their role in the aetiology of NGU in the homosexual men (Table 15.2). Although Bowie et al (1978) and Stamm (1984) cultured chlamydiae from the urethras of homosexual men less frequently than from those of heterosexual men with urethritis, the isolation rates reported by Oriel et al (1976) were similar. Munday et al (1981b) did not detail prevalence of chlamydiae from the urethras of homo- and heterosexual men with non-gonococcal urethritis, but stated that there was no significant difference in isolation rates between

these groups of patients. However, using a micro immunfluorescent antibody method with L_2 as antigen, Munday et al (1981b) detected IgG chlamydial antibody in the sera of 26% of 146 homosexual men. This finding was similar to that of Quinn et al (1981) who found antichlamydial IgG in the sera of 27% of 173 homosexual men, and contrasts with the higher prevalence (about 60%) of serum chlamydial antibody in a venereal diseases clinic population (Wang et al, 1977). The data presented by Stamm (1984) on the prevalence of antichlamydial antibodies in the sera of homosexual (52% of 114) and heterosexual patients (46% of 329) indicate that chlamydial infection of both groups of men is equally common. Because of the disparity between the urethral isolation rates and the presence of serum chlamydial antibodies, he concludes

Table 15.2 Isolation rates of Chlamydia trachomatis from the urethras of homosexual and heterosexual men with gonococcal and non-gonococcal urethritis

Sexual Orientation	Type of urethritis	Isolation rate	Reference
Heterosexual men	Gonococcal	30/118 (25.4%)	Oriel et al, 1976
		22/95 (23.2%)	Bowie et al, 1978
	Non-gonococcal	118/240 (49.2%)	Oriel et al, 1976
	Undefined	46/329 (14.0%)	Stamm 1984
Homosexual men	Gonococcal	5/23 (21.9%)	Oriel et al, 1976
		0/18 (0.0%)	Bowie et al, 1978
	Non-gonococcal	7/22 (31.8%)	Oriel et al, 1976
	Undefined	6/114 (5.3%)	Stamm 1984

that homosexual men acquire these antibodies from infections at areas of their body other than the urethra, the rectum being the most likely site. However careful prospective case-control studies with sampling from possibly-infected mucous membranes will be required before this hypothesis can be accepted.

Goldmeier & Darougar (1977) isolated *C. trachomatis* of undertermined serotypes from the rectums of two asymptomatic homosexual men, one of whom had a congested rectal mucosa containing many follicles when viewed with the operating microscope. Chlamydiae were cultured from the rectums of 4% of 150 homosexual men who attended an STD clinic in Glasgow (McMillan et al 1981); none of these men had ano-rectal symptoms but one patient was a sexual contact of a male with chlamydial urethritis. Two patients had concomitant gonococcal rectal infection. In a series of 180 homosexual men who consecutively attended a London clinic Munday et al (1981a) recovered chlamydiae (again, as in McMillan's study (1981) of undetermined serotype) from the rectums of 10 (5.6%); four of these patients had concomitant rectal gonorrhoea; of the other six men, three had no anorectal symptoms and three had clinical features of proctitis. The prevalence of *C. trachomatis* associated non-gonococcal proctitis was three of 51. From these studies it appeared that chlamydial proctitis was uncommon and that many individuals with chlamydial infection of the rectum had no symptoms or abnormal physical signs. Quinn et al (1981) working in Seattle investigated a group of 96 homosexual men who had symptoms suggestive of proctitis — anorectal pain and/or anal discharge, anorectal bleeding or a change in bowel habit — and compared the findings with a group of 75 homosexual men who attended the same clinic during the study period. *Chlamydia trachomatis* was isolated from the rectums of 14 (11.5%) of the 96 men with proctitis but from only 4% of the asymptomatic patients. Three of the 11 chlamydial isolates which had been typed were of serotype

L_2. These patients, one of whom had a concomitant Campylobacter infection, had more severe proctitis, with systemic symptoms, in comparison with those from whom non LGV serotypes had been cultured.

In this study (Quinn et al 1981), the inflammatory changes in the rectal mucosa of men from whom non-LGV serotypes of *C. trachomatis* were isolated were generally mild and confined to within 6 cm of the dentate line. Moderate leucocyte infiltration of the lamina propria with, in one case, crypt abscess formation was found in only two men, both of whom had concomitant rectal infection — one with *N. gonorrhoeae* the other with *E. histolytica*. Mild proctitis is a common finding in rectal biopsies taken from homosexual men in whom specific anorectal infection has not been detected (McMillan & Lee, 1981). The use of controls is essential if conclusions are to be made regarding the pathogenicity of oculogenital serotypes of chlamydiae, or, indeed, of any organisms isolated from the rectum.

In general, rectal infection with LGV serotypes of *C. trachomatis* is thought to be associated with severe proctitis, although this is often limited to within 12 cm of the dentate line (Geller et al, 1980; Levine et al, 1980; Quinn et al, 1981; Bolan et al, 1982; Mindel, 1983). As the prevalence of rectal LGV chlamydial serotypes in asymptomatic homosexual men is unknown and as several of the reported patients have had other concomitant infections it is difficult, as with the other organisms discussed, to ascribe with certainty an aetiological role for this organism.

The rectal mucosa from men infected with LGV serotypes of *C. trachomatis* always shows a diffuse infiltration of the lamina propria with neutrophils, plasma cells and lymphocytes. Crypt abscesses and the formation of granulomas with multinucleate giant cells are common, giving a histological pattern closely resembling that of Crohn's disease (Geller et al, 1980; Quinn et al, 1981; Mindel, 1983).

The serological diagnosis of chlamydial infection of the rectum has presented diffi-culties. Using a micro IF test Schachter (1981) demonstrated chlamydial IgG antibodies at titres of more than 1000 in the sera of 18 homosexual men with proctitis, from six of whom *C. trachomatis* was isolated. Two isolates were LGV type L_2, the other four were non-LGV serotypes (two DE, two not typed). Also, he noted that the IgG was broadly reactive. In this study, IgM antibodies were found in the sera of 18 of 24 men with presumed LGV. Using a similar fluorescent antibody test, Quinn et al (1981) found broadly reactive IgG antibodies at high titre (>512) in the sera of three men with LGV serotype associated proctitis, but low titre (<128) antibody in the acute phase sera from three of six men with non-LGV serotype rectal chlamydial infection. Paired serum samples showed a fourfold rise in antibody titre in four of these six patients. Serum IgM antibody was found in only one of 12 men from whose rectums chlamydiae had been isolated; that patient was infected with a non-LGV serotype. The discrepancy between the results obtained by Schachter and Quinn is difficult to explain. It is possible that Schachter examined sera from patients with earlier infection than those investigated by Quinn. However, antichlamydial IgM antibodies persist in the sera from one to five months (Wang et al, 1977) and this seems an unlikely explanation: variation in the antigen used in the micro IF test seems more likely.

Titres of >16 in the lymphogranuloma venereum complement fixation test (LGVCFT) are generally regarded as positive (Phillip et al, 1971). However, Schachter (1981) found complement fixing antibodies at a titre of >16 in the sera of four men with non-LGV chlamydial infection of the rectum. This finding clearly raises doubts as to the diagnostic value of the LGVCFT in patients with proctitis.

The best treatment of patients with proctitis associated with chlamydiae is clearly a difficult question to answer unequivocally. Tetracycline, 500 mg by mouth every eight hours for two to three weeks, proved effective in the elimination of the organism and in the resolution of the proctitis in the 14 patients treated by Quinn et al (1981) and in the cases reported by Geller et al (1980); Bolan et al (1982); and Mindel (1983). Doxycycline in an oral dose of 100 mg every 12 hours was effective in one patient (Bolan et al, 1982).

Mycoplasma hominis and ureaplasma urealyticum

The role of these organisms in the aetiology of non-gonococcal urethritis is uncertain; the subject has been well reviewed by Robertson, McMillan, Young (1980). Few studies comment on differences in isolation rates between homo- and heterosexual men. Bowie et al (1978) isolated *U. urealyticum* from the urethras of seven of 18 homosexual and 35 of 95 heterosexual men with untreated urethral gonorrhoea. Munday et al (1981a) cultured *U. urealyticum* and *M. hominis* equally often (41 and 39% respectively) from rectal material from 49 men with non-gonococcal proctitis, and cultured the organisms equally often (28%) from men without evidence of proctitis. Similarly Quinn et al (1983) found no difference in the isolation rates of *M. hominis* and *U. urealyticum* between men with proctitis and asymptomatic patients. It is difficult to believe that these organisms play any prominent role in the aetiology of proctitis.

Herpes simplex virus (HSV)

In any discussion of anogenital HSV infection, the terminology adopted should be clearly stated. Here the term *primary* infection is used for an acute one which may remain localised or become generalised; an *initial* infection is the first clinically obvious one occurring in an individual who has serum herpes antibodies; virus can be 'reawakened' from the nerve cells and initiate a peripheral lesion (*recrudescence*) or pass to a peripheral site and multiply without producing lesions (*recurrence*); from these latter cases HSV can be cultured (Wildy, Field, Nash, 1982).

The clinical features of primary perianal herpes are well documented, but there have been few reports on proctitis associated with HSV and most of these have concerned primary infections. Goldmeier et al 1975 recorded two cases of perianal herpes (one with HSV Type 1 and the other with Type 2) associated with acute urinary retention and intestinal obstruction. In both cases there was diffuse proctitis; no other pathogenic microorganisms were identified. Waugh (1976) described 13 men with anal herpes; five were described as having proctitis on naked-eye assessment. Samarasinghe et al (1979) described 11 homosexual men with anorectal herpes (HSV was isolated from seven men) associated with presumed sacral radiculomyelopathy. Proctitis of variable severity was noted in each patient, but frank ulceration of the rectum was found in only four men. Within 21 days the symptoms had resolved spontaneously, but HSV was still being excreted by one man.

Curry et al (1978) reported a case of herpetic proctitis (HSV Type 2) in a young homosexual man. They found that the proctitis, with severe ulcerative and haemorrhagic lesions, was confined to the distal 15 cm of the rectum, the most pronounced changes being within 4 cm of the anal margin: a rectal biopsy of affected mucosa showed an acute infective proctitis pattern.

Goldmeier (1980) investigated the prevalence of HSV infection in homosexual men who had had recent anal intercourse and who consecutively attended an STD clinic in London. A diagnosis of proctitis was made on the basis of the operating microscope appearance. HSV was cultured from rectal material from five (6%) of 77 men with non-gonococcal proctitis, but from none of the other men; two of the three isolates which were typed were of HSV type 1. Similar findings were reported by Munday et al (1981a) who cultured HSV (untyped) from the rectum of one (2%) of 46 men with non-gonococcal proctitis (as defined by clinical features and Gram-stained smear microscopy) and from two of 24 men with rectal gonorrhoea; HSV was isolated from three of 85 asymptomatic homosexual men who attended during the same study period. Both groups of workers concluded that HSV was an uncommon cause of proctitis in homosexual men.

Markedly different results were obtained by Goodell et al (1983) working in Seattle. They isolated HSV (all Type 2) from rectal material from 23 of 102 men who consecutively attended an STD clinic on account of symptoms of proctitis; eight of these men had some concomitant rectal infection. HSV was cultured from the rectums of three of 75 asymptomatic men; as judged by serological testing, one man had a primary and the other two men recurrent infections. Goodell et al (1983) reported the clinical and histological features of their patients with HSV infection. Anorectal pain, tenesmus, constipation, pruritus ani, neurological symptoms, fever, perianal lesions and inguinal lymphadenitis were more commonly found in patients with rectal herpes than in men with proctitis caused by other organisms. In most cases (eight of 10 men from whose rectums only HSV was isolated) the inflammatory changes were confined to the distal 10 cm of the rectum; diffuse ulceration of the distal rectum was found in four of these 10 men. Histologically, the pattern was that of an acute infective proctitis, with the additional features of multinucleated cells, intranuclear inclusions and perivascular cuffing of submucosal blood vessels. The histology of the rectum was normal in only one of 10 men.

An interesting case of herpetic proctitis associated with meningitis in a 24-year-old homosexual man was reported by Heller et al (1982). They isolated HSV types 1 and 2 from rectal material and, as judged by restriction endonuclease analysis, two different isolates of HSV1 from the cerebrospinal fluid, one of which was identical to the HSV1 rectal isolate.

Shigella spp and Campylobacter spp

Sporadic cases of infections with these organisms in homosexual men have been reported (Drusin et al, 1976; Carey & Wright, 1979; Quinn et al, 1980). In Seattle Quinn et al (1984) isolated *C. jejuni* from the faeces of 6% of 158 homosexual men with symptoms of proctitis or proctocolitis, from 3% of 75 asymptomatic homosexual men and from none of 150 heterosexual men and women. These findings differ from those of Simmons & Tabaqchali (1979) who did not isolate *Campylobacter* spp from the rectal material of 50 homosexual men who attended a London STD clinic. In a seroepidemiological study of patients attending a sexually transmitted disease clinic, McMillan et al (1984b) found antibodies against *C. jejuni* in the sera of 10% of 187 homosexual and 9% of 169 heterosexual men. Although the prevalence of antibody in both groups of men was similar, it was higher than in a group of women who attended an antenatal clinic in the same city.

Infection with species of *Shigella* and *Campylobacter* may be associated with a self-limiting diarrhoeal illness. As the disease process is not confined to the rectum, at sigmoidoscopy the inflammatory changes in the rectum are seen to continue into the sigmoid colon. In the acute phase of the illness, rectal biopsy specimens show the typical but non-specific changes of infective proctitis with a predominantly poly-morphonuclear leucocyte infiltration of the mucosa (Morson, 1974; Lambert et al, 1979). The diagnosis of proctocolitis associated with these bacteria rests on the isolation of the organism from the faeces or, in the case of campylobacter infection, by the demonstration of a significant change in antibody titre in acute and convalescent sera (Watson & Kerr, 1982).

Quinn et al (1983) isolated Campylobacter-like organisms from rectal material from homosexual men. These were motile, microaerophilic, Gram negative curved rods which, like known *Campylobacter* spp, were oxidase and catalase positive and did not utilise glucose. However, several other biochemical requirements distinguished them from other Campylobacter species (Fennell et al, 1984). Campylobacter-like organisms were cultured from rectal exudate of 26 of 158 men with proctocolitis and six of 75 asymptomatic men who attended a sexually transmitted diseases clinic (Quinn et al, 1984): 69% of symptomatic men had concomitant gastrointestinal infec-tions. Six of the eight men with only Campylobacter-like infection had symptoms of proctitis and proctocolitis; the sigmoidoscopic appearance of the rectal mucosa was abnormal in four of six men and in three the inflammatory changes continued into the sigmoid colon. Histologically, the mucosa showed a non-specific infective proctitis pattern. By immunofluorescence, antibody against the homologous isolate of Campylobacter-like organism was found in the sera of 15 of 25 infected men; a significant rise in titre of antibody, or the presence of IgM against the infecting strain was found in the paired sera of six of 12 men. This study strongly supports the hypothesis that Campylobacter-like organisms can be pathogenic. Further preva-lent data are needed to assess the extent of such infection in the homo- and heterosexual community.

Enterovirus
Echovirus 11 was demonstrated in the faeces of three of 119 homosexual men with proctitis and of one of 75 asymptomatic homosexuals (Quinn et al, 1983). The signifi-cance of this finding is not clear.

Entamoeba histolytica
The sexual transmission of *E. histolytica* amongst homosexual men is now well docu-mented (Felman & Ricciardi, 1979). However, although there have been several reports on its prevalence in men attending sexually transmitted diseases clinics, most studies have been incomplete for a variety of reasons (Editorial, Lancet 1981) and the data presented must be considered carefully before conclusions can be drawn.

Phillips et al (1981) in New York City demonstrated *E. histolytica* in the faeces of 10 of 51 homosexual men, one of 48 bisexual men and none of 64 heterosexual men; they showed a significant relationship between the presence of protozoa and the practice of oral-anal sexual intercourse. Ortega et al (1984) found *E. histolytica* in the stools of 36% of 150 homosexual men who attended a private practice in San Francisco. In homosexual males attending STD clinics in London and in Edinburgh, cysts of *E. histolytica* were found in the faeces of 12% of 83 men and 14% of 345 men respectively (Chin & Gerken, 1984; McMillan & McNeillage, 1984a).

For many years it has been known that many individuals who excrete cysts of *E. histolytica* in their stools have no symptoms referrable to the gastro-intestinal tract, and the existence of virulent or avirulent strains of the amoeba is recognised. However, the conditions responsible for pathogenicity in man have not been resolved. Recently McGowan et al (1982) have isolated a heat-labile cytotoxin from axenically cultured strains of *E. histolytica* which are considered virulent on the basis of the production of liver abscesses in hamsters; avirulent strains did not possess this cytotoxin. The relevance of this finding to human amoebiasis awaits further investigation.

Sargeaunt et al (1980) have analysed the electrophoretic patterns of four enzymes produced by *E. histolytica*; glucose phosphate isomerase, phosphoglucomutase, L-malate NADP + oxidoreductase and hexokinase. They were able to classify isolates of *E. histolytica* into 18 groups (zymodemes) on the basis of their isoenzyme pattern. From a consideration of the reports of clinical features, Sargeaunt et al (1982) thought that only amoebae with certain zymodemes were pathogenic. The isoenzyme patterns of *E. histolytica* isolated from the faeces of 52 homosexual men in London were determined and shown to be types not considered to be associated with pathogenicity (Sargeaunt et al, 1983). This view was challenged by McMillan et al (1984c) who analysed the clinical and rectal biopsy findings in 35 homosexual men with *E. histolytica* infection; 18 isolates were examined electrophoretically and shown to be of zymodeme types also not considered to be pathogenic. Clinical and histological findings were compared with those of a group of 35 non-infected homosexual men. Although the prevalence of gastro-intestinal symptoms was similar in both groups of patients, the histology of the rectal mucosa was abnormal in 17 (63.0%) of the 27 men with amoebic infection only and in two (7.4%) of the 27 control subjects, a highly significant difference. As amoebae were not observed in tissue sections and as antibodies reactive with *E. histolytica* were not detected in the patients' sera it is unlikely that tissue invasion had occurred. Burnham et al (1980) reported a case of amoebiasis with tissue invasion in a young homosexual man who had probably acquired his infection in England; unfortunately the zymodeme type of the amoeba was not determined and other causes of rectal ulceration had not been excluded. Interestingly, the occurrence in a homosexual man of a hepatic amoebic abscess has been reported (Thompson et al, 1983); the zymodeme type was not determined.

This is a great variation in the response of the rectum to infection with *E. histolytica* and the histopathology of intestinal amoebiasis has been well reviewed by Prathap & Gilman (1970). In many cases the histological changes are non-specific, and amoebae can be demonstrated in tissue sections in only some 50–60% of patients. The characteristic amoebic ulceration is seldom found on sigmoidoscopy in homosexual men with *E. histolytica* infection; most commonly there is a diffuse proctitis extending into the sigmoid colon.

The diagnosis of amoebiasis rests with the demonstration of (1) trophozoites in saline mount and/or stained smear proportions of faeces (2) cysts, concentated from faeces by the formol ether method, and (3) culture of the organism in Robinson's medium. McMillan & McNeillage (1984a) have compared the sensitivity of these methods and have shown the value of culture in the routine examination of faeces for *E. histolytica*: nine of 48 infected men would not have been identified if culture had not been undertaken. Although of value in invasive amoebiasis and in epidemiological studies, serological tests are of limited value in the diagnosis of intestinal disease (Ambroise-Thomas, 1980).

Cryptosporidium spp

Cryptosporidia are coccidian parasites which can infect man and other species of mammals, birds and reptiles (Angus, 1983). The various stages of the life cycle of the organism take place within the epithelial cells of the small and large intestine and occasionally the biliary and respiratory tracts; oocysts are excreted in the faeces and can be transmitted to members of the same or other species by the faecal-oral route (Current et al, 1983). Infection of immunocompetent individuals with *Cryptosporidium* spp is associated with self-limiting diarrhoeal illness, usually with fever lasting for one to 11 days with excretion of oocysts for a similar or slightly longer period (Anderson et al, 1982; Current et al, 1983). The importance of the organism in the aetiology of diarrhoea in different populations is not known with any degree of certainty. Jokipii et al (1983) from Finland detected oocysts in 9.1% of 1545 stool specimens submitted for examination from patients with gastro-intestinal symptoms. Casemore & Jackson (1983) working in Rhyl, Wales, found cryptosporidia in seven (1.4%) of 500 faecal samples from patients with diarrhoea; five of these infected patients were under 11 years of age. In a study of Liberian children aged five years and under 22 (7.9%) of 278 diarrhoeal stools contained cryptosporidia. McMillan & McNeillage (1984a) did not demonstrate cryptosporidia in any of the stools of 130 men (85 of whom were homosexual), who attended an STD clinic in Edinburgh.

In contrast to the self-limiting infection in otherwise healthy individuals, cryptosporidia produce severe persistent gastro-intestinal disease in patients with humoral or cellular immunodeficiency, including the acquired immunodeficiency syndrome (Lasser et al, 1979); Soave et al, 1984).

Histologically, non-specific inflammatory changes are found within the lamina propria of the small intestine, colon and rectum (Nime et al, 1976; Lasser et al, 1979). In tissue sections cryptosporidia appear on the epithelial surface of the lumen and crypts as small (2–3 µm) round or oval nucleated bodies which are basophilic on staining by Giemsa's method (Bird & Smith, 1980). The organisms are most numerous in the jejunum. Electron microscope studies of biopsy specimens show clearly the various stages in the life cycle of the coccidian (Bird & Smith, 1980). The diagnosis of cryptosporidiosis is made by (1) finding the oocysts in faecal smears stained by a modified Ziehl-Neelsen or Safranin stain (Henriksen & Pohlenz, 1981; Baxby & Blundell, 1983) (2) the demonstration of oocysts concentrated from faeces by Sheather's method (Ma & Soave, 1983) (3) the detection of stages of the life cycle of the organism in biopsy specimens, preferably jejunal.

Cryptosporidiosis in immunocompetent individuals is self-limiting, and treatment is not indicated and in the immunocompromised there is no known effective specific therapy yet and treatment is not indicated.

Strongyloides stercoralis

Strongyloides is a helminth which can be transmitted by the faecal-oral route. Rhabditiform larvae may metamorphose in the gut or in the perianal skin to filariform (infective) larvae which may infect partners during oral-anal sexual contact. Phillips et al (1981) detected *Strongyloides* in the faeces of two of 51 homosexual men who attended a sexually transmitted diseases clinic and Sorvillo et al (1983) reported the probable sexual transmission of the helminth. Although the larvae most commonly infect the upper intestine, the rectum may be involved. The larvae penetrate the submucosa and induce a chronic inflammatory cell reaction with eosinophilic infiltration (Carvalho-Filho, 1978).

Overwhelming infection may occur in immunocompromised individuals, producing massive invasion of the GI tract and lungs and extensive invasion of other organs such as the heart, adrenals and CNS (Scowden et al, 1978). The diagnosis of strongyloidiosis is made by the detection of larvae in stool samples by microscopy after concentration or by culture (Garcia & Ash, 1979).

Cytomegalovirus (CMV)
CMV has been documented as a cause of colitis in men with the acquired immune deficiency syndrome (Tapper et al, 1984). Intranuclear and intracytoplasmic inclusion bodies may be found within the cells of colonic or rectal biopsies in such cases.

Non-specific proctitis
Despite careful and extensive microbiological examination of rectal material or faeces and serological investigation for recognised pathogens there remains a group of homosexual patients with clinical and histological evidence of proctitis — so-called non-specific proctitis. McMillan & Lee (1981) could not detect pathogenic infection in 15 of 29 men with proctitis diagnosed histologically. Quinn et al (1983) in a more extensive investigation of 119 men with symptomatic proctitis found no organismal cause in 20%.

Undoubtedly many cases of so-called non-specific proctitis are caused by organisms which for a variety of reasons have not been identified. Trauma (Weinstein et al, 1981) and the use of enemas (see above) may also contribute to the development of proctitis in homosexual men. Many homosexual men suffer from repeated infections for which antibiotics are indicated. The use of these agents may themselves be associated with proctocolitis of varying severity (Price & Davies, 1977). In most cases non-specific proctitis is a self-limiting condition (Gilmour & McMillan — unpublished observations); the inflammatory changes resolve over a period of several weeks, as described by Kumar et al (1982).

REFERENCES

Adler M W 1978 Diagnostic, treatment, and reporting criteria for non-specific genital infection in sexually transmitted disease clinics in England and Wales. 1: Diagnosis. British Journal of Venereal Diseases 54: 422–427

Akdamar K, Martin R J, Ichinose H 1977 Syphilitic proctitis. Digestive Diseases 22: 701–704

Ambroise-Thomas P 1980 Amoebiasis and other protozoal diseases (ed) Houba V. Immunological investigation of tropical parasitic diseases. Churchill Livingstone, Edinburgh, p 75–83

Anderson B C, Donndelinger T, Wilkins R M, Smith J 1982 Cryptosporidiosis in a veterinary student. Journal of the American Veterinary Medical Association 180: 408–409

Angus K W 1983 Cryptosporidiosis in man domestic animals and birds: a review Journal of the Royal Society of Medicine 76: 62–70

Antonakopoulos G, Newman J, Wilkinson M 1982 Intestinal spirochaetosis: an electron microscopic study of an unusual case. Histopathology 6: 477–88

Baron J H, Connell A M, Lennard-Jones J E, 1964 Variation between observers in describing mucosal appearances in proctocolitis. British Medical Journal i: 89–92

Baxby D, Blundell N 1983 Sensitive, rapid, simple methods of detecting Cryptosporidium in faeces. Lancet ii: 1149

Bird R G, Smith M D 1980 Cryptosporidiosis in man: parasite life cycle and fine structural pathology. Journal of Pathology 132: 217–233

Bolan R K, Sands M, Schachter J, Miner R C, Drew W L 1982 Lymphogranuloma venereum and acute ulcerative proctitis. American Journal of Medicine 72: 703–706

Bowie W R, Alexander F R, Holmes K K 1978 Etiologies of post gonococcal urethritis in homosexual and heterosexual men: roles of Chlamydia trachomatis and Ureaplasma urealyticum. Sexually Transmitted Diseases 5: 151–154

Burnham W R, Reeve R S, Finch R G 1980. Entamoeba histolytica infection in male homosexuals. Gut 21: 1097–1099

Carey P B, Wright E P, 1979 Campylobacter jejuni in a male homosexual. British Journal of Venereal Diseases 55: 380

Carlson B L, Fiumara N J, Kelly J R, McCormack W M 1980 Isolation of *Neisseria meningitidis* from anogenital specimens from homosexual men. Sexually Transmitted Diseases 7: 71–73

Carvalho-Filho E 1978 Strongyloidiasis. Clinics in Gastroenterology 7: 179–188

Casemore D P, Jackson B 1983 Sporadic cryptosporidiosis in children. Lancet ii: 679

Chin A T L, Gerkean A 1984 Carriage of intestinal protozoal cysts in homosexuals. British Journal of Venereal Diseases 60: 193–195

Current W L, Reese N C, Ernst J V, Bailey W S, Heyman M B, Weinstein W M 1983 Human cryptosporidiosis in immunocompetent and immunodeficient persons. New England Journal of Medicine 308: 1252–1257

Curry J P, Embil J A, Williams C N, Manuel F R 1978. Proctitis associated with *Herpesvirus hominis* Type 2 infection. Canadian Medical Association Journal 119: 485–486

Day D W, Mandal B K, Morson B C 1978 The rectal biopsy appearances in Salmonella colitis. Histopathology 2: 117–131

Deheragoda P 1977 Diagnosis of rectal gonorrhoea by blind anorectal swabs compared with direct vision swabs taken via a proctoscope. British Journal of Venereal Diseases 53: 311–313

Dickinson R J, Gilmour H M, McClelland D B L 1979 Rectal biopsy in patients presenting to an infectious disease unit with diarrhoeal disease. Gut 20: 141–148

Douglas J G, Crucioli V 1981 Spirochaetosis: a remediable cause of diarrhoea and rectal bleeding? British Medical Journal 283: 1362

Drusin L M, Genvert G, Tofj-Olstein B, Levy-Zombek E 1976 Shigellosis: another sexually transmitted disease? British Journal of Venereal Diseases 52: 348–350

Drusin L M, Singer C, Valenti A J, Armstrong D 1977 Infectious syphilis mimicking neoplastic disease. Archives of Internal Medicine 137: 156–160

Editorial 1981 Sexual transmission of enteric pathogens. Lancet ii: 1328–1329

Felman Y M, Ricciardi N B, 1979 Sexually transmitted enteric diseases. Bulletin of the New York Academy of Medicine 55: 533–539

Fennell C L, Totten P A, Quinn T C, Patton D L, Holmes K K, Stamm W E 1984 Characterization of Campylobacter-like organisms isolated from homosexual men. Journal of Infectious Diseases 149: 58–66

Fluker J L, Deheragoda P, Platt D, Gerken A 1980 Rectal gonorrhoea in male homosexuals: presentation and therapy. British Journal of Venereal Diseases 56: 397–399

Garcia L S, Ash L R 1979 Diagnostic Parasitology Clinical Laboratory Manual C V Mosby Company, St. Louis

Geller S A, Zimmerman M J, Cohen A 1980 Rectal biopsy in early lymphogranuloma venereum proctitis. American Journal of Gastroenterology 74: 433–435

Gluckman J B, Kleinman M S, May A G 1974 Primary syphilis of rectum. New York State Journal of Medicine 74: 2210–2211

Goldmeier D, Bateman J R M, Rodin P 1975 Urinary retention and intestinal obstruction associated with anorectal Herpes simplex virus infection. British Medical Journal 1: 425

Goldmeier D, Darougar S 1977 Isolation of *Chlamydia trachomatis* from throat and rectum of homosexual men. British Journal of Venereal Diseases 53: 184–185

Goldmeier D 1980 Proctitis and Herpes simplex virus in homosexual men. British Journal of Venereal Diseases 56: 111–114

Goodell S E, Quinn T C, Mkrtichian E et al 1983 Herpes simplex virus proctitis in homosexual men. Clinical, sigmoidoscopic and histopathological features. New England Journal of Medicine 308: 868–871

Harkness A H 1948 Anorectal gonorrhoea. Proceedings of the Royal Society of Medicine 41: 476–478

Harland W A, Lee F D 1967 Intestinal spirochaetosis. British Medical Journal 3: 718–719

Heller M, Dix R D, Baringer J R, Schachter J, Conte J E 1982 Herpetic proctitis and meningitis: recovery of two strains of herpes simplex virus type 1 from cerebrospinal fluid. Journal of Infectious Diseases 146: 584–588

Henriksen S A, Pohlenz J F L 1981 Staining of cryptosporidia by a modified Ziehl-Neelsen technique. Acta Veterinaria Scandanavica 22: 594–596

Højlyng N, Mølbak K, Jepsen S, Hansson A P 1984 Cryptosporidiosis in Liberian children. Lancet i: 734

Hovind-Hougen K, Birch-Andersen A, Henrik-Nielsen R et al 1982 Intestinal spirochetosis: morphological characterization and cultivation of the spirochete *Brachyspira aalborgi* gen. nov, sp. nov. Journal of Clinical Microbiology 16: 1127–1136

Janda W M, Bohnhoff M, Morello J A, Lerner S A 1980 Prevalence and site-pathogen studies of *Neisseria meningitidis* and *N. gonorrhoeae* in homosexual men. Journal of the American Medical Association 244: 2060–2604

Jokipii L, Pohjola S, Jokipii A M M 1983 Cryptosporidium: a frequent finding in patients with gastrointestinal symptoms. Lancet ii 358–361

Judson F N, Ehret J M, Eickhoff T C 1978 Anogenital infection with Neisseria meningitidis in homosexual men. Journal of Infectious Diseases 137: 458–463

Kaplan L R, Takeuchi A 1979 Purulent rectal discharge associated with a nontreponemal spirochete. Journal of the American Medical Association 241: 52–3

Kreutzer E, Hansbrough J 1979 Superimposed traumatic and gonococcal proctitis: report of two cases. Sexually Transmitted Diseases 6: 75–76

Kumar N B, Nostrant T T, Appelman H D 1982 The histopathologic spectrum of acute self-limited colitis (acute infectious type colitis). American Journal of Surgical Pathology 6: 523–529

Lambert M E, Schofield P F, Ironside A G, Mandal B K 1979 Campylobacter colitis British Medical Journal 1: 857–859

Lasser K H, Lewin K J, Ryning F W 1979 Cryptosporidial enteritis in a patient with congenital hypogammaglobulinaemia. Human Pathology 10: 234–240

Lebedeff D A, Hochman E B 1980 Rectal gonorrhea in men: diagnosis and treatment. Annals of Internal Medicine 92: 463–466

Lee F D, Kraszewski A, Gordon J, Howie J G R, McSweveney D, Harland W A 1971 Intestinal spirochaetosis. Gut 12: 126–133

Levine J S, Saeed M 1979 Herpes virus hominis type 1 proctitis. Journal of Clinical Gastroenterology 1: 225–227

Levine J S, Smith P D, Brugge W R 1980 Chronic proctitis in male homosexuals due to lymphogranuloma venereum. Gastroenterology 79: 563–565

Ma, P, Soave R 1983 Three step stool examination for cryptospridiosis in 10 homosexual men with protracted watery diarrhea. Journal of Infectious Diseases 147: 824–828

Mandal B K, Schofield P F, Morson B C 1982 A clinicopathological study of acute colitis: the dilemma of transient colitis syndrome. Scandanavian Journal of Gastroenterology 17: 865–869

Marino A W M 1964 Proctologic lesions observed in male homosexuals. Diseases of the colon and rectum 7: 121–128

McGowan K, Deneke C F, Thorne G M, Gorbach S L 1982 Entamoeba hystolitica cytotoxin: purification, characterization, strain virulence and protease activity. Journal of Infectious Diseases 146: 616–625

McMillan A, Young H 1978 Gonorrhea in the homosexual man: frequency of infection by culture site. Sexually Transmitted Diseases 5: 146–150

McMillan A, Lee F D 1981 Sigmoidoscopic and microscopic appearance of the rectal mucosa in homosexual men. Gut 22: 1035–1041

McMillan A, Sommerville R G, McKie P M K 1981 Chlamydial infection in homosexual men: frequency of isolation of *Chlamydia trachomatis* from the urethra, anorectum and pharynx. British Journal of Venereal Diseases 57: 47–49

McMillan A, Gilmour H M, Slatford K, McNeillage G J C 1983a Proctitis in homosexual men. A diagnositic problem. British Journal of Venereal Diseases 59: 260–264

McMillan A, McNeillage G, Gilmour H M, Lee F D 1983b The histology of rectal gonorrhoea in men with a note on anorectal infection with *Neisseria meningitidis*. Journal of Clinical Pathology 36: 511–514

McMillan A, McNeillage G J C, 1984a Comparison of the sensitivity of microscopy and culture in the laboratory diagnosis of intestinal protozoal infection. Journal of Clinical Pathology 37: 809–811

McMillan A, McNeillage G J C, Watson K C 1984b The prevalence of antibodies reactive with *Camphylobacter jejuni* in the serum of homosexual men. Journal of Infection 9: 63–68

McMillan A, Gilmour H M, McNeillage G J C, Scott G R 1984c Amoebiasis in homosexual men. Gut 25: 356–360

Meisel J L, Bergman D, Graney D, Saunders D R, Rubin I E 1977 Human rectal mucosa: proctoscopic and morphological changes caused by laxatives. Gastroenterology 72: 1274–1279

Mindel A, 1983 Lymphogranuloma venereum of the rectum in a homosexual man British Journal of Venereal Diseases 59: 196–197

Morson B C, 1974 The technique and interpretation of rectal biopsies in inflammatory bowel disease (ed) Sommers S C, Pathology Annual Appleton — Century — Crofts New York 209–230

Munday P E, Dawson S G, Johnson A P et al 1981a A microbiological study of non-gonococcal proctitis in passive male homosexuals. Postgraduate Medical Journal 57: 705–711

Munday P E, Thomas B J, Johnson A P, Altman D G, Taylor-Robinson D 1981b Clinical and microbiological study of non-gonococcal urethritis with particular reference to non-chlamydial disease. British Journal of Venereal Diseases 57: 327–333

Nazemi M M, Musher D M, Schell R F, Milo S 1975 Syphilitic proctitis in a homosexual. Journal of the American Medical Association 231: 389

Nime F A, Burek J D, Page D L, Holscher M A, Yardley J H 1976 Acute enterocolitis in a human being infected with the protozoan cryptosporidium. Gastroenterology 70: 592–598

Oriel J D, Reeve P, Wright J T, Owen J 1976 Chlamydial infection of the male urethra. British Journal of Venereal Diseases 52: 46–51

Ortega H B, Borchardt K A, Hamilton R, Ortega P, Mahood J 1984 Enteric pathogenic protozoa in homosexual men from San Francisco. Sexually Transmitted Diseases 11: 59–63

Parr L W Intestinal spirochetes 1923 Journal of Infectious Diseases 33: 369–83

Philip N W, Hill D A, Greaves A B et al 1971 Study of Chlamydiae in patients with lymphogranuloma venereum and urethritis attending a venereal diseases clinic. British Journal of Venereal Diseases 47: 114–121

Phillips S C, Mildvan D, William D C, Celb A M, White M C 1981 Sexual transmission of enteric protozoa and helminths in a venereal diseases clinic population. New England Journal of Medicine 305: 603–606

Prathap K, Gilman R 1970 The histopathology of acute intestinal amebiasis. A rectal biopsy study. American Journal of Pathology 60: 229–239

Price A B, Davies D R 1977 Pseudomembranous colitis. Gut 30: 1–12

Quinn T C, Corey L, Chaffee R G, Schuffler M D, Holmes K K 1980 Campylobacter proctitis in a homosexual man. Annals of Internal Medicine 93: 458–459

Quinn T C, Goodell S E, Mkrtichian P-A C et al 1981 *Chlamydia trachomatis* proctitis. New England Journal of Medicine 305: 195–200

Quinn T C, Lukehart S A, Goodell S, Mkrtichian E, Schuffler M D, Holmes K K, 1982 Rectal mass caused by *Treponema pallidum*: confirmation by immunofluorescent staining. Gastroenterology 82: 135–139

Quinn T C, Stamm W E, Goodell S E et al 1983 The polymicrobial origin of intestinal infections in homosexual men. New England Journal of Medicine 309: 576–582

Quinn T C, Goodell S E, Fennell C et al 1984 Infections with *Campylobacter jejuni* and *Campylobacter-like* organisms in homosexual men. Annals of Internal Medicine 101: 187–192

Robertson D H H, McMillan A, Young H 1980 Clinical practice in sexually transmitted diseases. Tunbridge Wells, Pitman Medical p 203–222

Salit I E, Frasch C E 1982 Seroepidemiologic aspects of *Neisseria meningitidis* in homosexual men. Canadian Medical Association Journal 126: 38–41

Samarasinghe P L, Oates J K, MacLennan I P B, 1979 Herpetic proctitis and sacral radiomyelopathy — a hazard for homosexual men. British Medical Journal 2: 365–366

Sargeaunt P G, Williams, J E, Kumate J, Jimenez E 1980 The epidemiology of *Entamoeba histolytica* in Mexico City. A pilot survey I Transactions of the Royal Society of Tropical Medicine and Hygiene 74: 653–656

Sargeaunt P G, Jackson T F H G, Simjee A 1982 Biochemical homogeneity of *Entamoeba histolytica* isolates especially those from liver abscess. Lancet i: 1386–1388

Sargeaunt P G, Oates J K, MacLennan I, Oriel J D, Goldmeier D, 1983 *Entamoeba histolytica* in male homosexuals. British Journal of Venereal Diseases 59: 193–195

Schachter J 1981 Confirmatory serodiagnosis of lymphogranuloma venereum proctitis may yield false-positive results due to other chlamydial infections of the rectum. Sexually Transmitted Diseases 8: 26–27

Scowden E B, Schaffner W, Stone W J 1978 Overwhelming *strongyloidiasis*: an unappreciated opportunistic infection. Medicine 57: 527–544

Selby W S, Janossy G, Goldstein G, Jewell D P 1981 T lymphocyte subsets in human intestinal mucosa: the distribution and relationship to MHC derived antigens. Clinical and Experimental Immunology 44: 453–458

Shera A G Specific granular lesions associated with intestinal spirochaetosis 1962. British Journal of Surgery 50: 68–77

Simmons P D, Tabaqchali S 1979 Campylobacter species in male homosexuals. British Journal of Venereal Diseases 55: 66

Soave R, Danner R L, Honig C L et al 1984 Cryptosporidiosis in homosexual men. Annals of Internal Medicine 100: 504–511

Sorvillo F, Mori K, Sewake W, Fishman L 1983 Sexual transmission of *Strongyloides stercoralis* among homosexual men. British Journal of Venereal Diseases 59: 342

Stamm W E, 1984 Proctitis due to *Chlamydia trachomatis*. In: Ma P, Armstrong D (eds) The acquired immune deficiency syndrome and infections of homosexual men. Yorke Medical Books, USA, p 40–47

Takeuchi A, Jervis H R, Nakazawa H, Robinson D M 1974 Spiral-shaped organisms on the survace colonic epithelium of the monkey and man. American Journal of Clinical Nutrition 27: 1287–1296

Tapper M L, Lerner C W, Rotterdam H Z 1974 Four cases of acquired immune deficiency syndrome (AIDS) in the United States. Opportunistic infections complicating acquired immune deficiency syndrome. In: Ma P, Armstrong D (eds) The acquired immune deficiency syndrome and infections of homosexual men. New York. Yorke Medical Books, USA, p 225–239

Thompson J E, Freischlag J, Thomas D S 1983 Amebic liver abscess in a homosexual man. Sexually Transmitted Diseases 10: 153–155

Tompkins D S, Waugh M A, Cooke E M 1981 Isolation of intestinal spirochaetes from homosexuals. Journal of Clinical Pathology 34: 1385–7

Voinchet O, Guivarc'h M 1980 Chancre syphilitique simulant un cancer du rectum. Gastroenterologie Clinique et Biologique 4: 134–136

Wang S-P, Grayston J T, Kuo C-C, Alexander E R, Holmes K K 1977 Serodiagnosis of *Chlamydia trachomatis* infections with the microimmunofluorescence test. In: Hobson D, Holmes K K (eds) Nongonococcal urethritis and related infections. American Society of Microbiology. Washington DC, p 237–248

Watson K C, Kerr E J C 1982 Comparison of agglutination, complement fixation and immunofluorescence tests in *Campylobacter jejuni* infections. Journal of Hygiene 88: 165–171

Watts J McK, Thompson H, Goligher J C 1966 Sigmoidoscopy and cytology in the detection of microscopic disease of the rectal mucosa in ulcerative colitis. Gut 7: 288–294

Waugh M A 1976 Anorectal Herpesvirus hominis infection in man. Journal of the American Venereal Diseases Association 3: 68

Weinstein M A, Sohn N, Robbins R D 1981 Syndrome of pelvic cellulitis following rectal sexual trauma. American Journal of Gastroenterology 75: 380–381

William D C, Felman Y M, Ricciardi N B 1981 The utility of anoscopy in the rapid diagnosis of symptomatic anorectal gonorrhea in men. Sexually Transmitted Diseases 8: 16–17

Wildy P, Field H J, Nash A A 1982 Classical herpes latency revisited in Mahy B W J, Minson A C, Darby G K (eds) Virus Persistence. Cambridge University Press, Cambridge, p 133–167

16. Provision of services for sexually transmitted diseases in developing countries

André Meheus   Peter Piot

SEXUALLY TRANSMITTED DISEASES AS A PUBLIC HEALTH PROBLEM

The epidemiology of sexually transmitted diseases (STD) in developing countries differs in three major respects from the situation in industrialised nations:

1. In developing countries, STD are a much more frequent health problem, and have a very high incidence and prevalence in some population groups; for example, female prostitutes are an important high risk group for STD infection and transmission, while male homosexuals are not a significant group.
2. There is a higher relative frequency of the so-called tropical STD which cause genital ulcers: chancroid, lymphogranuloma venereum and granuloma inguinale.
3. There is a much higher incidence of complications and sequelae.

Data on the frequency of STD are available from recent reviews (WHO, 1978b, 1981, 1982; Osoba, 1981; Piot & Meheus, 1983). These data indicate that STD are endemic in many developing countries, including the rural areas where there are few facilities for diagnosis and treatment. Complications are frequent, and particularly severe in women. In developing countries women are the main victims of STD, and they should be considered much less as transmitters (McCormack, 1982). Both sexes are equally important as reservoirs and transmitters of STD (Potterat et al, 1980).

Data on the prevalence of STD in antenatal attenders are a good indication of potential complications in puerperal women and neonates. Table 16.1 summarises data on the prevalence of gonorrhoea and a positive serological test for syphilis in antenatal attenders in African countries. The prevalence of gonorrhoea ranges from 3.9–15%. As the rate of transmission of gonorrhoea from mother to infant at birth is 30–40%, the data indicate that at least 1.3–5% of neonates are likely to acquire gonococcal conjunctivitis, which carries a risk of blindness unless adequately treated. Now that 20–50% of gonorrhoea infections are due to penicillinase-producing *N. gonorrhoeae* (PPNG), treatment of gonococcal ophthalmia in the developing world has become a considerable problem (Rajan et al, 1978; Thirumoorthy et al, 1982; Fransen et al, 1983; WHO, 1984a) and prophylaxis of ophthalmia neonatorum with 1% silver nitrate eye drops is a necessary strategy in these countries (Meheus & Causse, 1983; WHO, 1984a; Galega et al, 1984). The interpretation of the data on the prevalence of a positive serological test for syphilis is more difficult, as this may be due to venereal syphilis (infectious or non-infectious), past infection with a non-venereal treponematosis or to biological false-positive reactions. Nevertheless, it has been reported from Zambia that there is a considerable risk of congenital syphilis and of stillbirths due to this infection (Ratnam et al, 1982).

The incidence of pelvic inflammatory disease (PID) was estimated in Kenya as 360 per 100 000 population (Muir & Belsey, 1980). In Africa, between 17% and 44% of admissions to gynaecology wards are for the treatment of PID (Lithgrow & Rubin, 1972; Grech et al, 1973; De Clercq, 1982). Between 8% and 10% of gonococcal or chlamydial infection of the cervix is complicated by PID. A large proportion

Table 16.1 Prevalence of gonorrhoea and a positive serological test for syphilis in antenatal attenders

Country	Reference	Gonorrhoea prevalence (%)	Positive serology (%) VDRL/RPR (1)	TPHA/FTA-ABS (2)
Cameroon	Nasah et al, 1980	15.0		
Ethiopia	Friedman & Wright, 1977		12.7	10.9
Gabon	Yvert et al, 1984	5.5		
Gambia	Mabey & Whittle, 1982	6.7		
Kenya	Lagae, 1984	13.0		
Central African Republic	Widy-Wirski & D'Costa 1980	9.5	9.5	
Rwanda	De Clercq, 1982		4.4	
Swaziland	Meheus et al, 1980	3.9	10.0	33.3
Zaire	Kakiesse Musumba, 1983		20.0	2.0
Zambia	Ratnam et al, 1982		14.3	12.5

(1) Venereal disease research laboratory test/rapid plasma reagin test
(2) Treponema pallidum haemagglutination assay/fluorescent treponemal antibody test with absorption

of postabortal and postpartum endometritis and PID is related to STD. Infertility due to STD has serious consequences for the individual woman, the marriage, and the community as a whole. In the World Fertility Survey, it was found that the average level of involuntary childlessness among married women aged 40–49 years was 3.4%, but much higher levels have been reported from the Sudan (10%), the Central African Republic (14%), parts of Zaire (18%) and Gabon (32%) (Belsey, 1976; Sherris & Fox, 1983). Bilateral tubal occlusion due to PID is responsible for 44–86% of cases of female infertility in African studies (Sherris & Fox, 1983; Meheus, 1984b).

In men, urethral stricture and infertility are important complications of STD. Urethral stricture was shown to be an important health problem in Uganda (Bewes, 1973), but no recent data from other countries are available. A male factor is responsible for 30–40% of infertile couples; the commonest is azoospermia caused by sperm duct blockage following epididymitis (Lee, 1970; Burgos, 1981). The epididymes are also infected in 25–30% of men with urethritris (Berger, 1981).

Carcinoma of the cervix has a high incidence in developing countries (Gigase, 1982; Standaert et al, 1985), which is consistent with a high incidence of STD, early marriage, and low socio-economic status leading to poor genital hygiene.

CONTROL OF STD

STD are a public health problem because of the high incidence of acute infections, and the frequency and seriousness of their complications and sequelae, which include PID, puerperal infections, congenital syphilis, neonatal infections such as ophthalmia neonatorum, urethral stricture and male and female infertility. In most developing countries, the morbidity from STD is one of the top three health problems in the age group 15–34 years. In these countries the health budget per capita is between 5 and 10 US dollars. The economic consequences of STD are considerable: costs of medical examinations and treatment, consultations at different levels of the health services and for hospitalisation. In one central African country, the medical costs related to gonorrhoea alone were estimated to take 17% of the budget for medicines,

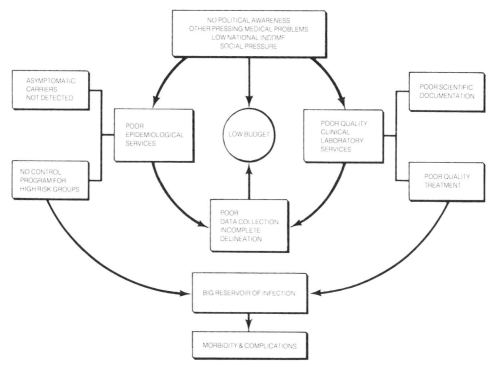

Fig. 16.1   Factors contributing to the vicious circle of poor control of STD (Source: Rajan, 1980).

and 4.3% of the overall health budget. The economic cost from loss of productivity was estimated as 10 500 days lost per 1000 inhabitants (Jancloes, 1984). Because of the increasing prevalence of PPNG strains, which is approaching 50% in most areas, the cost of treatment is rapidly increasing; the alternatives to penicillin are 3–10 times more costly, which means that a very large proportion of the budget for drugs will be needed to treat gonorrhoea and other STD. This fact may be the reason why many governments tend to ignore STD rather than face the real magnitude of the problem: this is the basis of the vicious circle in which STD control is entangled in most developing countries (Osoba, 1980; Rajan, 1980; and see Fig. 16.1).

In national control programmes, much emphasis is placed on the prevention of STD, the main goal being to decrease the incidence of uncomplicated STD and thereby to diminish the incidence of complications. STD are behavioural diseases which are related to sexual promiscuity. In general, it is very difficult to change behaviour, and control programmes based on health education have not been very successful, for example in changing smoking and eating habits, and in reducing the use of drugs. For the prevention of STD we have no vaccines or other efficacious prophylactic measures, so prevention has to be based mainly on health education. But it is not realistic to expect significant changes in sexual behaviour to come about by this means. Such behaviour depends mainly on what a person prefers or values in life, and much less on what that person knows. Furthermore, health education in this area can easily develop moralistic or repressive undertones and become counterproductive. Clear priorities in health education must be chosen, such as the integration of education on STD, together with contraception, into sex education, and STD education directed at high risk groups (WHO, 1976).

A realistic goal for STD control is a reduction in the incidence of their complications. This means that in the implementation of a control programme the medical services have a major role. Priority activities to be considered are (Meheus, 1984):

1. Adequate management of patients with STD and their contacts.
2. Case finding for syphilis, and eventually for gonorrhoea as well, in antenatal populations.
3. Screening and case finding for gonorrhoea and syphilis in high risk groups which are known to have a high prevalence of infection. As an alternative to this strategy, mass treatment might be considered.
4. The adoption of systematic prophylaxis for ophthalmia neonatorum.

The starting point of the programme is certainly the adequate management of patients with acute STD and their complications, and of their sex partners. In the United Kingdom and Singapore, and in some other countries, the control of STD is organised mainly through special STD clinics (Catterall, 1976), but in most areas financial resources and medical manpower are so restricted that STD control must be integrated into the general health system.

ORGANISATION OF HEALTH SERVICES IN DEVELOPING COUNTRIES

The organisation of health services in most developing countries is outlined in Table 16.2. The hospital sector, from district level up to the national reference (teaching) hospital, caters for the health problems of 10–20% of the population, who are mainly living in the urban areas (King, 1966; Bryant, 1969). The services delivered are predominantly curative, modelled on those in industrialised countries; they involve diagnostic investigation followed by treatment. This can be called the 'diagnostic approach' to disease. The health budget is almost entirely consumed by the hospital sector, which leads to a severe maldistribution of services between the 'haves' (mainly in

Table 16.2 The organisation of health services in many developing countries

Health facility	Type of personnel
Ministry of Health	Senior administrative staff
National Reference Hospital	Specialists, laboratory experts and technicians
Regional Hospital	Some specialists and laboratory technicians
District Hospital	Mostly general medicine only, laboratory technicians
Health Centre	Paramedicals with variable supervision by doctors; laboratory auxiliaries
Dispensary	Paramedical or auxiliary workers only
Community	Community health workers

Source: adapted from Arya & Bennett, 1976

the towns) and the 'have nots' (in the outskirts of towns and in rural areas). Some countries also have a private medicine system, but this is available to only a tiny fraction of the population.

The health centre, dispensary and community facility comprise the primary health care system. This system caters for the health needs and demands of 80–90% of the population in the urban and rural areas. The services provided are not only curative medicine but also preventive health services such as family planning, maternal and child health care, nutritional programmes, sanitation, communicable disease control and health education. The staff at primary health care level consists mostly of paramedicals and auxiliaries, but in some countries doctors are available to lead the health team in a health centre (Fendall, 1972, Mercenier & Van Balen, 1979).

In order to have an adequate coverage of the population, health planners aimed at one health centre for every 10 000–30 000 inhabitants (King, 1966). But wide coverage of the population was not achieved by these static health services. This was due to non-existent or insufficient participation of the community in health matters, and to a failure to reallocate resources to peripheral health services. Because of this, a new concept of primary health care was developed in which the local community organisation has to be actively involved in health matters (Ebrahim, 1975; Newell, 1975; WHO, 1978a; King, 1983). A new element is the use of a community health worker, who is often a villager selected by the community and trained locally. He or she can be an unpaid volunteer, or be partly or totally supported by the official health service or by the village people in cash or kind. The work of the community health worker covers both health care and community development. He has to serve a population of between 500 and 2000 people (WHO, 1980). The new primary health care system is composed of the dispensaries and health centres, together with the peripheral community activities implemented by the community workers. Some criticism has been expressed of the actual state of primary health care in many developing countries — is this care rhetorical or a reality (Smith, 1982)? But all control programmes have to be implemented within that system, and proposals and guidelines have been developed for the control of treponematoses (Hopkins, 1985; Meheus, 1985), and of STD (Arya et al, 1980; WHO, 1984a, 1984b, 1985; Meheus, 1984a).

Characteristics of primary health care

The confidence which a patient has in a health service is determined by the effectiveness of the management of his health problem at the first consultation. The management of patients at the primary health care level has the following characteristics (Essex, 1980; Equipe de Kasongo, 1982):

1. It starts with the presenting symptoms and signs which define the health problem to be solved, i.e. this is a problem-orientated approach. The diagnosis must be based on the history, physical examination and simple laboratory tests, if available.
2. Investigations should be performed routinely only if they are important to decide the management of the health problem.
3. Correct management should take less than 5 minutes.
4. The choice of treatment should be rational, and treatment regimens standardised.
5. Referral of patients should be exceptional: preferably less than 5% of the total.

It must be emphasised that in many developing countries referral is a real problem owing to lack of time, distance to travel, or financial and socio-cultural barriers between peripheral and more sophisticated levels of care. Therefore practical, useful guidelines for simplified approaches to STD control, such as simple management protocols, are of the utmost importance.

Problem-orientated approach to STD management
STD of public health importance generally present in their acute stages as one of the following health problems:

Urethral discharge.
Gynaecological complaints such as vaginal discharge, dysuria or low abdominal pain.
Genital ulceration.
Inguinal bubo.

As the consequences of the complications of STD are often so severe, adequate management of the following health problems is also very important:

Swollen scrotum.
Low abdominal pain with fever of more than 38°C and an abnormal vaginal discharge.
Conjuctivitis in the newborn.

STD management protocols have been developed and evaluated during the last five years (Meheus et al, 1979; Arya et al, 1980; Sherris & Fox, 1983, Meheus, 1984a). The general principles for the design of these protocols have been outlined (WHOa, 1985). The most important are knowledge of the local etiology of the health problem, information on the laboratory tests available for diagnosis (sensitivity, specificity, cost, operational value in local circumstances), and treatment efficacy. The standardisation of treatment is essential, and this can be established by controlled and uncontrolled clinical trials, knowledge of antimicrobial sensitivity patterns, information from neighbouring countries or international recommendations (WHO, 1983). Furthermore, the current STD care practices and policies in the community should be assessed, and the intended users of the protocols should be clearly defined. Once a protocol has been designed for a country, it is very desirable to test and evaluate its performance in a small demonstration or pilot project.

Early detection of STD in high risk groups
The strategy of early detection can take two forms:

1. Screening: the ascertainment of the probability of disease in populations not seeking health care — for example, screening bar girls with a VDRL test.
2. Case-finding: the use of clinical and/or laboratory tests to detect STD in individuals seeking health care for other reasons — for example, performing a VDRL test on women attending for an antenatal consultation.

Detection programmes for early STD concern individuals who are nearly always asymptomatic, so much emphasis must be placed on laboratory tests. These tests should be available in sufficient quantity, but in addition the quality of performance should be regularly checked. Cost-effectiveness and possible operational problems should be thoroughly evaluated before the introduction of large-scale early detection programmes (Hart, 1980; Meheus, 1982).

EARLY DETECTION OF GONORRHOEA

In women, the first manifestation of gonococcal infection is often salpingitis, because the cervical infection is often symptomless, or passes unnoticed. Case-finding for gonorrhoea in antenatal or family planning attenders, or screening of high-risk groups such as prostitutes, can be considered. For early detection, culture for *N. gonorrhoeae* must be used. Unfortunately, in most developing countries facilities for culture are very limited, so they should normally be used for the diagnosis of gonorrhoea in women with genital symptoms. In groups with a high prevalence of gonorrhoea, e.g. above 10%, early detection could be introduced once the laboratory facilities are better developed. But besides the prevalence of infection, many other factors affect the cost-effectiveness of an early detection programme. For instance, a culture for *N. gonorrhoeae* is read after 48 hours, and persons checked should then return for these results, and receive treatment if they are positive. In Southern Africa, treatment rates for positive cases in early detection programmes were only 30–46% (Weissenberger et al, 1977; Hall & Whitcomb, 1978). The efficacy of treatment for gonorrhoea should also be considered, and should be at least 95%.

The use of Gram-stained cervical smears for the early detection of gonorrhoea in women is controversial. Under good conditions the sensitivity of this technique is around 50% and its specificity 90%. If these validity estimates are applied in situations where the prevalence of gonorrhoea is 5%, 15% and 25%, the positive predictive value of the smear is 29%, 47% and 63% respectively (Meheus & Piot, 1983); the positive predictive value of the cervical smear being the percentage of those with a positive test who actually have gonorrhoea. It is clear from these data that it is only in high prevalence situations that the Gram-stained cervical smear is acceptable for the early detection of gonorrhoea. The validity of the test should always be regularly assessed in the local situation.

EARLY DETECTION OF SYPHILIS

The early detection of syphilis is an important strategy in the prevention of congenital syphilis. It can also be considered for non-pregnant high risk groups. A qualitative or quantitative reagin test such as the VDRL or RPR card test may be used, but the interpretation of a positive result may not be easy (see above). If a treponemal test such as the TPHA is available, biological false positive reactions to reagin tests can be excluded by applying a TPHA to all sera which give positive reactions in the VDRL or RPR tests. Alternatively, if both tests are available they can be applied together to all sera (WHO, 1982). But this approach considerably increases cost, and detects cases of past, non-active treponematosis; in some countries the numbers of these are considerable, and as most of them do not need to be treated these VDRL-negative TPHA-positive cases are troublesome for both the health worker and the patients themselves.

Selective mass treatment

Under certain circumstances, such as a high prevalence of STD, insufficient or non-existent laboratory facilities and highly mobile populations, mass treatment of high risk groups can be a substitute for early detection. In California, mass treatment of prostitutes for syphilis diminished the incidence of the infection by 51% in the prostitutes and by 27% in seasonal workers (Jaffe et al, 1979). In Kenya, mass treatment of prostitutes for gonorrhoea decreased the prevalence of the infection considerably, but after 4 weeks the rate had returned to its initial level (Plummer, 1984). It was concluded that this was not an effective strategy under such circumstances.

STD CONTROL CENTRE

STD surveillance and control should be integrated into the primary health care system, and not implemented as a 'vertical' programme. But in each country a specialised STD centre remains necessary, and in this centre expertise in clinical, laboratory, epidemiological and social science skills related to STD control should be brought together (WHO, 1956). This centre should propose, evaluate and adapt different strategies for STD control for use in the primary health care system. Its main functions are to improve clinical care, improve laboratory diagnosis, develop programmes for the training of health care personnel, and perform relevant operational research.

Clinical care can be improved by identifying current providers of STD care in the community and reviewing their current practices. Standards and simple guidelines can be developed for history taking, physical examination, specimen collection, and the recording and interpretation of results. Treatment recommendations should be elaborated and evaluated by the centre, and based on available international recommendations, local clinical trials and regular surveillance of the antibiotic susceptibility of STD micro-organisms. Approaches to patient counselling and contact tracing which are appropriate to local culture should be determined. The centre should identify the laboratory tests which should be routinely available for patient care at different levels of the health system. The tests which influence clinical decisions are particularly important.

The centre has an important role in developing training programmes for all levels of health workers. These programmes relate to standards for clinical services and laboratory procedures, contact tracing and health education. The development of health education material adapted to the country for both patients with STD and the general public is very important.

The STD centre should identify, conduct and analyse special operational studies needed to support the control programme. Particular emphasis should be placed on studies of the etiology of STD problems as they occur in patients, because these are the basis of the problem-orientated approach to the management of STD. Studies of the prevalence of infection in high risk groups are also useful, e.g. in pregnant women, attenders at family planning clinics, prostitutes, students and military personnel. These allow some assessment of the size of the STD problem, and where the priorities for intervention lie.

To fulfill the functions described above, an STD clinic should be a part of the STD control centre. Patients seen in the clinic should represent STD patients in the area; therefore, patients should have direct and easy access to the clinic, and patients who have been referred should be only a small proportion of the total. In practice, the clinic is best situated in a large town in a densely populated area, where problems of STD are most prevalent.

REFERENCES

Arya O P, Bennett F J 1976 Role of the medical auxiliary in the control of sexually transmitted diseases in a developing country. British Journal of Venereal Diseases 52: 116–121

Arya O P, Osoba A O, Bennett F J 1980 Tropical Venereology. Churchill Livingstone, Edinburgh

Belsey M A 1976 The epidemiology of infertility: a review with particular reference to sub-Saharan Africa. Bulletin of the World Health Organisation 54: 319–341

Berger R E 1981 Acute epididymitis-Editorial. Sexually Transmitted Diseases 8: 286–289

Bewes P C 1973 Urethral stricture. Tropical Doctor 3: 77

Bryant J 1969 Health and the developing world, Cornell University Press, Ithaca

Burgos A A 1981 Estudio sobre 100 historias clinicas de infertilidad. Revista Colombiana de Obstetricia Y Ginecologia 31: 235–242

Catterall R D 1976 The system in Britain. In: Catterall R D, Nicol C S (eds) Sexually transmitted diseases, Academic Press, London, p 61–67

De Clercq A 1982 Problèmes en obstétrique et gynécologie. In: Meheus A, Butera S, Eylenbosch W, Gatera G, Kivits M, Musafili I (eds) Santé et Maladies au Rwanda, Administration Générale de la Coopération au Développement, Bruxelles, p 627–656

Ebrahim G J 1975 A model of integrated community health care in a rural area. Tropical and Geographical Medicine 28 suppl

Equipe de Kasongo 1982 Stratégies de diagnostic-traitement à la consultation curative primaire. In: Meheus et al (eds), Santé et Maladies au Rwanda, Administration Générale de la Coopération au Développement, Bruxelles, p 217–237

Essex B J 1980 Diagnostic pathways in clinical medicine, Churchill Livingstone, Edinburgh

Fendall N R 1972 Auxiliaries in health care: programs in developing countries, Johns Hopkins Press, Baltimore

Fransen L, Piot P, Nsanze H, Ndinya-Achola, Hazlett D T, D'Costa L, Ronald A, Brunham R 1983 Aetiology and management of ophthalmia neonatorum in Nairobi Kenya. In: Nsanze H, Widy-Wirski R, Ellison R (eds) Proceedings Third African Regional Conference on STD, Nairobi, 139–144

Friedmann P S, Wright D J 1977 Observations, on syphilis in Addis Ababa. 2. prevalence and natural history. British Journal of Venereal Diseases 53: 276–280

Galega F P, Heymann D L, Nasah B T 1984 Gonococcal ophtalmia neonatorum: the case for prophylaxis in tropical Africa. Bulletin of the World Health Organisation 62: 95–98

Gigase P 1982 Aspects épidémiologiques du cancer en Afrique. In: Meheus A, Butera S, Eylenbosch W, Gatera G, Kivits M, Musafili I (eds) Santé et Maladies au Rwanda, Administration Génerale de la Coopération au Développement, Bruxelles, 497–515

Grech E S, Everett J V, Musaka F 1973 Epidemiological aspects of acute pelvic inflammatory disease in Uganda. Tropical Doctor 3: 123–127

Hall S M, Whitcomb M A 1978 Screening for gonorrhoea in family planning acceptors in a developing community. Public Health, London 92: 121–124

Hart G 1980 Screening to control infectious diseases: evaluation of control program for gonorrhoea and syphilis. Reviews of Infectious Diseases 2: 701–712

Hopkins D R 1985 Yaws and other endemic treponematoses — Vertical and/or integrated programs. Reviews of infectious diseases 5: S338–S342

Jaffe H W, Rice D T, Voigt R, Fowler J, St John R 1979 Selective mass treatment in a venereal disease control program. American Journal of Public Health 69: 1181–1182

Jancloes M 1984 Conséquences économiques des MST dans les pays en développement. Paper presented at the General Assembly of the International Union against Venereal Diseases and Treponematoses, Montréal

Kakiesse Musumba 1983 La syphilis à Kinshasa. Thesis Université Nationale du Zaire, Kinshasa

King M (ed) 1966 Medical care in developing countries, Oxford University Press, London

King M (ed) 1983 An Iranian experiment in primary health care. The West Azerbaijan project, Oxford University Press, London

Lagae M 1984 unpublished data

Lee H Y 1970 Studies on male infertility (in Korean). Journal of the Korean Medical Association 13: 1008–1017

Lithgrow D M, Rubin A 1972 Pelvic inflammatory disease. In: Greenwood G P (ed) Gynaecology in Southern Africa, Witwatersrand University Press, Johannesburg, 177

Mabey D, Whittle H C 1982 Genital and neonatal chlamydial infection in a trachoma endemic area. Lancet 2: 301–302

McCormack W N 1982 Sexually Transmitted Diseases: women as victims, Editorial. Journal of the American Medical Association 248: 177–178

Meheus A 1982 Epidemiologic issues for STD screening and case finding, WHO-PAHO Scientific Working Group on STD control, Washington DC, Background document

Meheus A 1984 a Management of patients with STD problems-practical approaches in developing nations. In: Holmes K K, Mårdh P A, Sparling P F, Wiesner P J (eds) Sexually transmitted diseases, McGraw Hill, New York, ch 81, 998–1008

Meheus A 1984b Fécondité et maladies sexuellement transmissibles. Proceedings of the Séminaire international sur fécondité humaine et MTS, Gabon, Franceville, in press

Meheus A 1985 Integration of yaws control and primary health care activities. Reviews of Infectious Diseases 5: S284–S288

Meheus A, Piot P 1983 Lutte contre les maladies sexuellement transmissibles dans les pays en développement. Annales de la Société belge de Médecine Tropicale 63: 281–311

Meheus A, Causse G 1983 Epidemiology and Control of ophtalmia neonatorum. Unpublished document

Meheus A, Dlamini M, Friedman F, Antal G, Causse G 1979 Gonorrhoea control based on simplified health technology. Unpublished document

Meheus A, Friedman F, Van Dyck E, Guyver T 1980 Genital infections in prenatal and family planning attendants in Swaziland. East African Medical Journal 57: 212–217

Mercenier P, Van Balen H 1979 International colloquium on basic health services in developing countries. Annales de la Société belge de Médecine tropicale 59 suppl

Muir D G, Belsey M A 1980 Pelvic inflammatory disease and its consequences in the developing world. American Journal of Obstetrics and Gynaecology 138: 913–928

Nasah B T, Nguematcha R, Eyong M, Godwin S 1980 Gonorrhoea, trichomonas and candida among gravid and non-gravid women in Cameroon. International journal of obstetrics and gynaecology 18: 48–52

Newell K (ed) 1975 Health by the people, WHO, Geneva

Osoba A O 1980 Microbiologic techniques for the diagnosis of pelvic inflammatory disease in developing countries. American Journal of Obstetrics and Gynaecology 138: 1091–1095

Osoba A O 1981 Sexually Transmitted Diseases in tropical Africa. British Journal of Venereal Diseases 57: 89–94

Piot P, Meheus A 1983 Epidemiologie des maladies sexuellement transmissibles dans les pays en développement. Annales de la Société belge de Médecine tropicale 63: 87–110

Plummer F 1984 Mass treatment for gonorrhoea in prostitutes in Kenya. Paper presented at the international conference on Tropical Diseases, Calgary

Potterat J J, Phillips L, Rothenberg R B, Darrow W W 1980 Gonococcal pelvic inflammatory disease: case-finding observations. American Journal of Obstetrics and Gynaecology 138: 1101–1104

Rajan V S, Pang R, Sng E H 1978 An evaluation of treatment in gonococcal ophtalmia neonatorum. Singapore Medical Journal 19: 86–88

Rajan V S 1980 Problems in the surveillance and control of sexually transmitted agents associated with pelvic inflammatory disease in the Far East. American Journal of Obstetrics and Gynaecology 138: 1071–1077

Ratnam A V, Din S N, Hira S K, Bhat G J, Wacha D S, Rukmini A, Mulenga R C 1982 Syphilis in pregnant women in Zambia, British Journal of Venereal Diseases 58: 355–358

Sherris J D, Fox G 1983 Infertility and sexually transmitted diseases: a public health challenge. Population Reports Series L No 4, John Hopkins University, Population Information Program, Baltimore

Smith R A 1982 Primary Health Care — rhetoric or reality? World Health Forum 3: 30–37

Standaert B, Meheus A 1985 Epidémiologie du cancer du col de l'utérus en Afrique. Médecine d'Afrique Noire 32: 407–415

Thirumoorthy T, Rajan V S, Goh C C 1982 Penicillinase — producing Neisseria gonorrhoeae ophtalmia neonatorum in Singapore. British Journal of Venereal Diseases 58: 308–310

Weissenberger R, Robertson A, Holland S, Hall W 1977 The incidence of gonorrhoea in urban Rhodesian black women. South African Medical Journal 57: 1119–1120

Widy-Wirski R, D'Costa J 1980 Prévalence des MST dans la population des femmes enceintes en milieu urbain en Centrafrique. In: Rapport final, 13e Conférence Technique OCEAC, Yaoundé, 655–660

WHO 1976 Social and health aspects of sexually transmitted diseases. Public Health Paper No 65, Geneva

WHO 1978 a Primary Health Care — The declaration of Alma Ata. WHO, Geneva

WHO 1978b Neisseria gonorrhoeae and gonococcal infections. WHO Technical Report Series No 616, Geneva

WHO 1980 The Primary Health Worker — working guide — guidelines for training — guidelines for adaptation, Geneva

WHO 1981 Nongonococcal urethritis and other selected sexually transmitted diseases of public health importance. WHO Technical Report Series No 660, Geneva

WHO 1982 Treponemal Infections. WHO Technical Report Series No 674, Geneva

WHO 1983 Current treatments in the control of sexually transmitted diseases. Document WHO/VDT/83.433, Geneva

WHO 1984a Prevention and treatment of conjunctivitis in the newborn at the primary level. WHO Document PBL/84.4, Geneva

WHO 1984b Prevention of infertility at the primary health care level. WHO Document in press, Geneva

WHO 1985a Simplified approaches for STD control at the primary health care level. Document WHO/VDT/85.437 Geneva

WHO 1985b Control of sexually transmitted diseases. Geneva

Yvert F, Riou J Y, Frost E, Ivanoff B 1984 Les infections gonococciques au Gabon — Haut Ogoué. Pathologie Biologie 32: 80–84

Index

Aquired immune deficiency syndrone (AIDS), 169,
180, 209–219, 223–238
  B cell lymphoma, 229, 232
  candidiosis, 225, 226, 231
  CDC surveillance definition, 209, 210–211
  children, transmission to, 215
  clinical aspects, 211, 216–218, 223–238
  CMV infection, 226, 227, 228, 256
  CNS infections, 227–228
  cryptococcal meningitis, 227, 231
  cryptosporidiosis, 217, 231, 255
  epidemiology, 211–213
  exposure to blood/blood products, 214–215
  gastrointestinal infection, 226–227
  herpes simplex infection, 226–227, 231
  high incidence groups, 211, 212, 213
  immune dysfunction, 216, 233–235
  immune reconstruction, 235–236
  immunopathogenesis, 235
  Kaposi's sarcoma, 217, 228–229, 231
  Legionella infection, 231
  Mycoplasma avium-intracellulare, 217, 227, 231
  Nocardia infection, 231
  opportunist infection, 216–218, 223–224, 225
  prevention strategies, 218–219
  Pneumocystis carinii, 216–217, 226
  prodromal, 224–225, 233, 236
  pulmonary infections, 225–226
  seroepidemiology, 213–214
  seropositive asymptomatic individuals, 213, 214
  sexual transmission, 211–213, 214, 215
  staff safety considerations, 218, 237
  systemic infections, 228
  therapy, 216–218, 230–232
  toxoplasmosis, 217, 228, 230
  tumours and, 228–230
  see also HLTV-III/LAV
Acyclovir, 35, 86, 91, 92, 93, 94, 96, 99, 149,
163–164, 231
Adenine arabinoside (ARA-A), 161–163, 171
Adriamycin, 231
Amoxycillin, 34, 42, 46, 178
Amphotericin, 225, 231
Ampicillin, 42, 46, 65, 66, 178, 190, 231
Anorectal warts, 129, 139
Ansamycin, 217, 231
Antimoniotungstate, 217
Azathioprine, 166, 167

B cell lymphoma, 229, 232
Bacterial vaginosis, 185–191

Bacterial vaginosis (*contd.*)
  aetiology, 186–188
  clinical syndrome, 185–186
  diagnostic criteria, 185–186
  epidemiology, 189–190
  management, 190–191
  pregnancy and, 191
Bacteroides spp., 186, 187
Bartholinitis, 46
Betadine, 96
Bleomycin, 149, 231, 232
Bowenoid papulosis, 135
Bowen's disease, 135

Campylobacter spp., 252–253
Candidiosis, oral, 225, 226, 231
Cefotaxime, 33, 34, 66
Cefoxitin, 33, 34, 49
Ceftriaxone, 66, 180
Cefuroxime, 33, 34
Cephalosporins, 24, 33, 34, 35, 49, 66, 190
Cephalothin, 65
Cervical dysplasia/intraepithelial neoplasia (CIN)
  chlamydial infection and, 47
  epidemiological aspects, 138
  genital warts association, 134
  HPV detection, 115
  HPV infection and, 130, 131, 136–138
  HPV types and, 119, 120, 132, 136, 137, 138
Cervical squamous-cell carcinoma, 136
Cervicitis
  HSV, 78, 85
  postgonococcal, 45
Chancroid, 59, 176, 179, 180, 181
  epidemiological aspects, 175, 176
  see also Haemophilus ducreyi
Chlamydia trachomatis infection, 39–55
  acute salpingitis and, 47–49
  asymptomatic infection, 44
  Bartholinitis and, 46
  cervical dysplasia and, 47
  cervical infection, 44–46
  cytology, 53–54
  DNA probes, diagnostic, 54
  endometritis and, 49, 50
  enzyme immunoassay, 54
  female infertility and, 48, 49–50
  inclusion conjunctivitis of the newborn and, 51
  isolation, 52–53
  laboratory diagnosis, 52–55
  life cycle, 39

Chlamydia trachomatis infection (*contd.*)
  LGV and *see* Lymphogranulorum venereum
  oral contraceptive use and, 50
  perihepatitis and, 49
  pneumonia syndrome in infants, 51–52
  postgonococcal urethritis and, 42
  pregnancy and, 50
  proctitis and, 43–44, 248–251
  prostatitis and, 43
  reactive arthritis and, 202–203
  risk factors, 50
  serology, 39, 54–55
  transmission, 40–41
  treatment, female, 50–51
  urethral, female, 46–47
  urethral, male *see* Nongonococcal urethritis
Chloramphenicol, 65, 66, 231
Chloropactin, 149
Chloroquine, 164
Chlorpromazine, 164
CHOP regime, 232
Cimetidine, 153
Ciprofloxacin, 66
Clavulanic acid, 34, 66, 178
Clindamycin, 49
Clofazmine, 231
Colchicine, 149
Colomycin, 231
Condylomata acuminata
  anorectal warts, 129
  associated infections, 128
  chemotherapy, 148–150
  children, 128–129
  CO_2 laser therapy, 151–152
  cryotherapy, 151
  emotional factors and, 147–148
  general management, 147–148
  giant condyloma, 134, 139
  HPV detection, 115
  immunotherapy, 152–153
  incidence, 127–128
  infectivity, 128
  penile, 129, 138
  perianal, 139
  pregnancy, 133, 148, 151
  see also Human papilloma virus
Cotrimoxazole, 180, 230
Cryptosporidiosis, 217, 231, 255
Cytomegalovirus (CMV) infection, 226, 227, 228, 256

2-Deoxy-D-glucose, 92, 95
Developing countries, 261–268
  community health workers, 265
  control of STD, 262–264
  early detection strategies, 266–267
  epidemiological aspects, 261
  management protocols, 266
  ophthalmia neonatorum, 261, 264
  organisation of health services, 264–268
  primary health care, 265
  problem-orientated approach, 266

Developing countries (*contd.*)
  selective mass treatment, 267–268
  STD control centre, 268
Donovanosis, 176, 177
Doxycycline, 42, 231, 251

Endometritis, 49
Enoxacin, 66
Entamoeba histolytica, 253–255
Enterovirus, 253
Epidermodysplasia verruciformis (EV), 122, 134
Epidophyllotoxin, 231
Erosive balanoposthitis, 178, 180
Erythromycin, 41, 42, 51, 52, 66, 178, 231

Female infertility, developing countries, 262
Fitz-Hugh-Curtis syndrome, 49
5-Flucytosine, 231
5-Fluorouracil (5FU), 149

Gardnerella vaginalis, 185, 186
  sexual transmission, 189–190
  taxonomy/identification, 188
  see also Bacterial vaginosis
Genital ulcers, tropics, 175–181
  aetiology, 176–179
  epidemiology, 175–176, 261
  presentation/diagnosis, 179–180
  standard management, 180
Gentamicin, 34, 231
Giant condyloma, 134, 139
Giardia lamblia, 246
Gonococcal ulcers, 178, 179
Gonorrhoea, 268
  clinical spectrum, 1
  detection strategies in developing countries, 267
  epidemiological aspects, 261, 264
  epididymitis and, 43
  proctocolitis and, 246–247
  reactive arthritis and, 204
  vaccine, 1–2, 13
  see also Neisseria gonorrhoeae

Haemophilus ducreyi, 59–67, 178–179
  antimicrobial profile, 65–67
  biochemical characteristics, 60–61
  colonial morphology, 64
  cultural environment, 64
  epidemiology, 60
  historical aspects, 60
  indications for culture, 64–65
  media, 61–63
  positive culture, predictive value, 65
  specimen collection, 61
  staining, 61
  taxonomy, 60–61
Heck's disease, 139
Hepatitis B infection, chronic, 157–171
  acyclovir and, 163–164
  adenine arabinoside (ARA-A) and, 161–163
  anti-HBe positive phase, 157, 160
  autoimmune reaction, 166–167

Hepatitis B infection, chronic (*contd.*)
  BCG therapy, 165–166
  HBe Ag-positive phase, 157, 159
  hepatitis B immune globulin (HBIG)
    prophylaxis, 170
  hepatocytes containing integrated HBV-DNA,
    166
  immune response manipulation, 164–166
  interferon, 160–161
  liver damage, 158–159
  prevention, 167–170
  reactivation of infection, 159–160
  treatment, 159–167
  vaccine, 168–170
Hepatitis D virus (HDV), 159, 160
Herpes simplex (HSV), genital, 71–99
  acyclovir and, 91, 93, 94
  AIDS and, 226–227, 231
  antibody prevalence, 73–74
  antiviral agents, 91, 94–96
  asymptomatic infection, 72, 88
  cellular immune response, 89–90
  cervical infection, 78
  cervicitis, 78, 85
  chemotherapy, 91–97
  chronicity of infection, 86–88
  CNS complications, 79–82
  disseminated infection, 82
  extragenital lesions, 82
  first episodes, 75
  genital ulceration, 86
  goals of therapy, 90–91
  heterologous vaccines, 93, 97
  humoral immune response, 89
  local extension of disease, 82–83
  non-specific immune modulators, 96–97
  pharyngeal infection, 78–79
  photodynamic inactivation, 96
  prevalence, 71–75
  primary genital herpes, 75–83
  prior HSV-1 infection and, 75
  proctitis, 86, 251–252
  prophylaxis, 97–98
  recurrent, 83–84
  sexual transmission, 88
  signs, 77–78
  superinfection, 83
  symptoms, 75–77
  topical surfactants/antiseptics and, 96
  'triggers' of recurrence, 88
  tropics, 176, 177, 178, 179, 180
  urethritis and, 85–86
  vaccine, 91, 98
  viral shedding, 78
  vulvar infection, 78
HLTV-III/LAV, 223
  AIDS and *see* Acquired Immune Deficiency
    Syndrome (AIDS)
  idiopathic thrombocytopenic purpura and, 225,
    233, 236
  immune dysfunction and, 216, 235
  minor clinical disorders and, 233

HLTV-III/LAV (*contd.*)
  natural history of infection, 214–215
  persistent generalised lymphadenopathy (PGL)
    and, 224–225, 232–233, 236
  screening, 236–237
Human papilloma virus (HPV), 109–123
  anal/anal canal infection, 119, 139
  antibody detection, 121
  associated lesions, 110, 120
  cell transformation in vitro, 113
  cervical infection, 119, 128, 130–133 *see also*
    Cervical dysplasia/intraepithelial neoplasia
    (CIN)
  DNA-DNA hybridisation, detection and,
    115–119, 121
  genital neoplasia and, 133–138
  genome, 110–112
  immune responses to, 121–123
  immunochemical detection, 114–115
  laryngeal lesions, 120, 128, 134, 139–140
  male genital tract manifestations, 129
  oncogenic potential 113–114
  oral cavity infection, 139
  penile warts, 119, 129, 138
  pregnancy and, 133, 148, 151
  replication, 113
  structure, 110, 111
  treatment, 147–153
  types, 109–110
  types associated with dysplasias/malignant
    disease, 119–121
  vaginal warts, 129–130
  virus coded proteins, 112–113
  vulval warts, 119, 129–130
  see also Condylomata acuminata

Idiopathic thrombocytopenic purpura, 225, 236
Idoxuridine, 95, 149
Immunosuppressed patients, 114, 121–122, 138
Inclusion conjunctivitis of the newborn (ICN), 51
Infertility, female, 48, 49–50
Interferon, 93, 97, 149–150, 160–161, 171, 217, 231
Isoprinosine, 97

Kanamycin, 34, 65, 178
Kaposi's sarcoma, 217, 228–229, 231
Ketoconazole, 231

Laryngeal squamous papilloma, 139–140
Laryngeal warts, 120, 128, 134
Levamisol, 96, 164
L-lysine therapy, 92, 95
Lymphogranuloma venereum, 176, 179–180
  proctitis and, 43–44, 250–251

Mass treatment, selective, 267–268
Mecillinam, 231
Methotrexate, 149
Metronidazole, 190
Minocycline, 42
Mobiluncus sp., 187, 190
  taxonomy/identification, 188–189

Mobiluncus sp. (*contd.*)
  see also Bacterial vaginosis
Moxalactam, 34
Mucopurulent endocervicitis, 45
Mycobacterium avium-intracellulare, 217, 227, 231
Mycoplasma genitalium, 204
Mycoplasma hominis, 48, 178, 251
Mycoplasma pneumoniae, 203

Neisseria gonorrhoeae, 1–16
  antigenic variation, 12
  auxotyping, 13–14
  colony morphology, virulence and, 4–5
  columnar epithelium invasion, 2–4
  cytoplasmic membrane, 7
  electronmicroscopy, 5–6
  hydrolysases, 13
  LgA protease, 13
  lipopolysaccharides, 7–9
  opacity of colonies, 6, 12
  outer membrane, 7–9
  outer membrane proteins, 10–13
  pathogenic mechanisms, 2–4
  penicillinase-producing *see* Penicillinase-
    producing *Neisseria gonorrhoeae* (PPNG)
  peptidoglycan layer, 7
  pilation, 6, 9
  pilus vaccine, 10
  serodiagnosis, 8
  serological classification, 11–12, 14–16
  see also Gonorrhoea
Neisseria meningitidis, 247
Non-gonococcal urethritis (NGU), 39–40, 248–249
  epididymitis complicating, 43
  reactive arthritis and, 196
  specific diagnosis, 42
  transmission, 40–41
  treatment, 41–42
  urethral stricture and, 43
Nystatin, 225, 231

Ophthalmia neonatorum, 13, 32, 261, 264
Oral cavity condylomata acuminata, 139
Oral contraceptives, 50
Oral epithelial hyperplasia, 139

Pelvic inflammatory disease, developing countries,
  262
Penicillin, 34, 35, 40, 45, 65, 180
Penicillinase-producing *Neisseria gonorrhoeae*
  (PPNG), 23–35, 261, 263
  African data, 26, 30
  antibiotic treatment, 32–34
  control, 34–35
  development, 31–32
  European data, 30–31
  Far East data, 25–26, 30
  historical aspects, 23
  initial reports, 23–24
  plasmid types, 24–25
  prevalence, 25–31
  UK data, 27–30, 32

PPNG (*contd.*)
  US data, 26–27
Penile neoplasia, 135
Penile warts, 129, 138
Pentamidine isethionate, 217, 230
Perianal warts, 139
Persistent generalised lymphadenopathy (PGL),
  224–225, 232–233, 236
Phosphonoacetic acid, 96
Phosphonoformate, 92, 96, 164
Pneumocystis carinii, 216–217, 226
Podophyllin, 148–149, 153
Postgonococcal cervicitis, 45
Postgonococcal urethritis, 42
Prednisolone, 166, 167, 171, 232
Primacrine, 164
Proctocolitis/proctitis, 243–256
  Campylobacter spp., 252–253
  Chlamydia trachomatis, 43–44, 248–251
  Cryptosporidium spp., 255
  cytomegalovirus (CMV), 256
  diagnosis, 244–245
  Entamoeba histolytica, 253–255
  enterovirus, 253
  Giardia lamblia, 246
  histopathology, 243–244
  HSV and, 86, 251–252
  Mycoplasma hominis, 251
  Neisseria gonorrhoeae, 246–247
  Neisseria meningitidis, 247
  non-specific, 256
  rectal spirochaetosis, 247–248
  Shigella spp., 252–253
  Strongyloides stercoralis, 255–256
  transmissible enteric pathogens, 245
  Treponema pallidum, 247
  Ureaplasma urealyticum, 251
Prostatitis, 43
Pyrimethamine, 230

Reactive arthritis, 195–204
  acute enteric infection and, 202
  cardiovascular lesions and, 199
  chlamydial infection and, 202–203
  course, 199–200
  enthesopathies, 198
  epidemiology, 196
  eye lesions and, 198
  gonorrhoea and, 204
  inherited susceptibility, 200–201
  initiating infections, 201–204
  mycoplasmas and, 203–204
  peripheral arthritis, 197
  presentation, 196–197
  skin/mucous membrane lesions and, 198–199
  spondylitis, 197–198
  ureaplasmas and, 203–204
Reiter's syndrome *see* Reactive arthritis
Ribavarin, 92, 95–96, 217
Rifampicin, 178, 231
Rosaramicin, 34, 178
Rosoxacin, 66

Salpingitis, acute, 47–49
Seronegative spondarthritis *see* Reactive arthritis
Shigella spp., 252–253
Spectinomycin, 24, 32–33, 34, 35, 178, 180
Spiramycin, 217, 231
Streptomycin, 65, 180
Strongyloides stercoralis, 255–256
Sulphadiazine, 230
Sulphadoxine, 230
Sulphamethoxazole, 178, 180
Sulphametrole, 178, 180
Sulphonamides, 65, 66
Suramin, 217
Syphilis, 64, 65, 176, 177, 179, 180, 264, 268
   epidemiological aspects, 176, 261
   developing countries, detection strategies, 267

Tetracycline, 41, 42, 45, 46, 49, 51, 65, 66, 179,
   180, 190, 251
Thiamphenicol, 34
Thiotepa, 149
Tinidazole, 190
Tobramycin, 49
Toxoplasmosis, 217, 228, 230
Transfer factor, 96, 97, 164

Treponema pallidum, 64, 65, 247
Trichloracetic acid, topical, 149
Trifluorothymidine, 95
Trimethoprim, 34, 66, 178, 180, 217
Trisodium phosphonoformate, 164

Ureaplasma urealyticum, 41, 203, 251
Urethral condylomata, 129
Urethral stricture, 43, 262
Urethral syndrome, 47, 86
Urethritis
   HSV, 85–86
   NGU *see* Non-gonococcal urethritis (NGU)
   postgonococcal, 42

Vancomycin, 231
Vidarabine, 92, 95
Vinblastine, 231
Vaginal neoplasia, 134–135
Vaginal warts, 129–130
Vulval intraepithelial neoplasia (VIN), 120,
   134–136
Vulval warts, 119, 129–130

Warts, genital *see* Condylomata acuminata